L/N   c/a   H1/   E. Anne Whiteley.

DISEASES OF THE CHEST

First published April   1944
Reprinted September   1945
Reprinted July   1946
Second Edition February 1948
Reprinted January   1950
Reprinted October   1951

DISEASES OF THE CHEST

DESCRIBED FOR STUDENTS
AND PRACTITIONERS

BY

ROBERT COOPE
M.D., B.Sc., F.R.C.P.

Physician, Liverpool Royal Infirmary; Consulting
Physician, King Edward VII Sanatorium, Midhurst;
Physician, Liverpool Chest Hospital; Physician, Liver-
pool and North-Western Chest Surgical Unit; Visiting
Physician, Maghull Epileptic Homes; Lecturer in
Clinical Medicine, Lecturer in Applied Physiology and
Lecturer in Clinical Chemistry, University of Liver-
pool; Examiner in Medicine to the Conjoint Board
and in the University of Liverpool; and previously
Examiner in the Universities of London and Aberdeen

With a Foreword by

LORD HORDER

SECOND EDITION
REPRINT

EDINBURGH

E. & S. LIVINGSTONE, LTD.
16 & 17 TEVIOT PLACE
1951

" Do not imagine that the knowledge, which I so much recommend to you, is confined to books, pleasing, useful and necessary as that knowledge is. But I comprehend in it the great knowledge of the world, still more necessary than that of books. In truth, they assist one another reciprocally ; and no man will have either perfectly who has not both. The knowledge of the world is only to be acquired in the world, and not in a closet. Books alone will never teach it you ; but they will suggest many things to your observation which might otherwise escape you ; and your own observations upon mankind, when compared with those which you will find in books, will help you to fix the true point."

—CHESTERFIELD, "Letters to His Son" (4th October 1746).

" Take care not to fancy that you are physicians as soon as you have mastered scientific facts ; they only afford to your understandings an opportunity of bringing forth fruit, and of elevating you to the high position of a man of art. . . . Do not, therefore, fancy yourselves physicians because you have acquired the habit of applying to the diagnosis of diseases the ingenious proceedings by which science has become enriched since the beginning of this century. The admirable diagnostic methods—auscultation and percussion—given by Laennec to the public for the general good, and of which no one is allowed to be ignorant, are in our hands what the telescope and the magnifying-glass are in the hands of the astronomer and the naturalist —instruments intermediary between external objects and the mind ; but a magnifying-glass will no more make a Tournefort or a Galileo, than a stethoscope will make a Sydenham or a Torti."

—TROUSSEAU, "Lectures on Clinical Medicine," vol. ii, p. 42.

Made and Printed in Great Britain

PREFACE TO THE FIRST EDITION

MEDICAL students seem to "find chests difficult," just as they did a hundred years ago when the students at Guy's asked Marshall Hughes to write " a book that beginners could make use of : it really is much wanted for pupils." That was only a generation after Laennec had revolutionised this aspect of Medicine, with an authority founded upon pathological as well as clinical experience. Nowadays chest physicians are perhaps more devoted to the X-ray viewing box than to the post-mortem table, for in recent years radiology has brought exciting advances in diagnostic methods. Herein, however, lies a danger, for radiological interpretation needs to be controlled by knowledge of the normal, and subjected to the confirmation and correction of pathology. At the moment students are apt to pick up from their teachers (and in this matter actions speak louder than words) an undue scepticism about physical signs, a disproportionate reliance on radiograms, and too easy an acceptance of purely " radiological diagnoses " which have as yet no clearly proved pathological picture. Happily the advances in chest surgery are likely to do something to redress the balance. We are at a stage similar to that when surgeons first explored the abdomen and exposed to view " the pathology of the living." No physician will in future be adequately trained in this subject unless he has accompanied his patients to the operating theatre sufficiently often to learn what the chest surgeon can teach him. The radiologist, too, would be wise to spend more time in the post-mortem room and in the operating theatre.

This book is an essay in medical education, an endeavour to set forth, as I see it, how diseases of the chest should be taught. There is no attempt to say anything new or revolutionary, but rather to return to first principles. As Faraday said, a fundamental fact, like an elementary principle, never fails us.

In the same Royal Institution Lecture on Mental Education in 1854, Faraday said : " The education which I advocate will require patience and labour of thought in every exercise tending to improve the judgment." Learning to be a good doctor, like learning to be a good farmer, cannot be done in a hurry. There are no short cuts. The student will note that, pressed though he is for time, I have thought that he will read a somewhat lengthy book on one field only of Medicine. The right sort of student will always make time for " patience and labour of thought," provided that he can feel that it is not wasted.

That there are only two illustrations of radiograms in the text is deliberate—not because I am unappreciative of the indispensable help which radiology brings to the study of chest diseases, but because I feel that the student can only begin to understand its value under the guidance of the experts in his own hospital, and in relation to his own patients. At the end of the book, however, he will find a small collection of representative radiograms which may serve to whet his appetite.

Many friends and colleagues have helped me by their criticism, and I give them my grateful thanks. Dr R. E. Roberts and Dr J. H. Mather gave me advice on the chapter on Radiology, and have provided most of the films in the Appendix ; moreover, for many years I have had the benefit of their collaboration and instruction. Both Dr W. Allen Daley, Chief Medical Officer of the London County Council, and his colleague Dr Heaf read the chapter on Pulmonary Tuberculosis, and made many invaluable suggestions. Dr E. L. Middleton of the Factory Department, Home Office, read the chapter on Harmful Respiratory Dusts, and gave me the benefit of his authoritative experience. Dr C. V. Harrison, Senior Lecturer in the Department of Pathology of the University of Liverpool, has read most of the book, and has not only advised me on pathology but has also brought an interested and critical mind to bear on many of the clinical aspects of chest disease. From the very first, Professor D. M. Dunlop of Edinburgh has given me encouragement ; moreover, he has helped me in the tedious task of reading through the page proofs.

To two friends I am especially indebted. Professor Henry Cohen has read the manuscript and has been generous of time and interest in discussing it with me. His criticism has been all the more valuable in that it is the expression of exacting standards of medical education.

To Mr H. Morriston Davies I owe more than I can say, not only because he has read and discussed the book in detail, chapter by chapter as it was written, but also because it has been my good fortune to work with him in the Liverpool and North-Western Chest Surgical (E.M.S.) Unit and elsewhere. To him I dedicate this book in token of our friendship and as a tribute to one who is a pioneer in thoracic surgery and a most physicianly surgeon.

I have not always taken the advice of my friends, and for any errors, omissions and defects I am wholly responsible. I have to express my pleasure and thanks to Mr Douglas Kidd for his fine line drawings, and to Mr C. Shepley of the Department of Surgery at the University of Edinburgh who, after Mr Kidd went into the Army, continued the high standard of the illustrations.

I am grateful to those who have loaned blocks for illustrations : Professor Dunlop and his colleagues for Fig. 86, and Plates 3-6 ; Dr Robertson Ogilvie for his generosity in allowing me to use the beautiful coloured illustrations of Figs. 98-101, 106-109 ; Mr Hamilton Bailey for Fig. 132 ; Dr J. J. Conybeare for Plates 7-10, 15, 16, 21 ; and Drs R. E. Roberts and J. H. Mather for their X-ray films.

I thank also all those who have been concerned with the task of producing this book in spite of the difficulties of war time. I am especially grateful to Mr Charles Macmillan, who throughout the making of it has been a most helpful, patient and understanding collaborator.

ROBERT COOPE

LIVERPOOL
March 1944

PREFACE TO THE SECOND EDITION

IN the *Analects* of Confucius it is written : "Hui was not any help to me, he accepted everything I said." While I have naturally been pleased to find that this book has found favour with students and practitioners, I feel a special sense of obligation to reviewers and others who have helped me by their criticism. The main change in this new edition is the correction of certain errors in the description of the anatomy of the bronchial tree. Here I have had the benefit of authoritative advice from my friends Drs Clifford Hoyle and Foster-Carter, and Mr R. C. Brock. For detailed criticism and stimulating discussion of many points concerned with clinical teaching, I am grateful in particular to my sometime co-examiners Dr Hope Gosse and Sir Adolphe Abrahams. I am in constant debt, also, to my more intimate colleagues Mr H. Morriston Davies and Mr F. Ronald Edwards.

ROBERT COOPE

January 1948

CONTENTS

xi

LIST OF PLATES

xii

FOREWORD

MEDICAL books, when they are written by teachers of Medicine, provide a clear reflection of medical education generally : as men teach so they write. This being so, Dr Coope's treatise on Respiratory Disease strikes a clear note of hope in the breasts of those of us who look to the present generation of physicians to lift the teaching of Medicine out of the academic rut into which it has fallen on to the plane of a live and useful science and art that shall keep pace with the general march of human progress.

During the past few decades we have tried to make doctors by facing the student with a series of largely detached studies and experiences. During the preclinical stages of the curriculum, professors, each one staking out bigger and bigger claims in his particular field, have drugged their pupils' minds with maximum doses of more or less abstract science, largely obscuring the main purpose of their great adventure. Then we gave the doped brain a sudden jostle by arranging a close but quite unfamiliar impact of its senses with actual human beings in the form of patients in the wards, out-patient departments and the post-mortem room. And then, before the student could recover from the shock and begin to look closely at these strange objects, talk to them and examine them, we switched him off and submerged him in pathological techniques, X-ray shadows and the ritual of the operating theatre.

The writing of medical books has largely followed the lead given by this staccato method of tuition. Here and there an effort has been made to integrate the various view-points of the diseased person and stress the unity of pathology in terms of the patient, but in the main the trend has been in the other direction. The student must either read a catalogue of signs and symptoms, with appropriate prognosis and treatment, usually found in a condition to which the name of a disease is conveniently given (that is, a " textbook of medicine "), or he must do his best to trace his patient's disability and its consequences through a series of manuals, each one of which concerns itself with a part, but only a part, of the trouble.

To-day, however, we are—but very slowly—trying to relate the preclinical studies to the student's subsequent contacts with the patient, and we are also trying—again very slowly— to keep the patient in the forefront of the student's mind during the clinical period of his training—"les malades, toujours les malades." In our books the same wholesome tendency is becoming apparent. Therefore we may welcome, and heartily, this treatise on Respiratory Disease (called, by a concession to tradition, " Diseases of the Chest ") because of the valiant and successful effort it makes along these lines. The degree of the debt in which the author places us for his courage in following his conviction—that the principle just outlined is the one that should guide those who shoulder the great responsibility of writing books—will only be apparent later. The debt will probably be a considerable one.

This is a foreword and not a review. All the same, a few points call for brief comment. The range of the subject-matter is very wide, but all the sections are relevant. The inclusion of such topics as Asthma, Mediastinal and Diaphragmatic Lesions, Circulatory Disturbances of the Lungs and Chest Injuries will be found of much service. Since the overlap of Influenza and the Common Cold with the respiratory organs is so definite, we welcome sections on these infections.

The social and economic factors involved in a study of Respiratory Disease have received attention, not obtruding as a sop to the current interest shown in " Social Medicine " and " Health in Industry " but as displaying the author's purpose, followed uniformly throughout the book, to present disease in all its bearings and not in its academic aspects only.

Just as the teacher of Anatomy and Physiology should constantly take the forward view and envisage the actual work of the clinician-to-be, so should the teacher of Clinical Medicine take a step back and relate, as far as is possible, the morbid changes that face him and his pupil with the bedrock facts of Anatomy and Physiology. This process the author follows with admirable consistency throughout the book.

The insistence upon care and thoroughness in the assembling of the case-history, in the inquiry about symptoms and in the methodical collection of signs is noteworthy. The beginner should never be ashamed of being a slave to method : only facility—and that comes late—enables the observer to decide

what he may safely omit. Stress is laid upon the importance
of giving play to a healthy scepticism in regard to the claims
made for what the author calls " the unbiased precision of
objective science."

The very numerous diagrams, simple and elucidatory,
evince a quite unusual gift for clarity of expression and interpretation. The general format is admirable.

Altogether this is a very notable book and will surely take
a high place in medical literature.

HORDER

LONDON
March 1944

CHAPTER I

PHYSIOLOGICAL AND ANATOMICAL
CONSIDERATIONS

INTRODUCTORY

THE lungs are part of a complex mechanism for ensuring that the tissues of the body are adequately supplied with the oxygen they need. Their function, therefore, is bound up with that of the heart and circulation, and all the mechanisms are integrated and controlled through the nervous system. The student of thoracic diseases must constantly bear in mind this relationship.

The tissues obtain their oxygen from the air outside the body. This oxygen is made available for the circulating blood by the bringing of outside air into intimate contact with the blood over a vast surface, so that the red blood corpuscles pick up as much oxygen as they can carry. The essential structure of the lungs is that of tubes, leading to innumerable small air sacs lined by a thin membrane richly supplied with blood and exposed on both sides to the air. The blood bathing this membrane is kept in movement and renewed by the heart and other circulatory forces. A constantly renewed supply of air is ensured by the rhythmical bellows-like action of the thorax, controlled by nervous impulses from the respiratory centre, which itself is controlled by both nervous and chemical influences. At the same time as oxygen is thus taken into the body, waste products (particularly water vapour and carbon dioxide) are excreted.

Failure of proper respiration may arise, therefore, from defects in the supply or quality of blood to the lung membrane, from defects in the supply or quality of the air, or from defects in the lungs or of their nervous and chemical control.

The integration of heart and lungs is but one illustration of the fact that if one member of the body suffers, the other members suffer with it. In fibrosis of the lungs, for example,

1

the right side of the heart is likely sooner or later to become dilated. Moreover, if the student will keep in mind this integration of heart and lungs, it will remind him that clinical examination of the lungs must always be accompanied by examination of the heart and vice versa. In lung disease the condition of the heart, or in heart disease the presence of basal œdema, of lung infarction or of hydrothorax may greatly affect the prognosis. The purely anatomical relationships are important ; for the position of the apex of the heart may indicate whether the mediastinum is being displaced by a collection of air or of fluid in the pleural cavity, by fibrosis, or by collapse of the lung.

The inhaled air passes over the upper respiratory tract, with its spacious, warm and moist nasal sinuses. The warmed air is drawn through the larynx, trachea and bronchi into the depths of the lungs, where the interchanges with the blood can be made through the respiratory epithelium. On the journey the intermingling of the comparatively small amount of outside air which comes in with each respiration with that already in the lungs and respiratory passages (the proportion is roughly 1 in 7) is nicely adjusted to prevent any sudden and great differences in the composition of the alveolar air ; for the composition of the alveolar air must remain constant within fairly narrow limits, because it regulates the tension of gases in the arterial blood.

THE DEFENCES OF THE AIR PASSAGES

Harmful foreign material from outside cannot easily enter, much less remain in, the lower respiratory passages. Some 500 litres of air is inspired each hour, yet most of the microbes present in the air of a heavily populated town never even reach the trachea. A large number of them are trapped in the vestibules of the nose, being enmeshed by the hairs which are moistened with sticky, healthy mucus ; after arrest in the mucus the organisms are rapidly ejected by the action of the ciliated epithelium.

The mucus is spread in a thin, even, transparent layer, and is kept constantly on the move over the walls of the nasal sinuses, the greater part of the nasal cavities, the nasopharynx and the back of the soft palate. This activity of cilia and mucus extends also throughout the trachea and bronchi, as far down as the point where the smallest bronchioles expand into the terminal alveoli. It has been calculated that the movement of a particle by the cilia working *en masse* approximates to a velocity of about 12 ft. per hour.

The combination of the " mucus blanket " (acting rather like a sticky fly-paper) and ciliary movement is the prime defensive weapon of the air passages. If mucus collects and stagnates it may act as a nidus for a luxuriant growth of bacteria ; in the normal healthy individual, however, it is swept by the corkscrew-like motion of the mass of the cilia towards the outside world, carrying the invading organisms with it, and is replaced by fresh secretion.

The larynx protects the lower respiratory passages, when need arises, by its closure ; this is seen typically in exposure to irritant gases such as chlorine. Soiled mucus collecting in the interarytenoid region may excite the swallowing reflex, and so help to carry off invading organisms to the stomach, where most of them (but not tubercle bacilli) are killed by the acid secretion. If the exquisitely sensitive larynx is more seriously irritated, the *cough reflex* is brought into action (this is true also of irritation of the trachea or bronchi) ; thus foreign material is forcibly expelled—aided by the shortening and narrowing of the bronchial tubes, which is caused by the forced expiration characteristic of coughing.

Organisms passing beyond the larynx must still run the gauntlet of muco-ciliary activity in the trachea and bronchi ; some may be carried away by lymphatic drainage, but most will be swept back towards the mouth.

If all these defences fail against inhaled infective material, the battle must then be fought in the lung tissues themselves by means of inflammatory reaction. It is clear, therefore, that pneumonia or lung abscess may represent a battle on the last lines of defence, pitched on inconvenient ground.

There are several reasons why the primary defences may fail. The cilia may be damaged, as by an intense naso-pharyngeo-tracheitis such as occurs in certain " influenzal " infections, or by exposure to irritant gases or by poisoning by anæsthetics. There may be excessive mucus secretion with stagnation, and the resulting danger of heavy bacterial growth in it. Harmful foreign material may be overwhelming in amount or virulence, as in some types of upper respiratory tract suppuration or in prolonged exposure to harmful dusts. The normal cough reflex may be abolished by anæsthesia, coma or respiratory muscle paralysis. A combination of any or all of these factors may, by breaking down the primary defences, make the lung itself a battlefield.

THE MECHANISM OF THE THORAX

The lungs may be compared to two elastic balloons enclosed tightly in a box ; the two balloons have a common neck or outlet, outside the box, and kept open to the air (Fig. 1). If there is air inside the box as well as in the balloons then they will collapse limply ; but if there is a vacuum inside the box the atmospheric air will keep the balloons distended.

Replace the rigid box by a linen bag and both bag and balloons will collapse. A rigid box withstands the atmospheric pressure without and does not collapse like a linen bag. If there is a partial vacuum in the box the balloons inside it become inflated, not by forcibly blowing them up but by suction-traction on the outside of their walls. Thus there is produced a suction, or *negative pressure*, between the inside walls of the box and the wall of the balloons—a suction pressure which, if the walls of the box are completely rigid, can be expressed as the pull, or tendency to recoil, of the elastic stretched balloons. Puncture the box and let air in between its walls and the open-necked balloons, and they will collapse by their own elastic recoil.

Translating this analogy into anatomical terms, the balloons are the lungs and the box the thorax. The trachea, bronchi and nasal passages form the neck or outlet of the balloons, kept open to the atmospheric air. The lungs so fill the thorax that their outer lining pleura is in close contact with the parietal pleura of the thoracic cage ; if, however, these two pleural surfaces are separated—by air or by fluid, for example—then what was a potential space becomes an actual " pleural cavity."

The thoracic cage is formed partly by the rigid framework of ribs, sternum and vertebræ, and partly by soft structures—the diaphragm below, the intercostal muscles laterally, and the fascia, vessels and muscles at the root of the neck which close the upper opening. It is not a rigid box ; its capacity can be increased to cause an expansion of the lungs and draw air into them, or decreased to expel air. The lungs are elastic, and so not only does the thoracic wall exert suction-traction upon them, but they in their turn " pull " on the thoracic wall and on each other in the same way that a piece of elastic held stretched between the two hands pulls on them in its tendency to shorten. Between the two lungs and outside the " pleural cavities " lies the mediastinum, containing the trachea, heart

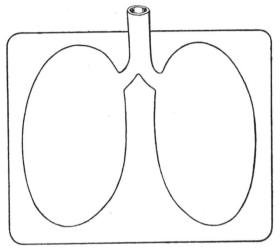

FIG. 1

Diagram of the " box and balloons " model of the thorax.

and other structures, held in position by the evenly balanced pull of the two elastic lungs ; above, it is somewhat loosely fixed in the root of the neck, but below it is firmly attached to the diaphragm. If the chest wall is suddenly perforated and air rushes in to separate the two pleural layers, the lung collapses to about one-fifth of its original size. If air or fluid collects in the pleural cavity, the lung on that side relaxes to accommodate it ; its elastic tension is lessened and its volume reduced. The elastic recoil in the opposite intact lung is then able to pull the mediastinum over towards its own side, always provided that the mediastinum has not been fixed by adhesions.

Inside the lungs the elastic tissue is intercepted by the bronchial tree, the bronchi having tough, strong walls into which the elastic fibres are inserted and on which they exert a continuous tension, increased as the lung expands with each inspiration. The trachea and bronchi are tubes which conduct the air to the air sacs of the lung. The larger tubes are kept open by hoops of cartilage; the smaller tubes have much smooth muscle in their walls, so arranged in a geodetic * pattern that they expand and contract rhythmically with respiration. In inspiration the tubes are elongated and dilated (Fig. 2); during expiration they contract down again. Around the orifices of the atria (see Fig. 11, p. 13) the muscle is arranged in a sphincter-like manner; beyond this, it ceases. Elastic fibres and muscle bundles follow very much the same geodetic pattern, and can be regarded as making up what has been termed the " myo-elastic sheet."

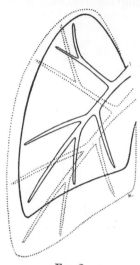

FIG. 2

Diagrammatic representation of the elongation of two main bronchi and divisions during inspiration. Note also the slight movement of the lung root.

Because of the elastic pull of the lungs within and the atmospheric pressure without the thoracic cage, the soft parts of the thoracic walls tend to be depressed inwards. In normal inspiration the thoracic cavity is increased in size, the lungs expand to follow its contours, the tension of the elastic tissue of the lungs is increased and the " negative intra-thoracic pressure " is greater than before. If a bronchus is obstructed, not only is the area of lung supplied by it unable to expand, but as the air contained in it is absorbed, it contracts. The corresponding portion of the thoracic cage remains in apposition to it. The collapsed zone acts as a focal point of strong elastic stresses between it and the thoracic wall, the rest of the lung, the mediastinum and the opposite lung. The most obvious results are a sucking-in of the ribs and intercostal spaces and a dragging displacement of the mediastinum towards the affected

* " Geodetic line : the shortest possible line that can be drawn from one point of a surface to another, the plane of curvature of which will be everywhere perpendicular to the surface." (Shorter Oxford English Dictionary.)

side, more obvious during inspiration, and particularly so if the thoracic wall happens to be soft and yielding as in children.

The respiratory movements of the thorax can be compared to the rhythmical action of a bellows. When the thoracic cavity is enlarged the lungs expand with it, for the pressure of the atmosphere transmitted through the trachea, bronchial tubes and air sacs keeps the walls of the lungs in close apposition to the walls of the thorax. In expiration the thoracic cavity diminishes in size and the lungs partially collapse—but not wholly, because at the end of expiration there is still a negative pressure inside the thorax.

The lungs and bronchial tubes normally contain about 3000 c.c. of air, of which about half can be forcibly expelled by a maximal expiratory effort. This 1500 c.c. is called *supplemental air*, and the remaining 1500 c.c. which cannot be so expelled is the *residual air*. This residual air can be got rid of only by opening the thoracic cavity and allowing the lungs to collapse completely. Each ordinary inspiration expands the lungs sufficiently to leave room for another 500 c.c. to enter, and an ordinary expiration expels the same amount. This is called the *tidal air*, for it ebbs and flows with each respiration. Of this, about 250 c.c. occupies the bronchial tree and does not immediately reach the alveoli—the *dead space air*, through which the diffusion of gases into and out of the alveoli takes place. Since the bronchi dilate and contract, the dead space air is variable in amount—it can be considerably increased, for example, by very deep breathing, and, pathologically, is much increased by the formation of emphysematous bullæ. A forced, maximal inspiratory effort will suck in *complemental air* to the amount of about another 1500 c.c. Remembering that ordinary quiet breathing introduces and expels 500 c.c. into and out of the lungs, some idea of the reserve capacity may be gained from the attempt to achieve the deepest breath possible. This can be made by emptying the lungs as far as possible by a maximal forced expiration, so getting rid of the supplemental air. Rebreathing 1500 c.c. of supplemental air, then taking in the usual 500 c.c. of tidal air, and then with a maximal inspiratory effort taking in the 1500 c.c. of complemental air—about 3500 c.c. in all—gives the deepest breath possible, which is thus about seven times as big as the normal-sized breath ; this is the **vital capacity**. It varies with the size of the individual and with the training or fitness of his respiratory mechanism. It is a measure of the efficiency of respiration, and is diminished in many diseases, especially in affections of the heart and lungs. On the figures given, it is clear that in ordinary quiet breathing only about one-seventh of the total lung capacity is used, so that there is a large reserve or margin of safety. Indeed it may be said that in round figures about one-tenth of the lung surface suffices for the resting man's respiratory exchange. Thus large parts of the lung can be put out of action by disease—

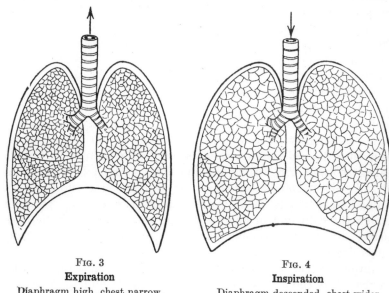

FIG. 3
Expiration
Diaphragm high, chest narrow.

FIG. 4
Inspiration
Diaphragm descended, chest wider.

pleural effusion or pneumothorax, for example—with no more serious result than shortness of breath on exercise (when the respiratory exchange may be increased from five to ten times the normal). If parts of the lung are poorly ventilated, yet with blood still circulating through them, then non-arterialised blood will enter the left heart, and there may be a distinct lack of adequate oxygen supply to the tissues in consequence. This sometimes happens in the earlier stages of bronchial carcinoma, with partial bronchial block, causing cyanosis which disappears later with complete bronchial block and collapse of the corresponding portion of lung. Usually when the air sacs are fully collapsed the blood flow is cut off.

The thoracic cavity can be enlarged downwards, forwards and transversely by the action of certain muscles. In inspiration the diaphragm contracts. It is a strong sheet of muscle with a central tendon to which the muscle fibres are attached. When the muscle fibres shorten they pull the central tendon downwards, and the whole diaphragm descends, rather like a piston in a cylinder ; this produces an increase in the intra - abdominal pressure, with consequent bulging of the abdominal wall (Figs. 3 and 4). The thoracic cavity is increased from the back forwards and from side to side by elevation of the ribs and sternum, the spinal column acting as a fulcrum (Figs. 5 and 6).

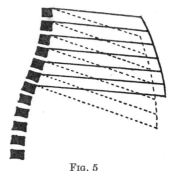

FIG. 5

To show enlargement of chest from back to front by means of elevation of ribs : spine fixed.

The ribs slant forwards and downwards ; they are raised rather as a bucket-handle is raised, the movement being possible owing to the articulations at one end and torsion of the costal cartilages at the other. The scalene muscles steady the first two ribs, and the external intercostal muscles raise the ribs both in front and at the side. In this way their oblique slant is lessened, the horizontal distance between the spinal column and the sternum is increased, and so the sternum is pushed forwards. Moreover, as the first seven ribs increase progressively in length, raising of a lower rib to take the place of the next higher one will increase the size of the thorax at this level both forwards and from side to side. Another factor in pro-

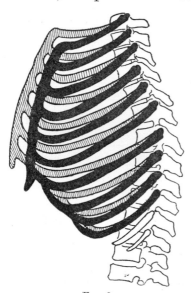

FIG. 6

More detailed drawing to show enlargement of chest as in Fig. 5.

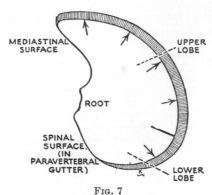

FIG. 7

Cross section, right lung

To show the excursion of the lung surfaces in inspiration. (*After Keith.*)

ducing enlargement depends on the twist of the ribs themselves. The raising of the ribs during inspiration involves a certain rotation of them, on an axis directed through their anterior and posterior ends, so that their outer surfaces are turned directly outwards instead of the expiratory position of outwards and downwards. These points will be more easily followed if the student studies them on the skeleton, handling one or two ribs in order to reproduce the movements which take place.

It is clear that the biggest expansion of the thorax during inspiration occurs in the lower and lateral parts, and that is where the lungs can expand most freely, for they cannot greatly expand backwards against the spine, upwards into the root of the neck or inwards against the mediastinum and each other (Figs. 7, 8 and 9). If inspiration has to be forced, then any muscles which can help to raise the chest wall are brought into action. These are *accessory muscles of respiration* — the

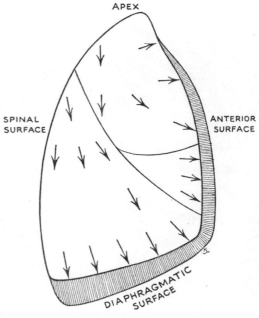

FIG. 8

Lateral view, right lung

To show the excursion of the lung surfaces in inspiration. (*After Keith.*)

scaleni, sternomastoids, trapezii, pectoral muscles, rhomboids and serrati antici. Ordinary expiration is mainly due to the elastic recoil of the lungs when the inspiratory muscles are not acting. In forced expiration the abdominal muscles are especially made use of in order to press the abdominal organs against the under surface of the diaphragm and so to reduce the size of the thoracic cavity. This helps to produce a pressure on the surfaces of the lungs from without inwards towards the central parts.

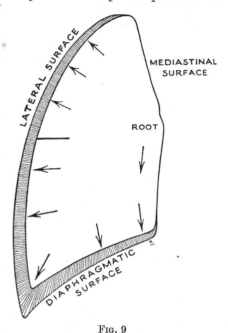

FIG. 9

Vertical section, right lung

To show the excursion of the lung surfaces in inspiration. (*After Keith.*)

During the movements of respiration the pleural surface of the lung slides over the pleural surface of the inner wall of the thorax, just as one hand can be made to slide over the other ; between the two pleural surfaces is a small film of fluid which acts as a lubricant. Inspiration is followed by expiration, with a slight pause between them, easily perceived if one listens with a stethoscope over the trachea. In the adult the number of respirations is ordinarily about fourteen to eighteen per minute—about 26,000 times in the day—but the frequency may be increased by muscular activity, emotion, or to a certain extent by a special act of will. The younger a person, the quicker he breathes ; thus a new-born child breathes about forty-four times a minute. It can be seen that the largely passive nature of expiration results in a great saving of muscular energy ; moreover, complete rest in bed will reduce the expenditure of energy on respiration to a minimum.

THE ESSENTIAL STRUCTURE OF THE LUNGS

The trachea and bronchial tree conduct air from the outside atmosphere to the air sacs of the lung. The larger bronchi divide and subdivide, eventually to become bronchioles,

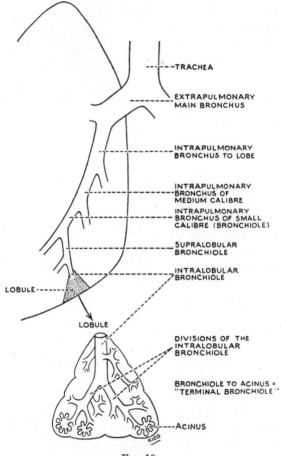

TRACHEA

EXTRAPULMONARY
MAIN BRONCHUS

INTRAPULMONARY
BRONCHUS TO LOBE

INTRAPULMONARY
BRONCHUS OF
MEDIUM CALIBRE

INTRAPULMONARY
BRONCHUS OF SMALL
CALIBRE (BRONCHIOLE)

SUPRALOBULAR
BRONCHIOLE

INTRALOBULAR
BRONCHIOLE

LOBULE

LOBULE

DIVISIONS OF THE
INTRALOBULAR
BRONCHIOLE

BRONCHIOLE TO ACINUS =
"TERMINAL BRONCHIOLE"

ACINUS

FIG. 10

To illustrate the lobular structure of the lung, each lobule
forming a " fundamental lung unit."

devoid of cartilage and mucous glands, but with a muscular coat relatively twice as thick as that of the larger bronchi. Each bronchiole ends in a " lobule," a sort of lung on a small scale enclosed in a fibrous capsule of its own (Fig. 10) with its own supply of blood vessels, nerves and lymphatics. The lobule forms, therefore, a fundamental lung unit, and it is the packing together of innumerable such units which, with the conducting tubes, make up the lung as a whole. Inside the lobule the bronchiole divides into still smaller tubes the terminal branches of which—the *respiratory bronchioles*—lead into an expanded space like the hall of a house (*atrium*) from which arise several short passages, each of which leads into two or three air sacs (*infundibula*). The air sacs are studded with minute finger-like protrusions, the *alveoli* (Fig. 11), which are

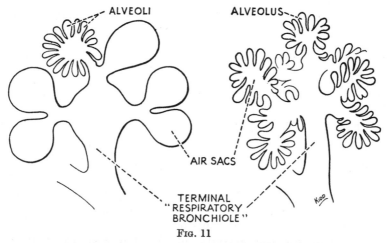

FIG. 11

Diagrammatic representations of the terminal lung unit. On the left is a simplified drawing to illustrate the terminal bronchiole leading into the atrium, from which open out the infundibular ducts. These lead to groups of two or three air sacs (infundibula), from the walls of which arise the alveolar protrusions.

lined by a single layer of large flattened cells. The air in these alveoli is separated from the blood capillaries only by this single layer of cells and the tenuous walls of the capillaries. The alveoli all over the lung are so packed together that any particular capillary lies between adjacent alveoli, so that the blood is in close contact with air on both sides. In the lung meshwork between the alveoli are large numbers of elastic fibres, nerve fibrils and lymphatic channels. It has been calculated that the area covered by the respiratory cells of all the alveoli in man—there are about 800,000,000 alveoli— corresponds to about one hundred times the surface area of the body. This represents roughly 1300 sq. ft. of respiratory surface, nearly half the area of a tennis court. The whole of this is not necessary for the proper oxygenation of the blood ; it allows for a large reserve of functional capacity.

The terminal bronchioles do not possess ciliated epithelium, so that if micro-organisms reach this part of the lung they will be sucked into the air sacs during inspiration, and the only defence left is an inflammatory reaction in the alveolar units. This is important in the pathology of pneumococcal pneumonia. Moreover, the lobules are so closely packed together that inflammation can easily extend to adjacent areas.

As a result of the interchange of gases through the respiratory membrane about 5 per cent. of oxygen is taken from the inspired air and about 4 per cent. of carbon dioxide is put out into the expired air. The latter is also saturated with water vapour.

THE REGULATION OF RESPIRATION

The respiratory centre in the brain extends through the upper part of the medulla oblongata and probably into the pons as well. Although one major and two minor centres have been described, it is wise to consider the central grey matter as a whole and to think of the whole " centre " acting normally as a co-ordinated unit. It possesses an inherent rhythmicity, just as does the sino-auricular node of the heart, and it controls the activity of the lower motor neurones supplying the respiratory muscles. It receives afferent impulses from the lungs via the vagus, and from the aortic arch and carotid sinus via the sino-aortic nerves. It is also influenced by impulses coming from the higher brain centres. It is, moreover, exquisitely sensitive to certain chemical variations in its *milieu*—alterations in the carbon dioxide tension or the hydrogen ion content of the blood, and also the presence of various poisons (Fig. 12).

A man breathes in order to get oxygen for his tissues and to get rid of carbon dioxide which has been formed in his body as a result of metabolism, during which heat is liberated. For every calorie of heat liberated in the body about 200 c.c. of oxygen is needed ; this can be obtained by breathing in 4 litres of air, for it has already been seen that 100 c.c. of inspired air provides about 5 c.c. of oxygen to the blood. An

average man, under the basal metabolic conditions of complete
rest, needs a pulmonary ventilation of about 5 litres per minute.
If the metabolism is increased in any way, more oxygen, and
therefore increased air intake, will be needed. In muscular
exercise, for example, the oxygen consumption (and therefore

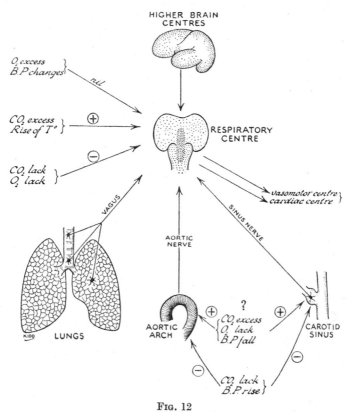

FIG. 12

Regulation of respiration. (*After Samson Wright.*)

the metabolic rate) may be increased tenfold or more, so that
50 or more litres of air must be breathed per minute.

Breathing, then (other things being equal), *is proportional
to the metabolic rate* ; the controlling mechanism here is almost
certainly the varying *carbon dioxide tension of the blood,* acting
mainly and directly on the respiratory centre. It is likely that
the increase of carbon dioxide tension in the blood also influences
the centre to a certain extent by stimulating sensory nerves

in the carotid sinus and the aortic arch, the impulses of which reinforce the main CO_2 stimulus to the respiratory centre. An excess of carbon dioxide in the inspired air produces first an increase in the depth and later an increase in the rate of breathing. If the CO_2 tension of the blood is lowered (as by voluntary over-ventilation, whereby too much CO_2 is expired), the breathing becomes shallow and apnœa is induced.

Apart from increased CO_2 formation in the tissues or excess CO_2 in the inspired air, *changes in hydrogen ion concentration of the blood* due to other causes influence the respiration in such a way as to preserve the normal reaction of the blood. An increase of blood hydrogen ion concentration (acidæmia) stimulates breathing, large quantities of CO_2 are eliminated from the blood via the lungs, and the hydrogen ion concentration is thus reduced to normal. For example, the accumulation in the circulation of abnormal acids such as β-hydroxybutyric acid and aceto-acetic acid in diabetes acts in this manner ; so also does the liberation into the circulation of hydrochloric acid following the ingestion of ammonium chloride, after the NH_3 portion has been split off, combined with CO_2 and converted into urea. On the other hand, in alkalæmia the breathing is depressed, so that CO_2 is retained in the blood to restore the normal reaction. This is seen after ingestion of sodium bicarbonate in excess, such as occurs sometimes during the course of treatment for peptic ulcer ; or after prolonged vomiting, by which the body loses too much HCl. Changes in the reaction of the blood influence the respiratory centre in the main directly, but also to some extent reflexly via the sino-aortic nerves.

The inhalation of pure oxygen by a normal person has no effect on respiration. The results of *oxygen defect* are somewhat complicated ; it depresses the respiratory centre directly, but stimulates the nerve endings in the carotid body and aortic arch and so reflexly increases breathing. In the healthy person the latter effect usually predominates (as in oxygen lack at high altitudes), even though the increased ventilation produces an alkalæmia ; nevertheless the total balance of the effects of oxygen deficiency depends largely on its rapidity and severity. Sudden and severe lack of oxygen causes failure of cerebral processes, especially those of the respiratory centre ; moderately severe deficiency, not too rapidly produced, may cause a hyperpnœa which is nothing like as marked as that due to excess of carbon dioxide, and which brings with it serious disadvantages such as alkalæmia (which in its turn depresses breathing). It is only in oxygen lack of very gradual onset that increase of breathing, together with fairly good compensation of the resulting disabilities, can occur for any considerable length of time.

Pulmonary ventilation can on occasion be increased in order *to eliminate more water vapour* and so maintain the normal temperature of the body when heat loss by evaporation and radiation from the skin is difficult. This is typically seen in the panting dog.

Afferent fibres from the substance of the lung pass via the *vagi* to the respiratory centre and take part in the regulation of the respiratory rhythm. They are sensitive to the amount of expansion of the lungs, inhibiting inspiration when it has proceeded to a certain extent ; expiration then follows (**Hering-Breuer reflex**). When the vagi are cut experimentally the rhythmic discharges of the respiratory centre produce long, deep inspirations with a prolonged rest period following each of them. The vagal reflexes interfere, therefore, with the rhythmic discharges of the respiratory centre, cutting short inspiration and therefore the consequent recovery period, so ensuring reasonably frequent and not too deep inspirations. The vagal nerve endings in the lung seem, therefore, to be analogous to stretch receptors in muscle.

It has been seen that *afferents from the carotid sinus and the aortic arch* pass to the respiratory centre. Their nerve endings are sensitive not only to chemical changes in the blood (CO_2 tension, changes in hydrogen ion concentration, oxygen lack) but also to changes in blood pressure. A rapid, severe rise of pressure reflexly depresses breathing and a fall stimulates it.

The chief *motor nerves* supplying the thoracic cage are the phrenic and intercostal nerves. *Intrinsic lung innervation* is by fibres from the vagus and the sympathetic. Vagal efferent fibres are broncho-constrictor ; the sympathetic fibres are broncho-dilator. Pilocarpine constricts the bronchi, while adrenaline dilates them. Nerve fibres to and from the pulmonary blood vessels are of no particular importance, for in the pulmonary circulation the blood pressure and the velocity

2

of blood flow are much smaller than in the systemic circulation. There is less peripheral resistance to the output of the right side of the heart, for the arterioles are wide, short and thin-walled, and there is an enormous capillary field. In consequence, pressure changes inside the thorax will appreciably affect the flow of blood, and the negative pressure helps the flow towards the great veins and the heart. In like manner there is free flow of lymph from the deeper and more distant parts of the lung towards the hilum.

SOME IMPORTANT ANATOMICAL LANDMARKS

When we examine a patient's chest we look at a thorax covered with soft tissues arranged in humps and hollows and hope thereby to discover something of the condition of the lungs and pleura underlying the bony cage. This involves a mental picture of what the thoracic contents would look like in health if an inspection window could be made in the thoracic wall, and then any divergences from the normal will be recognised.

Quite apart from any modifications in the general shape of the thorax, certain anatomical points are of real importance.

1. *The position of the apex of the heart*, which may be pulled or pushed out of its normal site.

2. *The trachea* should lie midway in the episternal notch ; if it is directed towards one side of the chest (owing, for example, to apical fibrosis or upper lobe collapse), the index finger, pushed straight into the notch just above the bone, will slide to the side of the trachea. In the normal person the finger hits the trachea " full on," deviating neither to right nor to left ; but if the trachea is pulled over to the left, the advancing finger hits it sideways on and so will slide to the opposite side in the notch (in this case, the right) from that towards which the trachea is deflected.

The bifurcation of the trachea is at the level of the second rib cartilage (and angle of Louis) in front (Fig. 13), and the lower border of the fourth dorsal vertebra behind. It is only a short way from the bifurcation of the trachea to the hilum of the lung, which is nearer the vertebral column than the front of the chest.

3. The first rib slopes downwards and forwards, so that

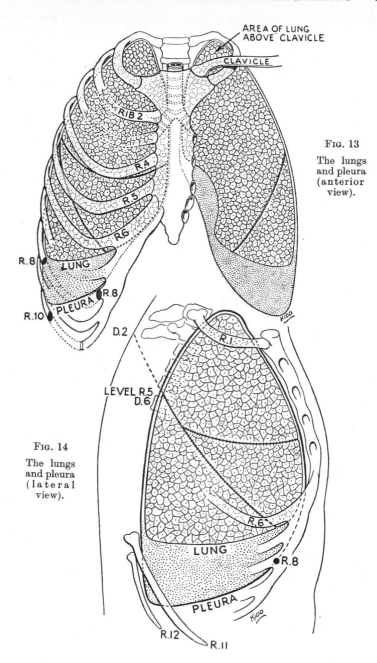

FIG. 13

The lungs and pleura (anterior view).

FIG. 14

The lungs and pleura (lateral view).

there is a *small portion of the lung apex*, behind and above the clavicle, going up into the root of the neck for about 1 to 1½ in. (Figs. 13 and 14).

4. It is of practical importance to know the boundaries of the *pleural sacs* and the surface markings, especially of the basal portion. At the sixth costal cartilage in front, by the

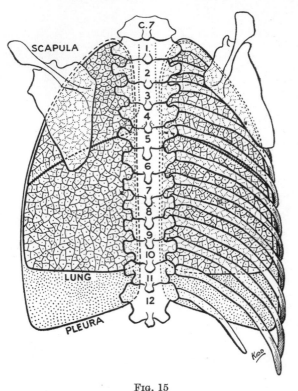

FIG. 15

The lungs and pleura (posterior view).

sternum, is the anterior end of the main lung fissure, dividing lower from upper lobes. In the mid-clavicular line the pleura reaches to the level of the eighth costal cartilage ; in the mid-axillary line, the tenth rib ; in the scapular line, the eleventh rib, whence it crosses the short twelfth rib to the outer border of the erector spinæ (Figs. 13, 14 and 15).

During expiration the lungs do not completely fill the pleural cavity, and the two layers of the pleura are in apposi-

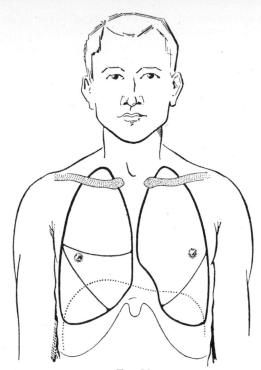

FIG. 16
Important anatomical landmarks (anterior view).

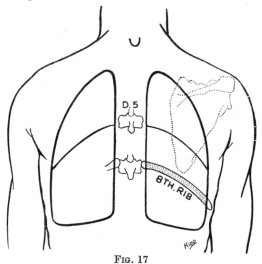

FIG. 17
Important anatomical landmarks (posterior view).

tion in the costophrenic angle. During inspiration the contraction of the dome-shaped diaphragm opens up this potential
space, sucking into it the thin tongue of the lung margins. For
expiration, therefore, there must be a different set of surface
markings for the lower borders of the lungs and of the pleura.

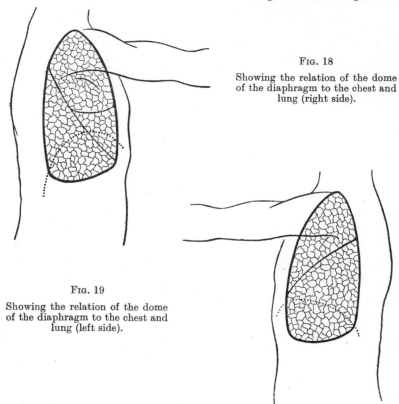

FIG. 18

Showing the relation of the dome
of the diaphragm to the chest and
lung (right side).

FIG. 19

Showing the relation of the dome
of the diaphragm to the chest and
lung (left side).

In medicine this is unimportant ; the surface marking of the
pleura is the one which the student should remember. In
surgery the difference is of importance in the operative approach
to a subdiaphragmatic abscess.

5. The position of the *fissures* separating the various lobes
of the lungs should be remembered ; the knowledge is useful,
for example, in the study of interlobar effusions and in collapse
of single lobes of the lungs. The two main fissures are marked
out by a line on each side from the spine of the second dorsal
vertebra (C7 is the " vertebra prominens "), passing down-

wards and outwards by following the fifth rib as it leaves the vertebral column, and reaching the sixth costochondral junction in front ; if the scapula is tilted by putting the patient's hand on his head, its vertebral border lies along the line of the fissure (Figs. 14 and 15).

On the right side an extra fissure passes horizontally from the level of the fourth costal cartilage to meet the main fissure at the mid-axillary line, at the level of the fifth rib or inter-space ; the middle lobe, then, is anterior, and is not to be pictured on the patient's back.

6. The patient may be induced to uncover a wider area of lung behind by displacing his scapula. If he puts his foot on a low chair and bends forward to tie the bootlace, a strip of between 1 and 2 in. is exposed by the forward movement of the scapula.

7. The liver and diaphragm on the right side extend up to the level of the lower border of the fourth rib.

8. Consideration of the lateral views of the thorax (Figs. 18 and 19) will show that the lateral aspect of the lower part of the upper lobe is accessible to examination in the axilla.

9. The intercostal nerves and blood vessels run in the sulcus at the lower and internal border of the ribs. They are therefore deliberately avoided in such manipulations as " putting a needle into the chest."

THE BRONCHIAL TREE

If the student or doctor is to " place " certain pulmonary lesions or to advise the best posture for the efficient drainage of a bronchiectasis, he must be able to visualise the distribution of the bronchi to the lung tissue and know which parts of the lung they supply. While, however, a general idea of the archi-tecture of the tree up to the finer bronchioles (" twigs ") and alveoli (" foliage ") is helpful, detail must not be allowed to obscure the outstanding picture of the trunk and main branches. As H. P. Nelson pointed out (*British Medical Journal*, 1934, ii, 251), from the standpoint of bronchial distribution there are four main zones in each lung (Figs. 20 and 21).

The " dorsal " lobe is the upper part of the lower lobe and is situated posteriorly ; a lesion there (tuberculosis, lung abscess) will appear to be hilar in site in a " straight " X-ray film, and may extend right across the middle zone of the lung, but the lateral film will show its real position (Figs. 22 and 23).

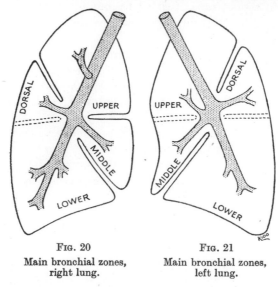

FIG. 20   FIG. 21

Main bronchial zones,   Main bronchial zones,
right lung.   left lung.

On the left side the anatomical upper lobe consists of the " true upper lobe " and the " middle lobe " or **lingular process.**

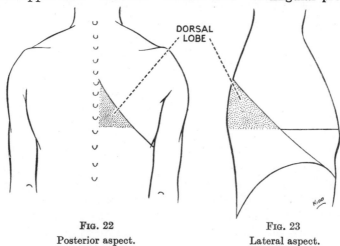

FIG. 22   FIG. 23

Posterior aspect.   Lateral aspect.

Though the bronchi for the left upper and " middle " lobes arise from a common stem, the *main bronchi* can be regarded as four in number on each side (Fig. 24), those on the left all coming off the main bronchus within a few millimetres of each other, whereas on the right side the upper lobe bronchus is more isolated. Each of these main bronchi divide into *segmental bronchi*, and so on to the finest ones (Fig. 10, p. 12).

The portions of the lung served by these principal branches of a lobar bronchus are known as *bronchopulmonary segments*, the geographical distribution of which is, for practical purposes, characteristic. Knowledge of this distribution is especially valuable in providing the key to many pulmonary shadows seen on the X-ray film—shadows which may result from obstruction of

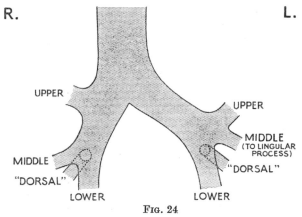

FIG. 24

The main bronchi and their divisions. (The "dorsal" bronchi
run directly backwards.)

one of these bronchi with resulting collapse of the corresponding pulmonary segment, or from localised inflammation such as marks a lung abscess. It is a guide, too, to the optimum position in which a patient must be placed to ensure adequate "postural drainage" of a localised zone of bronchiectasis, and it may determine the best approach for the surgeon when he comes to operate upon a pulmonary lesion.

The clinically important divisions of the bronchial tree (main and segmental bronchi) are shown in Figs. 25, 26, 32, and 33. For simplification, the relatively unimportant "cardiac" bronchus on the right side is omitted.

The right upper lobe bronchus divides into three segmental branches, to supply three main segments.

(a) *Right anterolateral segment.* Radiograms of this segment show opacities such as those drawn in Fig. 27.

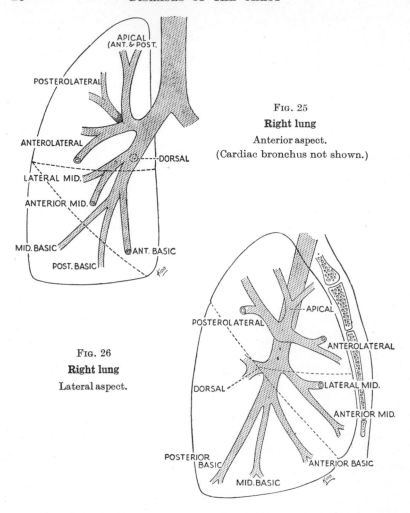

FIG. 25

Right lung

Anterior aspect.

(Cardiac bronchus not shown.)

FIG. 26

Right lung

Lateral aspect.

(b) *Right posterolateral segment.* Radiograms of consolidation of this segment show an opacity in the P.A. (or " straight ") film somewhat similar to that of the anterolateral segment (cp. Fig. 27), but as the lesion is posterior, the lateral film establishes the position of the lesion (Fig. 28).

(c) *Right apical segment.* This zone extends to the dome of the pleura above, to the mediastinum on its mesial side, and has a lateral border which is concave outwards. In the lateral X-ray film, it occupies a V-shaped wedge from apex to hilum, over which are superimposed the shadows of the right shoulder. Consolidation of this segment gives the shadowing seen in Fig. 29.

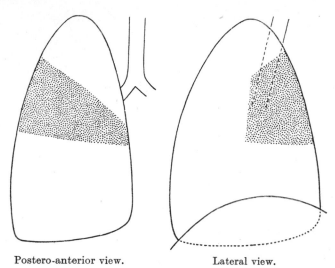

Postero-anterior view.   Lateral view.

Fig. 27

Consolidation of anterolateral segment, right upper lobe.

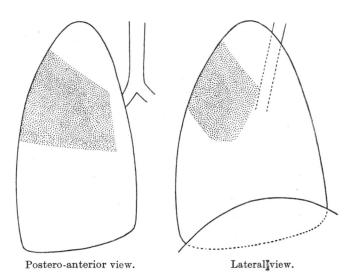

Postero-anterior view.   Lateral view.

Fig. 28

Consolidation of posterolateral segment, right upper lobe.

The **right middle lobe bronchus** divides into two major branches, which supply—

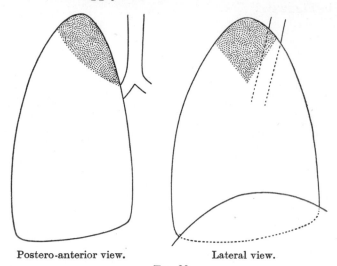

Postero-anterior view.   Lateral view.
FIG. 29
Consolidation, apical segment, right upper lobe.

(a) *the right anterior middle segment,* consolidation of which gives the following X-ray pictures :

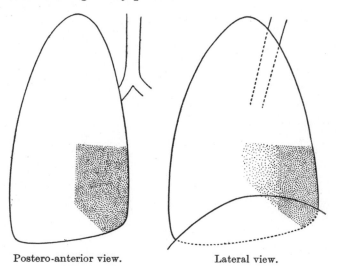

Postero-anterior view.   Lateral view.
FIG. 30
Consolidation, anterior segment of right middle lobe.

(b) the *right lateral middle segment*, consolidation of which gives the following X-ray pictures :

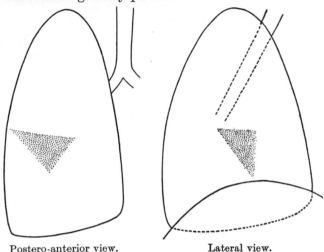

Postero-anterior view.   Lateral view.
FIG. 31
Consolidation, lateral segment, right middle lobe.

Because of the length of the middle bronchus before it divides into its segmental branches, consolidation or collapse usually

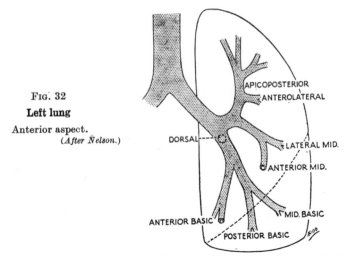

FIG. 32

Left lung

Anterior aspect.
(*After Nelson.*)

APICOPOSTERIOR
ANTEROLATERAL
DORSAL
LATERAL MID.
ANTERIOR MID.
ANTERIOR BASIC
MID. BASIC
POSTERIOR BASIC

involves the middle lobe as a whole, rather than its individual segments.

The important segments of both **lower lobes** are the *dorsal* (upper part of lower lobe) ; and the *anterior, posterior and middle basic segments*. These are supplied by the appropriate bronchi (Figs. 25 and 26).

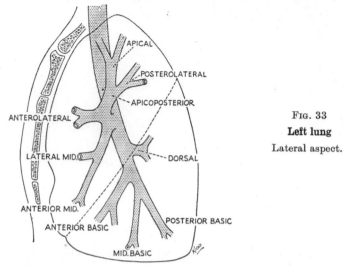

FIG. 33

Left lung

Lateral aspect.

" *Dorsal* " *segment.* Consolidation of this segment gives the following shadowing on the X-ray films :—

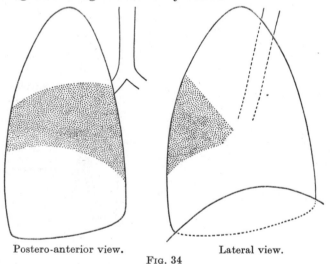

Postero-anterior view.   Lateral view.

FIG. 34

Consolidation of dorsal segment, right lower lobe.

Posterior basic segment. Consolidation of this segment gives the following X-ray pictures :—

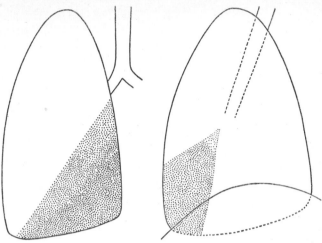

Postero-anterior view.   Lateral view.

FIG. 35

Consolidation of posterior basic segment, right lower lobe.
(In the left lung the corresponding shadow is often hidden by the heart shadow.)

Anterior basic segment. Consolidation of this segment gives the following X-ray pictures :—

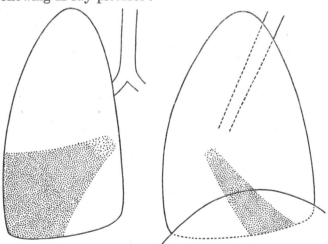

Postero-anterior view.   Lateral view.
Cardiophrenic angle clear (contrast with Fig. 35).

FIG. 36

Consolidation anterior basic segment, right lower lobe.

Note that when there is collapse of this segment, its shrinkage gives a narrow band of shadowing which may be mistaken for interlobar thickening or effusion : but the latter is usually fusiform in shape.

Middle basic segment. Consolidation of this segment gives the following X-ray pictures :—

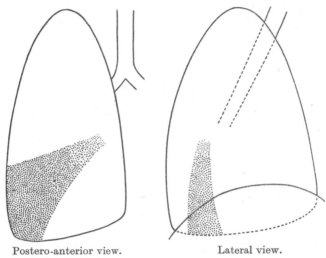

Postero-anterior view.   Lateral view.

FIG. 37

Consolidation of middle basic segment, right lower lobe.

Note that although on the lateral view the lesion might be confused with one involving the posterior basic segment (cp. Fig. 35), the P.A. view makes the situation of the lesion clear.

Similarly, while in the P.A. view it might be confused with a lesion of the anterior basic segment (cp. Fig. 36), the lateral view makes it possible to distinguish the segment involved.

The left upper lobe corresponds to the combined upper and middle lobes of the right lung. Its bronchus divides into two main branches, one supplying the " upper lobe " proper, the other (the left middle lobe bronchus) supplying the lingula, which corresponds to the right middle lobe.

The left **" upper lobe " bronchus** divides into two main divisions, the left anterolateral : and the left apicoposterior, which ascends and then divides in turn into an apical and a posterolateral branch, to supply a zone equivalent to the combined apical and posterolateral segments of the right lung.

(a) The *left anterolateral segment* corresponds closely in its X-ray appearances (for example, when consolidated) to the right anterolateral segment, though owing to the absence of a fissure between the " upper " and " middle " lobes, its lower border is usually not so sharply demarcated.

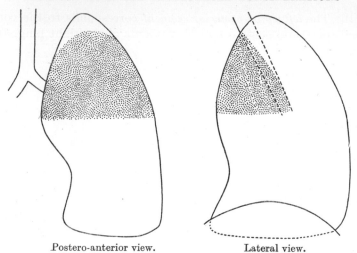

Postero-anterior view.   Lateral view.

FIG. 38

Consolidation of antero-lateral segment, left upper lobe.

Note that with absorption collapse, the shadow will shrink towards the hilum, and leave a clear area between it and the chest wall.

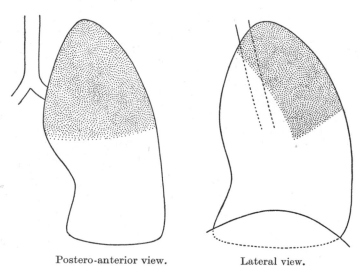

Postero-anterior view.   Lateral view.

FIG. 39

Consolidation of apico-posterior segment, left upper lobe.

Note how valuable the lateral view is in differentiating the apico-posterior segment from the antero-lateral segment, especially when the apico-posterior segment is collapsed, and the antero-lateral segment expands to compensate, so producing an aerated translucent zone on the mediastinal border of the apex of the lung.   Cp. Figs. 38 and 39.

3

(b) The *left apico-posterior segment* corresponds to the combined apical and postero-lateral segments of the right lung, and

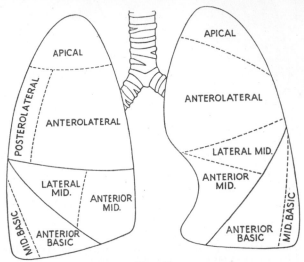

Fig. 40
Lungs—anterior aspect.

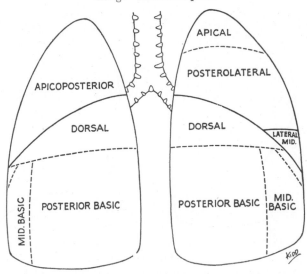

Fig. 41
Lungs—posterior aspect.

is supplied by a single ascending bronchus which later divides into apical and postero-lateral divisions.

The **lingula**. The left middle lobe or lingular bronchus corresponds to the right middle lobe bronchus, dividing into two segmental branches at some distance from the hilum.

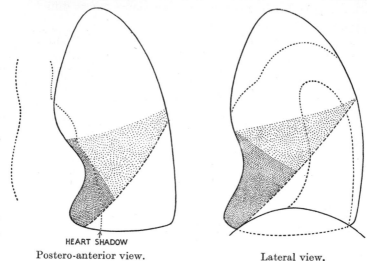

Postero-anterior view.   Lateral view.

FIG. 42

Lingula (middle and lateral segments) and its
relation to the heart shadow.

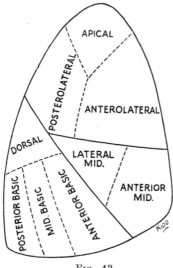

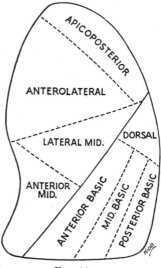

FIG. 43   FIG. 44

Right lung, lateral aspect.   Left lung, lateral aspect.

For this reason, segmental lesions are far less common than those of the lingula as a whole, and for most practical purposes the lingula can be regarded as a single unit. In X-ray films, the overlying heart shadow may at times cause difficulty by obscuring a lingular shadow.

The geography of the " respiratory districts " supplied by segmental bronchi is diagrammatically represented in Figs. 40, 41, 43 and 44. Chapter VII ("Collapse of the Lung") gives some practical clinical illustrations of the importance of these areas (see also Figs. 75 to 86). It should be already clear to the student that the discovery of a lesion involving one of these pulmonary segments may well be associated with some lesion in the bronchus which supplies it.

For further studies of the bronchial anatomy, the student should consult monographs by Foster-Carter and Hoyle, *Diseases of the Chest*, 1945, **11**, 511, and by R. C. Brock, *The Anatomy of the Bronchial Tree*, 1946, Oxford Med. Publications.

CHAPTER II

SYMPTOMS

INTRODUCTORY

SYMPTOMS are the obvious troubles noticed by the patient himself or his associates, or by the doctor who " looks him over " and asks him revealing questions. *Signs* are discoveries which the doctor makes by means of his trained technique.

Symptoms tell a patient that something is wrong ; they make him ask, " What is the matter with me ? " At times they may tell the doctor a good deal more, especially when a particular group of symptoms is present or if they have made their appearance in a particular chronological order. In any case, they define a problem which he must go on to solve by a study of physical signs and by certain special investigations. When that problem has been fully solved the explanation of each symptom will become clear.

Earlier physicians could study symptoms yet know little about the actual condition of the underlying diseased organs or the reasons why they were diseased. In 1761 Auenbrugger wrote his little book about a new way of examining the chest by percussion, and the same year Morgagni published his five volumes of cases in which history, clinical picture and post-mortem findings are all set out and correlated.* Henceforward the study of physical signs and of their correlation with the appearances of the organs after death was to go a long way towards enabling the doctor to see with the mind's eye the alterations of disease in organs hidden from view ; to " observe in physical signs and think in lesions."

It is true that symptoms are rarely pathognomonic ; nevertheless many an error of diagnosis is due to the failure to bring to light some symptom or to realise its importance. This is because a discerning appreciation of symptoms gives

* *De sedibus et causis morborum per anatomen indagatis.* Venice, 1761.

the doctor a lead in his whole examination, makes him ask himself the right questions about the illness, and leaves him dissatisfied unless he has found an answer which covers them all. Moreover, once the diagnosis is made, they may give much information about the course the disease is taking and so guide both treatment and prognosis.

Here is a common example which illustrates these points. A man in the thirties works in an office. For some time he has felt unduly tired. His wife has noticed it too ; she is worried and perhaps a little resentful, because when he comes home at night he sinks lethargically into an armchair and stays there. His friends notice that he looks pale and " seedy," and his face is thinner than it was. He feels " badly below the weather " and longs for the summer holiday which will put him right ; meanwhile his work is a burden and he has to force himself along duties which once he took easily in his stride. Then one day he gets a " dose of 'flu " and is distressed with a pain below his right shoulder blade. A day or two later the doctor is called in to hear the tale of all these symptoms and elicit others. Already a number of possible diagnoses come to his mind.

He proceeds to examine the patient according to a careful technique and discovers certain physical signs. He finds that the lower part of the right thorax does not expand so well as the left, and the apex beat of the heart is displaced into the left axilla. Percussion over the right base reveals an area of board-like dullness, and auscultation there shows that the normal voice and breath sounds are absent, whereas just above the dull area the voice sounds have a bleating quality. It is now almost certain that the pain was due to pleurisy and that an effusion has developed ; actual proof comes from inserting into the chest a needle attached to a syringe, and withdrawing fluid.

But what out of several possible causes is the actual cause of the pleurisy ? The fluid is serous, not purulent nor blood-stained. Is it a tuberculous pleurisy, or is it due to one of the less common causes of a serous effusion ? The doctor's own tools of hands and eyes and ears must be supplemented by certain special investigations. Examination of the fluid is called for, and if tubercle bacilli are found (and this is rare), or if the fluid when injected into a guinea-pig produces tuberculous lesions, then the tuberculous nature of the lesion is proved.

The diagnosis is still incomplete, for the doctor wants to know whether this tuberculous effusion is associated with obvious tuberculosis in the substance of the lung or whether it is due to a number of tiny tubercles dotted on or just under the visceral pleura ; to know this may guide him in his choice of whether to establish a replacement pneumothorax or not. So an X-ray examination of the chest must be made. It shows the shadow of the effusion and of the heart displaced away from the lesion, but there is nothing in the lung above it or in the other lung to suggest active parenchymatous tuberculosis. Later, when the fluid has been absorbed and the whole of the lung field is visible, it is clear that there is no obvious basal tuberculous lesion in the lung. Here at last is the complete diagnosis, always provided that there are no complications elsewhere. The young man is suffering from tuberculous pleurisy with effusion, of the type which used to be called idiopathic. It explains his tiredness, his " influenza," his pain and all his other symptoms ; it explains, too, the physical signs which the doctor discovered.

THE MEDICAL HISTORY OF THE ILLNESS

" Every man is of importance to himself." (SAMUEL JOHNSON.)

The first step in collecting the facts on which diagnosis can be based is to obtain a history of the patient's illness and any data of his past history or of his family history which may be relevant. This demands of the examiner a wide background of pathology, correlated with medicine, so that he may be in a position to appreciate the possible pathological meanings of what the patient " as a layman " tells him.

But to secure the data is in practice very largely an art— the art of dealing gently and wisely with one's fellows. Most patients come to the doctor in fear—fear of serious illness, of the economic consequences of illness, of the doctor whose decision means so much, and of the unknown. In the sphere of lung disease these terrors are often increased by newspaper clichés and by old accumulated traditions gathered round " consumption," including its social stigma. Many patients dare not face the truth, and hold back important facts, per-haps because they wish to persuade themselves that if the doctor fails to bring them to light they cannot be disturbingly

significant. Each patient, therefore, must be met as an individual, to be understood with kindness and sympathy, with
a quiet firmness if need be, and with the calm confidence
of the physician whose daily work is to assume the responsibility of making judgments. Some patients are talkative,
inconsequent, diffuse. Some are apparently casual or bom-
bastic—" whistling to keep up their courage." Some are dis-
trustful and reticent. But all are anxious in the presence of
the doctor ; they are troubled in body and mind by some
complaint which, however unimportant or otherwise it may be
to the physician, almost fills the screen of their attention. Let
them have their say about it, then, within reason ; to listen
seriously to their story will help them to give you a fuller trust
and confidence, and even if at first sight it may appear mainly
chaff, there is always the chance of finding grains of wheat
among it. Then ask your own questions, drawing out the
reticent and firmly keeping the talkative to the point. While
the patient has his present troubles in mind it is bad psychology
to switch away unnaturally to the family history or even to
his past history. Until you have convinced him that you
understand what he is trying to tell you, and that you are
ready to consider it carefully in assessing it for what it is worth,
you can hardly expect his full co-operation. Suppose, for
example, that he is worried by a pain in his side ; he comes
to the doctor to learn what it means and how it is to be relieved.
As the patient tells his tale the doctor thinks almost auto-
matically of the various pathological causes of pain in the
side, and how the pain may differ according to its cause, and
so he usually finds that he needs to know far more than
the patient volunteers. How long has he had the pain ?
How did it come on ? Is it always there ? What sort of a
pain is it, and how bad is it ? Does anything make it worse
or better ? Has he had anything like it before ? Any question
is useful which leads to a closer analysis and clarification of
the symptom.

   Tact, kindness and common sense go most of the way
towards obtaining a reliable and helpful history. This part
of the examination asks for a sense of leisure and of the value
of talk between two human beings. The doctor may with
advantage recall Samuel Johnson's complaint of someone who
was always in a hurry, " which is very disagreeable to a man

who loves to fold his legs and have out his talk." Provided
the talk is kept to the matter in hand, the time spent on
" history " can often be the most fruitful part of the doctor's
examination. Moreover, once the patient is satisfied in his
mind that the doctor is *au fait* with his present troubles it
will not seem illogical to delve into the past (his own or that
of his forbears) for possible influences on the onset and nature
of his immediate illness.

A patient suffering from a disorder of the respiratory tract,
then, may complain of various symptoms. These must be
integrated with the clinical picture as a whole ; the details are
elucidated as he tells the story of his illness and also as you
observe him while he is under your care.

It is important, therefore, to have in mind certain general
conceptions of the meaning of these symptoms as a background
to the study of the individual patient and of the particular
disease.

COUGH

It has already been pointed out that coughing is a defensive
reflex ; it helps to keep the lower respiratory passages clear
and to protect them against the entry of foreign material from
outside and the stagnation of secretions in the passages themselves. It consists essentially in a sharp, explosive expulsion
of compressed air from the tracheo-bronchial tree. It begins
with an inspiration—the deeper the inspiration the more air
in the lungs, and therefore the more effective the cough. The
glottis closes, the soft palate is raised, and both the ordinary
and the accessory muscles of expiration are tensed for a forced
expiration. At the moment of forced expiration against the
barrier of the closed glottis there is a marked rise of pressure
in the respiratory tract, as may be seen from the congestion
of the face and neck which is produced. Then the glottis
relaxes and the compressed air with its contents is violently
expelled through the mouth. In certain patients the marked
rise of intrapulmonary pressure is indicated by the tense bulging
of the apex of the lung into the root of the neck during a severe
bout of coughing.

The usual point of origin of the reflex is a stimulus to the
branches of the superior laryngeal nerve in the laryngeal area ;
it may take origin also from vagal afferents from the bronchial

mucosa (particularly at the bronchial bifurcations). There are
other afferents (from the pharynx, for example, in smokers or
whisky drinkers) ; but these are not very important, for in
nine cases out of ten cough is due to some stimulus from the
respiratory tract (Fig. 45).

Sensitivity varies in different parts of the tracheo-bronchial
tree, as is well seen during the passage of a bronchoscope in a
patient under light general anæsthesia. The larynx and the

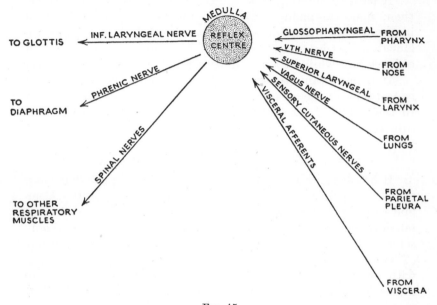

FIG. 45

The reflex arc for coughing.

bifurcation of the trachea are peculiarly sensitive ; the upper
mucosa is on the whole more sensitive than that of the deeper
tubes, but a tracheotomy tube can be worn quite comfortably
and secretions in the lower tubes may not excite cough until
a small change of position brings them in contact with the
more sensitive mucosa at the bifurcation of a bronchus.

The character of a patient's cough will depend on the factors
which go to make it up ; moreover, since in itself it is only a
symptom, its importance will depend largely on the clinical
signs and symptoms which accompany it.

If the respiratory muscles are weak, or if the reflex centre is poisoned, cough may be slight and ineffectual, or even absent ; this may happen in severe prostration or grave toxæmia. Moreover, a cough may be cut short voluntarily because it is painful, as in the short, restrained cough of the acutely painful stage of pleuro-pneumonia. Again, when a bronchial tube becomes obstructed by a foreign body or by a plug of sticky mucus, and the air has consequently been absorbed from the portion of the lung which it supplies, the collapsed portion of the lung " loses its power to cough," for there is now no air beyond the obstruction, to be compressed and forcibly expelled during the act of coughing.

The condition of the tracheal and bronchial mucosa will greatly influence the actual sound which is heard. Congestive catarrhal conditions of the pharynx or upper air passages will produce a hacking cough—short, dry, irritable, frequently repeated. With accompanying swelling of the tonsils blocking the pharyngeal outlet, it becomes thick and guttural. Slight catarrh of the vocal cords gives it a veiled, husky timbre ; a more serious laryngitis produces a harsh, hoarse cough (" croupy "). In destructive lesions of the vocal cords (as in tuberculous ulceration or neoplasm) the cough becomes toneless, whispering, aphonic. A cough is dry or moist, according to the presence or absence of secretions in the respiratory passages—productive when sputum is coughed up, unproductive otherwise.

Cough may be produced voluntarily, and, as with many reflexes, it may become a nervous habit. Occasionally a dramatic hysterical cough may be met with—a loud, painless, unproductive bark, distressing perhaps to the hearer but not to the patient himself.

In laryngeal paralysis due to involvement of the recurrent laryngeal nerve (through pressure, for example, by an aortic aneurysm or other mediastinal swelling) the tone and timbre are so modified as to produce a sound which may variously be described as " brassy," " gander," " bovine " or " leopard's growl." A somewhat similar modification may be caused by direct pressure on the trachea itself.

It is helpful, therefore, to know the answers to the following questions about the cough :—

    1. How does the patient describe it and what is its
        character?

2. How long has he had it ; how long does it last ; how often
   does it occur ?
3. When does it come on and what brings it on ?
4. Does it come in spasmodic attacks ?
5. Is it dry or moist ; does the coughing bring up sputum
   or not ?
6. Is it painful and distressing, accompanied by whooping
   or vomiting ?

Coughing may accidentally and occasionally end in vomiting, either because of its violence or because a piece of mucus
sticks in an over-sensitive pharynx and stimulates the vomiting
reflex.   There are certain patients, however, whose bouts of
coughing almost invariably end in vomiting, so that before long
their general nutrition is seriously compromised ; both cough
and vomiting are due to drag on the diaphragm, usually on
the left side, by adhesions or fibrosis. Relaxation of the traction
by means of phrenic paralysis brings relief.

HOARSENESS

In disease inside the thorax the larynx is often secondarily
affected, either by local inflammation or by paralysis due
to pressure on the recurrent laryngeal nerve.   The dysphonia
which ensues may vary from a mild huskiness to a complete
loss of voice. The extent of the loss of voice is not a measure
of the seriousness of the lesion ; a simple laryngitis, lasting
only a day or two, may prevent a patient from speaking in
anything but a toneless whisper.

Hoarseness may persist throughout life by reason of laryngeal maldevelopment or of changes due to congenital syphilis.
Acute laryngitis causes a dysphonia which passes off as the
inflammation resolves. Mucopus, which gets into the larynx
from the nasal sinuses above or the lungs below, causes the
voice to become muffled and " phlegmy," with a superadded
huskiness if actual laryngitis is present. On the other hand, a
dry laryngitis suggests that there is inadequate lubrication by
mucus and maybe a symptom of a general disease like diabetes.
The voice may be altered also by extrinsic factors—nasal obstruction, tracheal obstruction, pharyngitis ; the raucous voice
(" whisky voice ") of the chronic alcoholic is a good example.
" Functional aphonia " may occur in neurotic patients ; here
the voice is a soft whisper.

Hoarseness which persists—say for more than a month—calls for careful investigation. It may be due (especially if it comes on in persons over the age of forty) to a tumour, benign or malignant. It may be a presenting symptom of tuberculosis of the lungs. Laryngeal tuberculosis is never primary. It is characteristic of the lesion that the alteration of the voice may be out of all proportion to the degree of laryngeal congestion.

It is impossible to find out the cause of a dysphonia without

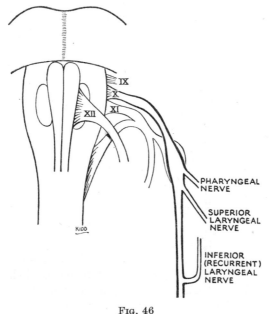

FIG. 46

Origin of laryngeal nerves.

making a laryngoscopic examination; whenever this has to be done, it is sensible to forbid the husky patient to talk at length about the story of his illness and so to fatigue his larynx. It is wiser to examine the larynx first and get his story later.

In laryngeal paralysis, laryngoscopic examination alone can reveal the lack of movement of one or both cords. Sometimes it is difficult to interpret the abnormal position of a cord; the real criterion of paralysis is its immobility, whatever its position. At times a relaxed, paralysed vocal cord may appear to move laterally, simply because it is slightly displaced to and fro by the inspiratory and expiratory currents of air ; observation of the corresponding arytenoid cartilage will show that it does not move at all.

In the presence of laryngeal palsy, diagnosis of the site of the lesion will go a long way to determining its ætiology. The derivation of the nerves supplying the larynx is seen in Fig. 46. With the exception of the cricothyroid muscle (innervated by the superior laryngeal branch of the vagus nerve), all the laryngeal muscles are supplied through the inferior (recurrent) laryngeal nerve. The characteristics of both intracranial and extracranial lesions will not be discussed here save for recurrent laryngeal palsies. They are the most frequent and the most important. This nerve has a long course, with particularly vulnerable relations on the left side with other organs. The cause of a paralysis of the nerve is usually to be looked for in the mediastinum or the lower part of the neck (there are rare instances of peripheral neuritis due to some systemic neurotoxin, such as diphtheria toxin, in which bilateral palsy is the rule). Aneurysm of the aorta and cancer of the œsophagus may compress the nerve, especially on the left side. Any form of mediastinal swelling (new growth, enlarged glands, pericardial effusion, dilated left auricle) may also compress it. In the neck the main causes are thyroid enlargements (especially malignant disease of the thyroid) and glandular enlargements of various types (Fig. 47).

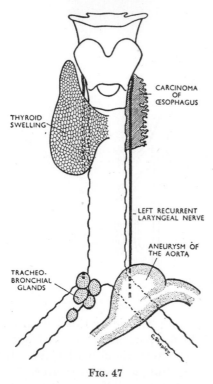

FIG. 47

Diagrammatic representation of the main causes of laryngeal palsy by compression.

Usually the earliest sign of a recurrent laryngeal lesion is abductor palsy. If it is unilateral there is no alteration in voice ; but the affected cord does not move outwards in inspiration like its fellow. On phonation the healthy cord meets the other in the middle line—as normally happens with two intact cords. Bilateral abductor palsy, which occurs in lesions affecting the cranial nuclei bilaterally, will also allow approximation of the cords in the middle line ; but as they do not move outwards on inspiration, there is respiratory obstruction, with laboured breathing and stridor.

In unilateral recurrent laryngeal palsy the voice does not alter until adductor palsy supervenes. The vocal cord on that side becomes fixed in the cadaveric position, half-way between abduction and adduction. Phonation is usually possible, because the healthy cord compensates by a movement of forced adduction, coming into contact with the paralysed cord beyond the middle line. If there is good contact the voice will not be altered ; often, however, approximation is not complete, and there is some huskiness of voice. Complete paralysis of both cords, when they are immobile in the cadaveric position, makes speaking impossible, because they cannot be approximated together.

Hysterical aphonia has certain special features. The patient's voice is reduced to a whisper. The onset is usually quite sudden and in relation to some strong emotion. On inspiration or on coughing the cords move normally, but phonation does not occur because the cords do not reach the middle line.

STRIDOR

Respired air passing in and out of a partially obstructed larynx or trachea may produce a harsh, vibrating noise which can be heard by the listener's ear ; to this noise is given the name stridor. It is a noise produced in the larger air passages in the same way as rhonchi are produced in the smaller ones ; it may occur during any part of the respiratory cycle, but naturally it will be most obvious when there is a strong current of air—ordinarily in inspiration. Clearly, therefore, it will also be particularly well heard during coughing, giving a stridulous quality to the cough. Even in so large a tube as a main bronchus, however, a noise due to obstruction is no longer a stridor ; it has become more like a wheeze. The obstruction of the larynx and trachea may be from within, as, for example, by a diphtheritic membrane ; or it may be due to pressure from without (such as an aneurysm, an enlarged thyroid, or mediastinal tumour), or from kinking (such as may be produced by localised fibrosis of the lung).

EXPECTORATION

Next to cough, expectoration is the commonest manifestation of affections of the respiratory tract ; by it the abnormal products of secretion, exudation or disintegration are emptied out of the tracheo-bronchial tree and the pulmonary alveoli. From the character of the sputum coughed up much information may be obtained about the nature of the underlying lesion. It may be made up of any or all of the following constituents : watery secretion, mucus, blood serum (in acute œdema of the lung or inflammations, for example), pus, blood (pure, or altered as in rusty sputum), epithelial cells from the respiratory tract, products of disintegration of lung tissue (elastic fibres, occasionally calcareous masses), bacteria and parasites. It is important to know how much sputum is being coughed up—in the twenty-four hour period, for example ; what it is like in colour, consistency and smell (is it fœtid ?) ; whether there is a considerable deposit on standing ; and whether it is coughed up in quantity at particular times or after changes of position. The more detailed characteristics of the sputum, with its macroscopic and microscopic features, will be dealt with later in relation to particular diseases.

DYSPNŒA

The word *dyspnœa* is used to cover difficult, painful or disordered breathing. *Hyperpnœa* is merely increased breathing and may not be noticed by the subject himself, for a healthy person is not conscious of any increase in respiration until the normal rate is doubled.

It has already been seen that there are two main factors in the control of respiration—one chemical, acting on the respiratory centre through its blood supply, and the other nervous, the Hering-Breuer reflex, acting through the vagus, the respiratory centre, and the phrenic and spinal nerve efferents to the thoracic cage. The respiratory centre is also influenced by impulses from the higher cerebral centres, as in emotion.

The obvious causes of dyspnœa are many—various diseases of the lungs and pleura, cardiac failure, anæmia, the effects of thyrotoxicosis, the acidosis of uræmia or diabetes, increased intracranial pressure and hysteria. The ultimate, fundamental causes, however, are (1) chemical alterations in the blood flowing through the respiratory centre ; (2) local conditions in the lungs which make them more rigid and less easily distensible, so increasing the excitability of the Hering-Breuer reflex and causing rapid and shallow breathing. Evidence grows that the latter is by far the more usual factor in the dyspnœa of ill patients. It determines the dyspnœa of pneumonia, of pulmonary œdema and of massive collapse of the lungs. Pulmonary congestion, with consequent rigidity of the lung tissue, is the cause of cardiac dyspnœa, whether from primary heart failure or from heart failure secondary to fibrosis of the lungs and the pneumoconioses, emphysema, thyrotoxicosis or arteriosclerosis. The chemical factor is paramount in profound anæmia, in conditions with deficient aeration of the blood (tracheal obstruction, bronchial asthma, uncomplicated emphysema) and in the acidosis of uræmia or diabetes ; but as soon as myocardial insufficiency complicates the picture, to produce some degree of pulmonary congestion, the lungs become less easily distensible, and the reflex, mechanical factor of dyspnœa is added.

Dyspnœa may also occur as a hysterical manifestation, either in the form of attacks of deep sighing respirations, usually following some emotional disturbance, or occasionally even as paroxysms of hyperpnœa, with deep and laboured breathing. If this persists long enough the hyperventilation may wash out enough carbon dioxide from the blood to cause alkalosis with tetany.

Certain clinical varieties of dyspnœa are commonly recognised. *Inspiratory dyspnœa* is due to obstruction (from within or without) of the larynx or trachea, which slows the respiratory rhythm by prolonging and deepening inspiration; it causes grave apprehension and indeed anguish to the sufferer, and is

4

accompanied by the sucking-in, during inspiration, of the soft parts above the sternum and below and between the ribs.

Expiratory dyspnœa is due either to serious loss of pulmonary elasticity (as in emphysema) or to generalised bronchial spasm (as in asthma). *Dyspnœa on exertion* (or dyspnœa of effort) is a symptom of many types of respiratory disease, as it is one of the principal signs of the disturbances of pulmonary circulation caused by cardiovascular diseases. *Orthopnœa* is the name given to dyspnœa which is present even when the patient sits up. On sitting up, blood collects into the splanchnic areas, with a resulting " decongestion " of the lungs, and therefore an increased vital capacity. Moreover, when the patient is lying down, the diaphragm rises into the thorax, so reducing the capacity of the lungs. When he is upright, the diaphragm descends and the capacity of the lungs, and therefore the vital capacity, is increased. Orthopnœa represents, therefore, a grave breakdown of the respiratory reserve.

Cheyne-Stokes breathing is the term given to a form of periodic breathing which was first described by Cheyne in 1818 and rediscovered by Stokes in 1857. It consists of a rhythmical waxing and waning of respiration—alternations of hyperpnœa and apnœa. Anoxæmia of the respiratory centre lowers its sensitivity and so abolishes the spontaneous rhythmical activity of breathing. The consequent apnœa results in the accumulation of carbon dioxide and acid metabolites in the blood, reawakening the centre and causing hyperventilation, which in turn removes the excess of carbon dioxide, whereupon the centre " goes to sleep again." During the period of breathing the depth of respiration may gradually increase to a maximum and then dwindle again to nothing ; or there may be no change in the level of respiration, with only a few uniform breaths in each group of respirations (Biot's irregular breathing). Anything which causes marked anæmia or anoxæmia of the respiratory centre may cause these types of periodic breathing — cerebral vascular disease or peripheral vasoconstriction associated with cardiorenal disease, cardiac failure, poisoning in uræmia and other conditions, and increased intracranial pressure from tumour, cerebral injury, hæmorrhage, or infection such as abscess or meningitis. Anæmia of the respiratory centre is accompanied not only by an increase of carbon dioxide in the blood but also by a rise of blood pressure, which helps to restore the activity of the centre by improving its blood supply. This type of respiratory embarrassment will be improved if the cerebral circulation is improved (by treating heart failure successfully), if poisons are eliminated (toxins in uræmia, morphia), if oxygen is given to cure the anoxæmia of the centre, or if carbon dioxide is administered to act as a respiratory stimulant (in carbon monoxide poisoning, for example).

It will be clear that respiratory disease which causes deficient aeration of the blood, so producing a need for oxygen and an accumulation of carbon dioxide in the blood, demands an increased depth of respiration ; this is obtained by prolonging and deepening respiration, with little or no increase in rate, and it occurs in laryngeal and tracheal obstruction, in the diffuse bronchial spasm of asthma and in the diffuse spasmodic obstruction of the earliest stage of bronchiolitis. On the other hand, in conditions of increased rigidity of the lungs, with exaggeration of the Hering-Breuer reflex, the breathing will be shallow and rapid ; this is seen in the pneumonias, in massive collapse of the lung, in all forms of pulmonary congestion or œdema (including that associated with pulmonary embolism, single or multiple), and in diffuse exudative or miliary tuberculosis.

CYANOSIS

The blue colour of the skin and mucous membranes, known as " cyanosis," is due to the presence of sufficient reduced hæmoglobin in the capillaries to give the dusky colour which shows through the integument. A minimum content of 5 gm. of reduced hæmoglobin per 100 c.c. of blood is necessary before the blue colour is apparent. In profound anæmia, however, with a hæmoglobin content of less than 30 per cent., the amount of reduced hæmoglobin cannot reach this minimum content, even in the presence of marked anoxia.* The greater the amount of reduced hæmoglobin the deeper the cyanosis.

* Normal blood contains about 15 gm. of hæmoglobin per 100 c.c. Now 0·75 gm. HB. takes up 1 c.c. of oxygen. Thus 100 c.c. of normal blood (= 15 gm. HB.) can take up, at full saturation, $\frac{15}{0.75} = 20$ c.c. of oxygen. 5 gm. of reduced HB. corresponds to $\frac{5}{0.75}$ or 6·7 c.c. of oxygen unsaturation. An anæmic patient with only 30 per cent HB. can only take up $\frac{30}{100}$ of 20 c.c. = 6 c.c. O_2. Which, even if wholly reduced, would not reach the minimum of about 6·7 c.c. O_2 unsaturation which is necessary to produce cyanosis.

It is best seen in the lips, nose, cheeks or extremities (ears, fingers, toes) ; it can be temporarily abolished by pressing out the dusky blood from the part. The intensity of the colour will depend also on whether the small peripheral vessels are dilated and " open," or contracted and " closed."

The blood in the capillary vessels may contain an excess of reduced hæmoglobin either because it left the heart in this condition, or because there is an abnormal, excessive change of oxyhæmoglobin to reduced hæmoglobin while the blood is passing through the peripheral capillary bed. Sometimes both causes are present in the same patient.

The most clear-cut form of cyanosis due to de-oxygenated blood leaving the heart is in congenital heart disease with some form of septal defect which allows the passage of un-aerated blood from the right heart direct into the systemic circulation. Here a marked diffuse blueness is (in the absence of congestive heart failure) accompanied by little or no distress in breathing, at all events when the patient is not exercising—an observation which emphasises the importance of " rigid lung " (as contrasted with deficiency of oxygen) in the production of dyspnœa. Deficient oxygenation of the blood in the lungs due to asphyxia, capillary bronchitis and other forms of acute or chronic pulmonary disease will also result in de-oxygenated blood leaving the heart ; very often, however, the cyanosis in patients with troubles such as these is to a greater or less degree associated also with heart failure and slowing of the peripheral circulation.

Abnormally slow passage of the blood through the peripheral capillaries allows the tissues to rob it of more oxygen than usual, and so to produce more reduced hæmoglobin. Slowing of the peripheral circulation is in any case a normal response to cold, and mild degrees of local blueness may therefore be compatible with good health. There are many instances, however, of capillary stasis or poor blood flow, associated either with general circulatory failure or with some form of local vascular paralysis where the cyanosis is indicative of serious disease.

It is not always easy to sort out the cause of cyanosis in a particular case, whether it is " respiratory " or " circulatory " or a combination of both. Roughly, it may be said that if the cyanosis is wholly relieved by the inhalation of oxygen, then deficient oxygenation of the blood in the lungs is the cause ;

if it is only partially relieved, then there is also a circulatory factor; and if it is not relieved at all, the trouble is wholly circulatory. Put this way, the rule is an over-simplification of a complex balance of phenomena, but it will serve as a guide. It is much more important when faced with a blue patient to recall the possible causes and to try to visualise the condition of the peripheral vessels—are they dilated or contracted ; are they full of blood or empty ; is the skin cold or hot ; is there sweating or not ? The capillaries may be engorged, the pulse full, the flow rapid ; often that means that in addition to the deficient oxygenation in the lungs there is associated carbon dioxide retention, with peripheral vasodilation and an inadequate circulation. The blueness is deep and "florid," and the patient is breathing heavily. On the other hand, the skin may be pale, cold and sweating, with leaden "*livid cyanosis*"—poorly filled capillaries in a patient with respiratory and circulatory failure, a rapid thready pulse and quick, shallow breathing. A bedside analysis of these various factors will contribute much to clinical judgment and is better than any merely descriptive impression in terms of colours such as plum, purple, mauve, lavender or heliotrope cyanosis.

Cyanosis may also result from the formation in the blood of certain derivatives of hæmoglobin. Methæmoglobin is a coffee-coloured pigment, and is produced by large doses of drugs such as chlorates, coal-tar derivatives and sulphonamides. The latter drugs may also determine the formation of sulph-hæmoglobin, a derivative of rare occurrence, which gives rise to a leaden type of cyanosis.

HÆMOPTYSIS

Bleeding from the lower respiratory tract may occur in a large number of conditions—acute and chronic infections, trauma, new growths, congestion, infarction and many more. The symptom will be considered in its appropriate contexts when individual diseases come to be studied ; but certain general observations may be made at this point.

Small hæmorrhages may arise from diapedesis through a congested mucosa, and the hæmoglobin may stain the sputum pink or red or (if the pigment is altered) "rusty." If there is more bleeding, the sputum becomes blood - streaked or may contain frank clots. Profuse bleeding may result from the rupture of a vein in an ulcerated patch or in the floor of a cavity, or from an artery (usually from a small miliary aneurysm in its wall) ; here the blood wells up and gushes into the mouth almost without a cough.

At times a patient may not know whether he has coughed up the blood or vomited it. Vomited blood is usually dark and acid in reaction ; blood from the lungs is alkaline, and bright and frothy from air bubbles. (If the hæmoptysis is severe, some of the blood coughed up may be swallowed and later vomited.) For some days after the bleeding from the lungs or bronchi the sputum will be streaked or stained with blood.

Every case of hæmoptysis must be carefully investigated, and the patient should be regarded as suffering from tuberculosis until the contrary is proved. Such a bias does not excuse the neglect of all possible aids to a proved diagnosis. However, in a patient of the cancer age who for the first time has hæmoptysis without any previous history of respiratory trouble, the cause of the bleeding is more likely to be ulceration of a bronchial carcinoma.

A sharp hæmoptysis may herald an acute general infection, revealing an intense pulmonary congestion. Pneumonia may begin in this way, as may typhoid fever or influenza, or the malignant " hæmorrhagic " varieties of any of the acute specific fevers.

PAIN IN THE CHEST

It does not need much experience in diseases of the lungs to be made aware that there may be extensive lesions in the lung with little or no pain whatever. There are many types of pain which may be felt in or about the thorax—muscular pains due to strain or even tearing of muscle fibres (aggravated by contraction of the affected muscles and accompanied with local tenderness on pressure) ; the boring pain of an eroding aneurysm ; root pains radiating round the trunk (caused by tabes dorsalis, syphilitic meningitis, tumours of the cord, herpes zoster, spondylitis and other lesions which involve the posterior nerve roots) ; substernal pain on swallowing (associated with œsophageal obstruction) ; the pains of angina or coronary ischæmia, or of aortitis ; pains in the breast ; occasionally, referred dyspeptic pains ; the pain of true intercostal neuritis, which must always be regarded as so rare that some other lesion must be diligently sought before true neuritis is accepted as the cause ; and, finally, the pains associated with disease of the lungs and pleuræ.

Lung tissue and the visceral pleura are entirely devoid of pain sense. The parietal pleura, on the other hand, is richly supplied with sensory (pain) nerves from the intercostals, and experiment has shown that pressure on the parietal pleura produces a sharp pain which can be located with fair accuracy over or near the point of stimulation. The diaphragmatic pleura is also sensitive, but stimulation of it never produces local pain ; the pain is always referred. The central part of the diaphragm is innervated by the phrenic nerve, and the afferents from here enter mainly the third and fourth cervical posterior nerve roots ; the peripheral part of the diaphragm is innervated by the lower intercostals, and the afferents enter the seventh to twelfth posterior nerve roots. Pain, therefore, from the central portion of the diaphragm is referred to the neck and the upper part of the shoulder ; from the outer parts of the diaphragm it is referred to the lower thorax, lumbar region and abdomen. The stronger the pleural stimulation the wider is the area of the referred pain, and it may even radiate to the other side of the body.

Pain in pleurisy is almost certainly due to the stretching of a tense, inflamed parietal pleura and not (as is usually accepted) to the friction of roughened pleural surfaces. The pain is usually severe on inspiration and absent on expiration, though the pleural surfaces rub against each other in both phases. Moreover, pain may be present without friction rub, and friction rub without pain. In the same way the pain of spontaneous pneumothorax is caused by the distension of the pleural cavity with air and consequent tension of the parietal pleura. It is clear that these pleural pains may vary greatly in intensity, according to the amount and rapidity of the pleural stretching and also to the condition of the pleura itself. If the parietal pleura is inflamed, the inflammatory products *in situ* may by their tension cause a severe pain stimulus in the nerve endings in contact with them.

There are unsolved problems of pleural sensibility ; for why should pleural pain be so common at the angle of the scapula and in the axilla outside the nipple line ? Why, on

the other hand, is apical pleurisy so seldom acutely painful—
the pain is usually a dull ache over the apex or the shoulder ?
It may be that the difference depends on the range of movement of the thoracic wall at these points. At all events the
physiological background of " pain in the chest " set out above
should always be kept in mind at the bedside.

CHAPTER III

PHYSICAL SIGNS : INSPECTION, PALPATION

THE routine of the doctor's examination of the patient is that consecrated by tradition and experience—" inspection, palpation, percussion, auscultation." Using his eyes and hands and ears, the doctor observes or brings to light signs which help him to determine lesions of the underlying lungs and pleura. Just as the painter cannot become a great artist without long experiment with paint and canvas, hard work and many a failure from which he buys his experience, so the student must live laborious days to learn by the bedside and in the post-mortem room what " normal " and " abnormal " findings really are, and what is their significance. Nowadays X-ray examination is also available for this study ; some modernists, indeed, regard radiology of the chest as an instrument which will largely replace the uncertainties of personal skill by the unbiased precision of objective science. Sooner or later we shall, no doubt, arrive at a properly balanced use of both these diagnostic methods, but at the moment we are in a phase where many clinicians and some radiologists accept an X-ray film as though it were a true likeness of the underlying tissues. Radiology offers a world of shadows ; and because it has been and can be so helpful in diseases of the chest, there is now a danger of asking it to solve problems which are outside its competence. So there are those who look at its shadows and confidently pin labels on to them without understanding or proving their actual pathological basis. For example, certain types of bronchopneumonia may give shadows on the X-ray film very similar to those of miliary tuberculous deposits ; here, obviously, radiology is not enough and needs (as it always should) a background of pathology. In the same way a new syndrome called " pneumonitis " has recently been invented—an attempt, doubtless, to give the name of a lesion to radiological appearances without the discipline of defining

57

its exact pathology. Just because radiology has already con-
tributed so much to the knowledge of lung diseases, it is now
more than ever necessary to "prove all things and hold fast to
that which is good"; for when it is properly correlated with
pathology it can do much to assess the value of many physical
signs, and can reveal lesions which otherwise might go unsuspected or misconceived.

INSPECTION

In a preliminary survey of the patient, the general appearance is noted, particularly the decubitus, the condition of the

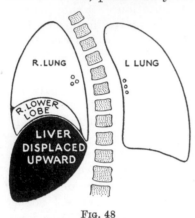

FIG. 48

To show distorting effect of scoliosis
on the lungs.

eyes, the state and colour of
the skin and lips, and the presence of emaciation or asthenia.
Next, with the patient completely stripped as far as the
waist, the doctor looks over his
chest with care from a position
directly in front of and then behind him. The general shape of
the thorax is noted, together
with the condition of the skin,
adipose tissue and musculature,
the presence of œdema, dilated
and projecting veins (collateral
circulation), operation scars and
rashes.

Alterations in the general shape of the chest are not of
particular importance, save for the barrel-shaped chest of
emphysema. Deformities from rickets in early life are not
usually apposite to adult disease, and " flat " and " phthinoid "
chests do not necessarily mark a patient down as a serious
candidate for pulmonary tuberculosis.

Scoliosis and kyphosis may raise problems for the examiner.
Primary scoliosis makes the chest asymmetrical, so that de-
ductions derived from comparison of one side with the other
may be misleading (Fig. 48) ; on the other hand, scoliosis
may be secondary to fibrosis of the lung, the concavity being
directed to the diseased side. Kyphosis may be the result of
emphysema ; angular kyphosis is usually the result of tuberculous disease of the spine.

Appreciable asymmetry of the chest is usually due to retraction of one side, though occasionally it may be due to enlargement. Obvious flattening (apart from the rare condition of unilateral wasting of overlying muscles) is caused by fibrosis of the lung—usually the pleural surfaces are also adherent, as a whole or in part—or by pulmonary collapse ; the intercostal spaces are narrowed, a fact which may be observed by the naked eye and also in the X-ray film. Unilateral increase in the volume of the chest, with the ribs more horizontal than normally and intercostal spaces enlarged and obliterated, is due usually to a large pleural effusion or to a pneumothorax, rarely to a diffuse neoplasm of the pleura. Localised alterations in the shape of the chest may be caused by aortic aneurysm, great enlargement of the heart, pericardial effusion, malignant tumours invading the chest wall, and rarely by the pointing of an encysted empyema.

During this observation of the patient the examiner is meanwhile watching the patient's breathing, noting its rate, rhythm and depth, and any activity or otherwise of the accessory muscles of respiration. He notices whether the alæ nasi are working. He takes the pulse rate (looking at the fingers as he does so for any clubbing or curving of the finger-nails) and notes the respiration rate as the patient's attention is drawn away from the act of breathing. He notes, too, if there is any asymmetry of movement during respiration, a point which he can explore more accurately by palpation. He should pay special attention to the lower intercostal spaces, for normally the soft tissues are sucked in slightly with inspiration though the ribs themselves become more widely separated. This sucking-in is diminished or abolished if there is a considerable pleural effusion or tension pneumothorax ; whereas it is exaggerated with fibrosis of the lung, and markedly so with pulmonary collapse due to bronchial obstruction.

Position of the apex-beat and trachea—Apart from alterations due to purely cardiac conditions, displacement of the apex beat and the trachea reveals displacement of the mediastinum towards the side of the lesion in fibrosis or collapse of the lung, away from it in pleural effusion and in certain cases of pneumothorax.

Clubbing of the fingers—Clubbed fingers can occur not only in patients with subacute or chronic pulmonary suppuration, but in many other conditions—for example, congenital heart disease, infective endocarditis, certain chronic diarrhœas, myxœdema following operation on the thyroid, cirrhosis of the liver and amyloid disease.   There is also a hereditary (" familial ") type unassociated with ill-health.   Unilateral clubbing occasionally occurs ; it may be associated with unilateral nerve lesions or with subclavian aneurysm.

Clubbing may vary in degree from the gross, blue " drumstick " fingers found in serious congenital heart disease or advanced chronic suppurative disease of the lungs, to the less

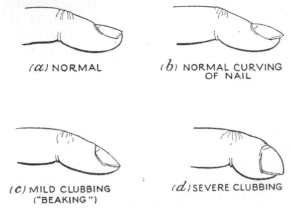

(*a*) NORMAL   (*b*) NORMAL CURVING
                                          OF NAIL

(*C*) MILD CLUBBING   (*d*) SEVERE CLUBBING
("BEAKING ")

Fig. 49

Normal and clubbed fingers.

severe " beaking " of the nails.   In all the cases, whatever the degree of clubbing or the disease causing it, the basic alteration lies in an overgrowth of the soft tissues of the nail bed ; and always it is revealed by the obliteration of the normal angle between the plane of the nail and the dorsum of the finger, seen in profile (Fig. 49).

In all the various diseases causing clubbing the mechanism is the same.   It depends on an exaggeration of a normal peculiarity of the vascular supply of the finger-tips.   When the vessels are dilated, the blood supply to the terminal phalanx is normally greater than that to the middle phalanx, greater to the finger than to the hand and greater to the hand than to the forearm.   Clubbed fingers differ from the normal in that with diminution of vasoconstrictor tone (as, for example, in raising the body temperature) the blood flow through the terminal phalanx is abnormally great and the fall of blood pressure from the brachial to the digital arteries is abnormally small.* These differences do not hold for the cases of familial clubbing unaccompanied by disease.

It is clear, therefore, that illnesses which produce clubbing of the fingers do not pick out the finger-tips for special damage ; the cause of the overgrowth of the nail bed lies in an increased blood flow to the finger-tips, whose blood supply in health is already somewhat different from that elsewhere. Hence the peculiar alteration in the extremities, for in severe cases the nail beds of the toes are similarly affected. The original excessive growth of the nail bed may be accompanied later by overgrowth of bone in the terminal phalanx, and eventually stasis of the local circulation may develop, so that under ordinary conditions the finger-tips become cyanotic.

PALPATION

Many of the observations of inspection can be confirmed or extended by means of palpation, especially the position of the apex beat and trachea, and the expansion of the two sides of the chest. Comparison of the expansion of the two sides of the chest is most important ; *often a diminution of expansion on one side is the only physical sign present to indicate underlying disease.* The student should draw with a skin pencil a line down the middle of the thorax, from the suprasternal notch in front, and over the vertebral spines behind. The hands are placed symmetrically with the palms of the hands gripping the sides of the chest firmly, and the thumbs just approximating to the mid-line in expiration and riding loosely over the skin so that they move easily as the chest expands. The patient breathes deeply in and out, and the respiratory excursion is noted by observing the distance over which the thumbs move from the middle line ; the pencilled line makes it easy to compare the movement on the two sides. The student should feel a sense of stretch in his thumbs so that he has actively to

---

* The possible importance of the amount of haemoglobin persistently present in the finger-tips is suggested by the following personal observation. A patient who for many months had allowed his hemiplegic arm to hang down constantly by his side was found to have advanced clubbing of the fingers in the diseased limb, although there was no clubbing in the healthy hand. I cannot recall a similar contrast in other sufferers from hemiplegia. This man, however, was also suffering from polycythæmia vera, the red-cell count being well over 8 million per c.mm.

bring them together to the mid-line in expiration ; but he must take care not to achieve this by pressing them too closely on to the chest wall and so increasing friction between them and the skin.   If he takes care to grip the sides of the chest with his palms, the manœuvre should not be difficult.

Expansion over the upper part of the chest may be studied either by noting the excursion of the thumbs from the middle line on the back, or with the thumbs in the same position over the

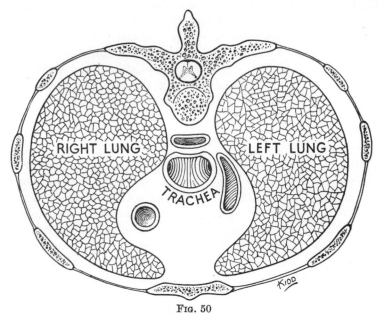

FIG. 50

To show the proximity of the trachea to the right lung at the apex.

vertebral column, placing the fingers over the clavicles in front and noting how far they are lifted up as the patient takes a deep breath.   Another way (a return to inspection) is to stand behind the sitting patient, after asking him to bend his head and neck forward, and to look down over the bent neck to the contour of the upper part of the front of the chest.   As he takes a deep breath any marked difference between the amount of expansion on the two sides is easily seen.   With palpation, sometimes one side of the chest is found to continue expanding after the other has ceased ;   the examiner's thumbs move symmetrically outwards from the mid-line for a certain distance, and then one thumb ceases to move altogether or lags behind the other. In the absence of a pencilled line down the middle of the chest, this difference is hard to detect.

The student should not forget to palpate the axillæ, the sides of the neck and the supraclavicular fossæ to detect if enlarged glands are present ; and he will also examine in detail any obvious localised tumours or swellings. Very occa-sionally he may detect small malignant or leukæmic deposits in the skin.

Vocal fremitus—If the examiner places the flat of his hand, or its ulnar border, on the patient's chest he can feel the vibra-tions of the man's voice as he says " ninety-nine." The chest, through the lungs and the chest wall, acts as a resonator of the sound produced in the larynx and conducted along the air passages. The adult thorax is better adapted as a resonator for the lower register of the male voice than for the high register of the female ; indeed, in most women, save for those with a deep contralto, the vocal vibrations are very difficult, often impossible, to feel. The smaller thorax of the child is, on the other hand, well adapted to the high pitch of the child's voice, and the vocal vibrations are in consequence easily felt.

Obviously the thickness of the chest wall will modify the effective transmission of the vibrations ; moreover, seeing that the trachea is in actual contact with the internal aspect of the right lung (Fig. 50), they will be felt better below the right clavicle than below the left. This is but one of the normal differences which ensue from this position of the trachea, and which make the right apex one of the diagnostic mare's nests of the body.

The presence of a pleural effusion or of a pneumothorax diminishes or abolishes the vocal fremitus on the affected side ; occasionally, pneumonic consolidation of the lung increases the intensity of the vibrations.

CHAPTER IV

PHYSICAL SIGNS : PERCUSSION

"If you must listen to his doubtful chest,
Catch the essentials, and ignore the rest."
—OLIVER WENDELL HOLMES.

FROM the time of Hippocrates, some five centuries before
the Christian era, up to the eighteenth century, only
inspection and palpation of the patient had really entered
into the body of general medical knowledge. Then an inn-
keeper's boy from Graz in Southern Austria was sent to Vienna
to study medicine. In 1761, when he was 39 years old, he
published a little book of ninety-five pages, his *Inventum
Novum*, describing the new method of percussion. As a lad
he must have tapped on many a cask of wine in his father's
cellar to see if it was full or empty ; years later the idea of
tapping on the chest of his patients led him to seven years of
observation and reflection, which came to fruit in his book.
Hardly anyone took notice of it until Corvisart in 1808 translated Leopold Auenbrugger's Latin into French and recalled
the beautiful invention to life.

Corvisart was a renowned Paris physician and teacher ;
one of his students was René Laennec, who in 1819 was
to publish the immortal *Traité de l'auscultation médiate*, ex-
plaining his own new method of examination, and mapping
out an entirely new country. So complete was Laennec's
mastery of this new terrain that his descriptions of the sounds
heard in normal and in diseased lungs largely stand to-day,
probably because he verified their significance by careful study
in the post-mortem room. Here is Laennec's own description
of his discovery :—

"In 1816 I was consulted by a young woman presenting general symptoms of
disease of the heart. Owing to her stoutness little information could be gathered by
application of the hand and percussion. The patient's age and sex did not permit
me to resort to the kind of examination I have just described—*i.e.*, direct application
of the ear to the chest. I recalled a well-known acoustic phenomenon, namely, if

64

you place your ear against one end of a wooden beam the scratch of a pin at the other extremity is most distinctly audible. It occurred to me that this physical property might serve a useful purpose in the case with which I was then dealing. Taking a sheaf of paper I rolled it into a very tight roll, one end of which I placed over the præcordial region, whilst I put my ear to the other. I was both surprised and gratified at being able to hear the beating of the heart with much greater clearness and distinctness than I had ever done before by direct application of my ear." *

Both percussion and auscultation are methods by which we examine the thoracic organs through the sense of hearing. Each provides information which the other cannot give, and so they are complementary techniques.

PERCUSSION

Percussion of the chest mediated through the bony and tissue mass of the percussed finger produces vibrations in the finger and sympathetic vibrations of the chest walls, lungs and other thoracic contents. The waves so set up pass through the air to the examiner's ear and produce a typical sound ; but soft, airless organs like the heart, the liver and the muscles do not thus vibrate anything like so well, nor does fluid, which has a damping effect on the sound. The " normal lung note " demands, therefore, an elastic thoracic wall and a healthy lung beneath it. Thus in old people with inelastic ribs and calcified costal cartilages, for example, the note is harder and more boxy.

In the technique of percussion certain things are important : (1) The percussed finger must lie in firm apposition to the chest wall. The student can test the alteration in note when his finger is crooked away from the chest wall. (2) Percussion should be done loosely from the wrist, just as the pianist produces " singing tone " ; and the student should practise this on all sorts of objects as often as he can, until he becomes proficient. (3) The strike must be short and decisive, the percussing finger being withdrawn immediately the blow is struck, so that it will leave the resulting note clear and not muffled.

One aim in percussion is to compare one localised area of the chest with another. While direct percussion by the whole hand over the bases may be done to compare broadly the large areas of the lower lobes of the lungs, as a rule more

* Hale White's translation.

localised percussion mediated through the index or second finger
of the left hand is preferable. Light as opposed to heavy
percussion will also ensure a sharper localisation ; one of the
best examples of this is seen over the edge of an enlarged liver
projecting well below the costal margin. If the student is
comparing similar areas on the two sides of the chest it is
obvious that he must place his hand in a similar position
on either side ; he must not percuss over rib on one side and
compare it with the note over an intercostal space on the
other, and he must percuss with the same force. Unequal
percussion may be confusing and misleading, because not only
is the note louder and less " localised " the heavier the percussion, but also the difference between the notes made by
light and heavy percussion over a resonant area is much greater
than between those over a dull area. The student can test
this for himself by trying light and heavy percussion over his
own chest and thigh respectively.

When he practises mediate percussion he is actually percussing his own finger ; he hears the note of his own finger,
altered to a greater or less degree by what is underneath it.
If he holds up his left hand, percussing the straightened second
finger which is supported underneath by the thumb, he will hear
a dull note, and will also *feel* a board-like or stony resistance.*
It is the note which he will often hear when he percusses over
a pleural effusion, and he will conclude that an underlying
effusion hardly alters at all the fundamental finger note. He
should percuss his own corpus in order to hear various types of
alteration of the note—convenient areas of lung, the air pocket
of the stomach, the liver, the skull ; and as a further example
he should observe that in the same patient he can get different
notes over the area of the pectoralis major, according to whether
the patient is relaxing it or contracting it into a hard mass.

Percussion helps us to delimit solid organs like the liver
and heart from the lungs, and it tells of alterations in the
underlying lungs and pleural spaces—consolidations or cavities
in the lungs, effusion or air in the pleural cavity. For any
particular patient there is a normal note for various areas of
the thorax ; the notes at the axillæ and bases and at the apices

* As Dr. Hope Gosse has reminded me, the term " dulness " is an absolute
one, and needs no adjectives. The frequently used terms " board-like dulness "
and " stony dulness " are obviously attempts to describe both the note heard and
the resistance felt.

behind and in front differ slightly from each other, and the student must come by experience to know whether the note at the right apex of Mr X., for example, can be regarded as normal or not. Obviously he must be content with a broad idea and not bother himself with finicky differences.

He does not need to be a skilled musician in order to be a sound " percussor." The elements in any percussion note are not difficult to understand. The first is the *intensity*, which depends on the amplitude of the vibrations produced. This in turn depends on the particular physical make-up of the object percussed (with equal force of stroke, the note over the lung is louder than that over the liver, because the lung with its contained air is a much more elastic organ and so vibrates more readily) ; on its mass (an adult chest gives a louder note than that of a child) ; and on the force of the percussing stroke. Moreover, the more elastic a tissue the longer it will vibrate ; so the dull note over the liver, other things being equal, is not only less loud than that over the lung but also it does not last so long.

Another factor is that of *pitch*, which depends on the rapidity of the vibrations.* The dull note when the bony and muscular mass of the finger is percussed by itself should be compared with the resonance when it is percussed as it lies on the normal chest. The dull note is high and treble, the resonant note low and bass. The student will recognise this if he seeks to copy the sound by trying to sing " Ah " to it ; the dull finger note is somewhere about two octaves above middle C, whereas the normal resonant chest note of the adult is about an octave and a half below middle C (it is about an octave higher in young children). It will help the student if he remembers that the more impaired (" duller ") the note the higher the pitch ; compare, for example, the note of the wooden xylophone with that of the big bass drum.

A further element is that of *timbre*,† which varies according to the combinations and permutations of the harmonics or overtones superimposed upon the simple fundamental note.

---

* The student should compare the different notes of a tuning fork which vibrates at 256 per second and one which vibrates at 128 per second.

† " Timbre : the character or quality of a musical or vocal sound (distinct from its pitch and intensity) depending upon the particular voice or instrument producing it ; caused by the proportion in which the fundamental tone is combined with the harmonics or overtones."—*Shorter Oxford English Dictionary*.

Here is obviously the basis for exceedingly complex differences of sound ; an illuminating illustration is given by the track of a gramophone record, which traces the complicated curve of all the tones and overtones of an orchestra. The vibrations determined by this curve strike the ear of the listener and are translated by his brain into the individual notes and

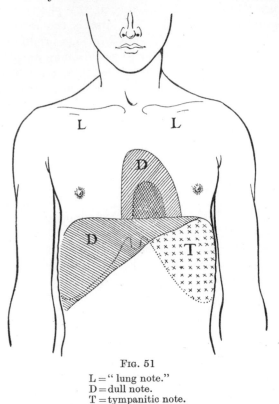

Fig. 51

L = " lung note."
D = dull note.
T = tympanitic note.

harmonics of the several instruments. So he hears not only a tune but also the notes of the violins, the French horns, the 'cellos and so on. If the student in his morning bath suddenly bursts into the first few bars of Beethoven's Fifth Symphony he knows only too well that his own " Pum-pum-pum-pom " is nothing like the grand " Fate knocking at the door " of the full orchestra ; nor can he fail to distinguish the difference between the same musical note played on an oboe and a violin. No book or teacher can adequately explain the difference ;

not until he has listened for himself will he understand and know. So it is with the difference between the normal percussion note and the tympanitic ; the latter is a more musical, simpler note. The student should percuss his own chest and compare it with the note over the air-pocket of the stomach, over the cæcum, or over his inflated cheeks with the lips shut. They are different, and by reason not of loudness or pitch but of timbre ; each is characteristic, and must be listened to time and time again until the student is familiar with them.

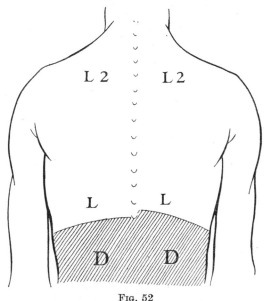

Fig. 52

L ="lung note."
L2=slightly less resonant " lung note."
D =dull note.

By contrast, timbre does not enter much into the difference between a dull note and a normal lung note ; here the difference is overwhelmingly one of loudness and pitch. If the student is listening at the end of the bed while his teacher percusses gently a chest with a right-sided pleural effusion he will hear the normal note on the left side, but he will not hear the dull note over the fluid. The resonant note is louder and carries, the dull note does not.

So he must practise percussion of the normal chest until he knows just what note he will hear in the various areas—

the normal lung note in the right axilla, for example, the dull note of the liver and the heart, the tympanitic note of the air-pocket of the stomach. He must learn also that the " normal lung note " is not always the same over the whole lung. If one takes the lung note in the right axilla as the normal, that in the left axilla is usually the same, though it may be more tympanitic if a distended air-pocket of the stomach projects upwards. The note is naturally rather more impaired (" duller ") over the scapula and its mass of muscles than over the corresponding upper area in front of the chest. Again, as the air-filled lungs are cone-shaped, so that there is more lung in the lower part of the thorax than in the upper, the note over the upper third will naturally be less resonant than that over the lower two-thirds—compare that of the apex in front, for example, with that of the base behind.

The student needs to familiarise himself with the three main percussion notes of dulness, normal lung note and tympany, and to know what to expect and where to expect it in the normal chest and its environs (see Figs. 51 and 52). Until he is quite at home with the " percussion-topography " of the normal chest, he will have no sure yardstick with which to measure the abnormal.

ABNORMAL PERCUSSION NOTES

The student will already be familiar with percussion of the heart, and with the significance of absolute and relative (" deep " and " superficial ") cardiac dulness, and of the in-crease in the area of cardiac dulness in enlargement of the heart and in pericardial effusion. From the point of view of lung diseases, displacement of the cardiac dulness to the right or to the left may be due to displacement of the mediastinum by a pleural effusion or pneumothorax, or by fibrosis or collapse of the lung. The liver dulness also has its absolute and relative zones, for a tongue of lung dips down into the space between the chest wall and the diaphragm, which is itself in close apposition to the upper surface of the liver. The alteration which theoretically takes place in the upper limit of liver dulness as the diaphragm moves up and down with expiration and in-spiration is not easy to percuss out in actual practice. Another difficulty is that even when the diaphragm is pushed upwards by a hepatic tumour or abscess or hydatid cyst, or by a sub-phrenic abscess, and the area of liver dulness is thereby in-creased in an upward direction, there may be complicating thoracic lesions also, such as pleural effusion (see Chap. XXIV) ; the dulness to percussion, therefore, cannot necessarily be assumed to be due wholly to subphrenic abnormalities.

The presence of a thin layer of fluid in the pleural cavity alters the normal lung note to one of diminished or impaired

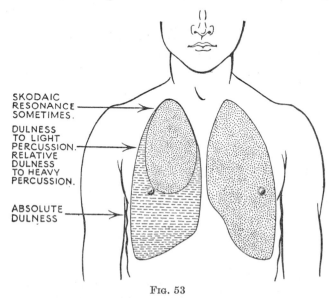

SKODAIC RESONANCE SOMETIMES.

DULNESS TO LIGHT PERCUSSION. RELATIVE DULNESS TO HEAVY PERCUSSION.

ABSOLUTE DULNESS

FIG. 53

To show various percussion notes over pleural effusion.

resonance. With a considerable amount of fluid the normal lung note is entirely abolished and replaced by dulness, similar both in note and feel (" board-like," " stony ") to that of the finger supported by the thumb. As the fluid collects between the two pleural layers (Fig. 53) the lung gradually relaxes towards the hilum, retaining at first a certain degree of its elasticity.

With the patient in the sitting position the fluid collects at the base ; as one percusses over it with the same force of stroke the absolute dulness at the base (Fig. 53) is replaced by impaired resonance towards the apex. The upper limit of the dulness of a medium-sized, free pleural effusion (non-encysted and not complicated by the additional presence of air in the pleura) is higher in the axilla. This depends on the particular way the lung retracts inside the somewhat conical thorax at the stage when the effusion amounts to somewhere about 800 to 1000 c.c.* In any case, the point is not of great diagnostic importance, and specially described "lines" such as Ellis' S-shaped line and Damoiseau's parabolic curve might now be retired from active service.

In hydropneumothorax the upper limit of dulness takes a horizontal position, whatever be the position of the patient ; this is well seen in the X-ray film, where, with the patient upright, the shadow of the effusion contrasts sharply with the translucency of the pneumothorax. As might be expected, the dulness of the fluid is sharply defined against the hyper-resonance of the air, and there is no area of impaired resonance above the dulness as in pleural effusion uncomplicated by pneumothorax.

Encysted effusions (for example, encysted empyema) of appreciable size usually give a round or oval area of dulness, according to their site.

If by reason of pneumonic or tuberculous consolidation, or of pulmonary collapse, a lobe or part of a lobe is rendered airless, the lung will not vibrate normally to the percussion stroke, and the note is impaired but not stony to the feel as in pleural effusion ; in the latter the vibrations of the chest wall as well as of the retracted lung are damped down by the mass of fluid. If the consolidation does not extend to the periphery of the lung, or if fibrosis or collapse does not deprive the lobe entirely of air, a lesser degree of impaired resonance will be found. Moreover, if there is about 2 in. depth of air-containing, healthy lung between the percussing finger and the lesion (as may happen in a central pneumonia), the percussion note will be the normal one of the overlying lung. A deep-seated abscess, therefore, or a central pneumonia, tuberculous focus, or cyst is beyond the reach of percussion ; students and teachers alike should beware, therefore, of percussing their own ideas into the chest, especially if they have first seen an X-ray film of it.

---

* Mr Morriston Davies suggests that the explanation is that at first the base of the lung can float upwards ; then, with the decrease in the intrapleural negative pressure, the retraction of the elastic tissue contracts the lung towards the hilum. The part of the lung below the hilum is, however, fixed by the ligamentum pulmonis. The fluid, therefore, tends to rise more in the axilla, as this part of the lung is more free to collapse.

The normal " percussion topography " can also be altered in the direction of increased resonance. Generalised pulmonary emphysema, by increasing the volume of the lungs, causes to a varying extent a diminution of the normal cardiac dulness, and lowers the upper limit of the normal liver dulness ; at the same time the normal lung note becomes hyper-resonant owing to the generalised alveolar distension.

A tympanitic note occasionally replaces the normal lung note. It may occur, but is a rare happening, when a large air-containing cavity (tuberculous, or following a lung abscess) is situated close to the thoracic wall. It may also be obtained over a pneumothorax when appropriate physical conditions of pressure of the air and tension of the pleural walls allow its production.

A special form of tympanitic note known as *Skodaic resonance* is due to relaxation of the interalveolar partitions. The note is a distinct one of " boxy " quality, and can be heard by percussing over healthy lung removed from the body at post-mortem. Here the lung is relaxed, but is still partially full of air. In life, Skodaic resonance is heard (though not always) over the upper lobe of the lung, under the clavicle, when a fair-sized pleural effusion occupies the lower part of the pleural cavity and causes the lung to relax upwards and towards the hilum (Fig. 53).

Krönig's bands, Traube's space, Grocco's and Garland's triangles and Wintrich's and Gerhardt's change of tone are all signs which should now be considered as of interest only to medical historians. Examiners might well agree to super-annuate them and so preserve their own and their students' sense of proportion.

CHAPTER V

PHYSICAL SIGNS : AUSCULTATION

AUENBRUGGER played on the thorax as though it were a set of percussion instruments ; Laennec added to the thoracic orchestra by using its wind instruments. His invention of the stethoscope was a great convenience, for it enabled the doctor to examine parts of the chest where he could not easily put his own ear and head—the axillæ, the subclavicular fossæ, and the breast areas in the female. It saved him from the difficulty of trying to listen accurately in awkward postures ; and the binaural stethoscope not only left him free to concentrate on the chest undisturbed by extraneous sounds, but allowed him also to see the chest easily as he listened.

THE NORMAL RESPIRATORY SOUNDS

" Neglect of a proper study of healthy signs is the secret of the failure of many who undertake to master auscultation and percussion."
—Austin Flint, 1881.

In a healthy subject, listen over the trachea and then over the right axilla. You will hear a more or less " rushing noise of wind " in both places, though the noises are vastly different one from another. Both of them have common elements. They last an appreciable time, during which they do not change in loudness or in pitch ; they are noises and not musical sounds ; and they have an inspiratory and an expiratory phase.

The sound in the axilla is something like the rustle of wind in the trees. No amount of description, however, can adequately convey the quality of these sounds ; they must be heard for themselves, and so become experiences rather than notions. The sound heard in the axilla is the *vesicular* breath sound. During inspiration it is a continuous murmur ; during expiration it is either absent altogether or at most it is a much briefer, softer murmur of lower pitch, which follows immedi-

74

ately on the end of inspiration. A series of breaths can be represented thus, therefore, in the time-honoured way :

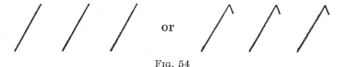

FIG. 54

or using *ad hoc* musical notation :

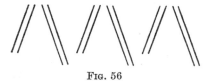

FIG. 55. (*After Rist.*)

The sound heard over the trachea is quite different ; inspiration gives a continued murmur of higher pitch than the vesicular, then there is a distinct pause, followed by an even longer murmur of higher pitch during expiration, seeing that normally expiration lasts longer than inspiration. It is the *laryngo-tracheal* or *glottic* sound, and can be represented thus :

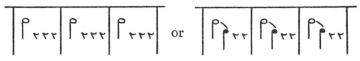

FIG. 56

or, in musical notation :

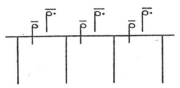

FIG. 57. (*After Rist.*)

The student must listen time and again to these two sounds until they are recorded indelibly in his memory ; * he will note that the outstanding difference between the two is in the expiratory phase.

* " To be able, in practice, to distinguish a vesicular murmur from bronchial breathing is the most essential step in auscultation."—HILTON FAGGE (1886).

How are they produced ? In respiration a wave of air
enters, and leaves, the lungs, past the larynx, through the
trachea and bronchi into the alveoli. The student has already
learnt that cardiac murmurs are produced by the passage of
blood from a narrower or narrowed tube into a wider one, and
that the intensity of the murmur so produced depends on the
relative narrowing of the orifice and of the speed of the flow of
blood. He may wonder if the same mechanism holds for the
production of these respiratory murmurs. It certainly does for
the **glottic sound** heard over the trachea, caused by the passage
to and fro of the respired air through the narrowed aperture

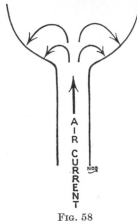

of the glottis. In inspiration the vocal
cords are more widely separated than
in expiration ; thus, because the orifice
is narrower in expiration, the pitch of
the expiratory sound is higher.

The *vesicular murmur* is, however, a
more complex sound, made up of tones
of different frequencies. Its pitch is
relatively low, because the components
with the lower frequencies are louder
and so contribute most to its characteristic quality. Though there is still
much argument about the physical
causes of this sound, it is probably right
to regard its inspiratory phase as due to
two factors : (i) the laryngeal sound,
altered and broken up as the vibrations are conducted along the bronchi

FIG. 58

To show the production of a
murmur as the air current
passes from terminal bronchioles into the atria.

and into the alveoli. The spongy lung parenchyma may be
thought of as acting somewhat like the baffles of the silencer
of a motor car, though the analogy must not be pressed too far ;
and (ii) the sum of all the murmurs produced at the site where
the wave of air passes from the narrow terminal bronchioles
into the wider vestibule leading to the alveoli (Fig. 58 ; see also
Fig. 11, p. 13). All these tiny murmurs, which if taken indivi-
dually could not be heard, add together to produce a considerable part of the inspiratory phase of the vesicular murmur,
in the same way as " the murmuring of innumerable bees "
can be heard at the bottom of the garden though a single bee
might go his way undetected.

Listening over the axilla with a stethoscope, a brief, soft expiratory phase of the vesicular murmur is sometimes but not always heard. It cannot under normal circumstances be produced at the junction of the terminal bronchiole with the vestibule, for the passage of a current of air from a wider tube to a narrower one does not produce a murmur. Nor is the expiratory glottic sound likely to be heard, for the direction of propagation is not towards the axilla, and the larynx is a long way from the stethoscope. The most likely explanation of the sound is that it originates at the orifices of the secondary bronchi where they come off the main bronchi, and is heard as the current of air sweeps through them during the earlier and relatively more forceful phase of expiration.

In any case, the important practical point to remember is that vesicular breathing is heard only over normally functioning, air-containing lung tissue. It indicates penetration of the air into the lung alveoli and its expulsion.

NORMAL VARIATIONS OF THE VESICULAR MURMUR

The vesicular murmur is the more obvious the stronger the respiration and the thinner the structures between the place of origin and the observer's stethoscope. Any thickening of the pleura or of the thoracic wall (muscle, fat, mammary gland) will absorb part of the sound. The thin chest of the child thus gives, other things being equal, a louder vesicular murmur than does that of the adult (*puerile breathing*). On the other hand, poor thoracic musculature may result in a weak vesicular murmur, because the respiration is comparatively feeble and superficial, while the strong breathers—muscular athletes and spacious *prima donnas*—produce a strong vesicular sound in spite of their covering of muscle or fat. So, too, deep breathing, whether voluntary or after exertion, enhances the intensity of the murmur ; as also does the exaggerated action of the healthy lung, which endeavours to make up for the deficiencies of its diseased fellow.

The vesicular murmur is modified in certain areas where the trachea and larger bronchi are near the surface of the chest wall. The tracheal (glottic) sound is normally heard over the larynx, trachea, neck and beneath the sternum. It can often be heard over the cervical and upper dorsal spine, well conducted through the bone. It is propagated along the main bronchi and can therefore be heard in the interscapular space ; the farther away from the spine the more likely is it to be mingled with the vesicular murmur of the lung tissue, giving a more or less degree of " bronchovesicular " breathing.

Now that the student is familiar with the breath sounds heard in the axilla and the trachea, the time has come for him to listen in a normal person over the subclavicular areas of both apices, in front. He will note that at the left apex the sound is not purely vesicular ; there is a slight element of tracheal sound also, though it remains more vesicular than tracheal. Over the right apex the sound has still more tracheal element in it, and can fairly be called *bronchovesicular* ; indeed, near the right edge of the sternum it may be wholly tracheal. So, apart from any question of loudness or intensity, he can distinguish four clear-cut differences of breath sounds, *all normal in their right place*, putting them in order of transition thus : trachea ; right apex and interscapular space ; left apex ; axilla and elsewhere. The modifications at the apices are due to the proximity of the trachea—in contact, on the right side, with the internal aspect of the lung, separated from it on the left by blood vessels and cellular tissue for the space of about an inch (see Fig. 50, p. 62).

PATHOLOGICAL MODIFICATIONS OF THE VESICULAR MURMUR

Anything which reduces the amount of, or makes the lung parenchyma impermeable to, inspired air diminishes the vesicular breath sound—partial bronchial obstruction, paralysis of the inspiratory muscles, loss of elasticity of the lung from emphysema or scarring, œdema of the lung, hyperæmia. So also does any obstruction to the transmission of the sound to the ear—thickening of the pleura, pleural exudate or pneumothorax (in the latter two cases the lung parenchyma is collapsed and the factor of diminution of air entry also comes into play).

The vesicular murmur is abolished and there is complete silence over the appropriate part of the lung if the bronchus to it is completely obstructed, or if the lobe is completely collapsed with the interposition between it and the chest wall of a large pleural effusion or a pneumothorax.

The student should beware of accepting slovenly expressions, such as " harsh respiration " ; often these betray the lack of a clear appreciation of what the auscultator is hearing. Sometimes the term represents nothing more than an exaggerated vesicular murmur or puerile breathing, sometimes it is used as a synonym for bronchovesicular breathing, sometimes it is even used because the listener does not recognise the presence of a continuous râle in a case of bronchitis. Nor should he worry about " cog-wheel breathing," an interrupted, jerking type of respiration, which by itself has no important significance.

ABNORMAL PROPAGATION OF THE GLOTTIC BREATH SOUND

As has already been seen, the laryngotracheal sound of the respiratory current of air fades away and is replaced by the vesicular murmur heard over the air cells of the lung. But if the lung parenchyma is consolidated and empty of air the vesicular murmur disappears. The homogeneous, airless lung acts as an excellent conductor of the glottic sound, *provided that the bronchi are patent* ; this sound then becomes conducted to, and is heard over, the chest wall in places where normally vesicular breathing alone is heard.

It differs from the laryngotracheal breath sound heard over the trachea only in being less loud and of higher pitch, the calibre of the bronchi being less than that of the trachea ; but it has the same fundamental characteristics of post-inspiratory pause, and the typical duration and loudness of the expiratory phase when contrasted with that of the vesicular murmur. Its most characteristic form is heard over pneumonic consolidation — a penetrating, blowing sound which can be imitated by breathing in and out with the tongue in the position to say " Kai," and to which the term " bronchial " or " tubular " is given. If the consolidation is not complete, so that in the same area there are patches of aerated lung and solid lung, the murmur is bronchovesicular, due to the mingling of the two types of breath sound.

Bronchial breathing may take on a different character if there is a cavity in the consolidated lung large enough to act as a resonating chamber ; a hollow, reverberating quality is then added to the murmur, and the breath sounds become *cavernous*. Cavernous breathing can be imitated by using the mouth as a resonating chamber, drawing the breath in and out through the open lips pursed into the shape of an O ; or by breathing into the hollow made by the two hands. It is not produced by the air entering and leaving the cavity, but by the production of overtones in the resonating chamber of the cavity which reinforce certain vibrations of the bronchial breath sounds, and so give an altered timbre to the original sound. The student should realise that all cavities will not necessarily act in this way as resonating chambers, and that cavities may be present without cavernous breathing ; moreover, unless there is consolidated lung present, neither bronchial breathing nor its cavernous modification will be heard. A cavity situated in the midst of healthy, aerated lung—and there are such—does not give cavernous breathing ; it is likely, indeed, to be completely " silent."

Bronchial breath sounds may also be altered if a pneumothorax with fairly rigid walls happens to act as a resonating cavity. The bronchial sound can be transmitted to it through a bronchopleural fistula, or very rarely even through adjacent collapsed or consolidated lung without any fistulous opening. The timbre takes on a metallic quality, and the resulting sound is called *amphoric breathing.* It is a sound like that made by blowing over the narrow neck of an amphora or bottle.

AUSCULTATION OF THE VOICE (" VOCAL RESONANCE ")

If the student listens over the trachea of a normal person speaking—usually the patient is asked to say " ninety-nine," or if a child, " one, two, three "—he will hear the words quite distinctly. If he then listens over some part of the thorax where the lung tissue is in contact with the chest wall, instead of distinct words he will hear a soft, confused murmur. The same physical reasons which prevent the unaltered propagation of the laryngotracheal respiratory sound through the lung parenchyma also prevent the unaltered propagation of the spoken voice ; and the same conditions which modify the normal vesicular murmur also modify the vocal resonance. Thus it is more marked in thin-chested persons than in those whose chest is covered with fat or muscle, and louder in people with penetrating voices than in those without. Such differences are normal and appropriate to the different persons concerned, and the examiner has to judge for himself what may reasonably be considered a normal vocal resonance for the particular individual.

Consolidation of the lung transmits the spoken word as effectively as it does the glottic respiratory sound. Listening over a lobar pneumonia at the base of the lung, for example, the spoken word is heard as distinctly as if the patient were speaking directly into the examiner's ear ; such transmission of the spoken voice is true *pectoriloquy*. On the other hand, there are conditions of disease in which the transmission is only partial ; the voice sounds are louder than normal, appearing to originate not under the bell of the stethoscope but in the very ear-pieces themselves, yet the actual words still cannot be distinguished. This abnormal reinforcement of the spoken-voice sound should be called *bronchophony*.

There is another alteration of the vocal resonance which is sometimes heard in certain cases of pleural effusion. The transmitted voice sound takes on a quavering, " nasal " quality, like the bleat of a goat—*ægophony*. More will be said about this in the chapter on pleural effusions.

The vocal resonance may be tested either by the patient's speaking or whispering voice. Like the glottic respiratory sound, the spoken or whispered word is formed in the larynx ; the conditions of transmission and the clinical significance are the same in both cases. It has already been made clear that the essential difference between the normal vesicular murmur and tracheal, or bronchial, breathing is in the expiratory phase ; therefore the transmission of the whispered voice is more useful and convenient to study even than that of the spoken voice. In the first place, the whispered voice is not so loud as the spoken voice, and is heard either very weakly or not at all over healthy lung. In the second place, to whisper " ninety-nine " is to produce a series of articulated, forced expirations —just the phase of respiration which is of special importance in auscultation. So *whispered pectoriloquy*, heard over con-solidated lung parenchyma, confirms and underlines the sig-nificance of bronchial breathing. If, therefore, the student is not sure whether he is hearing the transmitted glottic respira-tory sound or not (bronchial breathing) in an area where normally it should not be, he should listen for whispered pectoriloquy ; if this is present, he can be sure of the bronchial breathing and of the presence of consolidated lung parenchyma

6

under his stethoscope.* Where the bronchial breathing is altered to cavernous, whispered pectoriloquy takes on a cavernous quality ; if the breathing is amphoric, whispered pectoriloquy is amphoric too. Moreover, seeing that the whisper is a forced and not a normal expiration, it may come through to the ear at a stage when the bronchial breath sound is not audible ; this can happen, for example, when the lung is consolidated, but with just enough inflammatory thickening of the pleura to damp down the bronchial breath sounds while failing to abolish the stronger whispered sound.

ADVENTITIOUS SOUNDS

These are various noises produced in disease during the respiratory cycle, and superimposed upon the ordinary respiratory sounds. There is a great deal of confusion about them, because writers and teachers from Laennec onwards have introduced their own descriptive terms, without any agreement about the nomenclature. What Austin Flint said some sixty years ago still holds : " There have been over-refinements of description and of interpretation. The nomenclature has been open to criticism. Names have not been used by different writers with uniformity as regards signification. The names applied to some signs have conveyed not merely imperfect but erroneous ideas. . . . Hence it is that the study of auscultation and percussion, and their practical employment in diagnosis, have seemed to involve peculiar difficulties and to be necessarily restricted to a few practitioners."

The important thing for the student is to understand what is happening when these sounds are produced ; he can then use a simple nomenclature, knowing that he can readily " define his terms " both to himself and to others if occasion arises. He must accept the fact (as must his examiners) that whatever terms he uses have almost certainly been used by others in a different sense, and that even now there is no agreed terminology among those who guide his footsteps ; it would appear that in the past false prophets have risen and " shown signs and wonders, to seduce, if it were possible, even the elect."

* It should be borne in mind that if the trachea is displaced considerably to right or left, auscultation over the corresponding subclavicular area of the lung will actually be auscultation over the trachea—most misleading if the student is unaware of its abnormal position.

Râles, rhonchi and crepitations—Laennec introduced the word *râle*, which he derived from the " death-rattle " ; he deliberately widened its use, however, to " tous les bruits contre nature que le passage de l'air, pendant l'acte respiratoire, peut produire soit en traversant des liquides qui se trouvent dans les bronches ou dans le tissu pulmonaire, soit à raison d'un retrécissement partiel des conduits aériens." The following simple classification, then, covers all we need to know or express :—

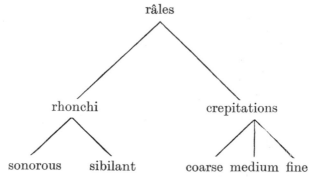

Rhonchi—Fig. 59 shows the three main ways in which these sounds may be produced.

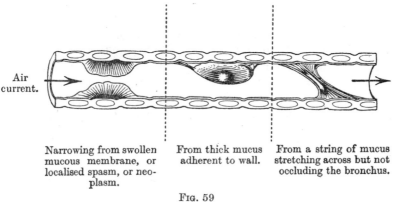

| Narrowing from swollen mucous membrane, or localised spasm, or neoplasm. | From thick mucus adherent to wall. | From a string of mucus stretching across but not occluding the bronchus. |

FIG. 59

They are produced in the bronchi, of low pitch (*sonorous*) in the larger tubes, or high pitch (*sibilant*) in the smaller ones. Obviously they will occur during both inspiration and expiration, as the current of air passes to and fro. When a rhonchus

is caused by the narrowing effect of mucus or mucopus, a
bout of coughing displacing that mucus will alter the site of
the rhonchus, and will finally abolish it if the mucus is successfully coughed up. The student should hold fast to the two
descriptive terms " sonorous " and " sibilant," even though
he may admire the accounts by others of rhonchi which wheeze
or whistle or squeak or snore or even guggle.

Crepitations—These are sounds due to the explosion of
bubbles of air which are formed during respiration in fluid
exudate present in the bronchi or in diseased lung tissue.
They are *coarse, medium* or *fine,* according to the size of the
tube in which they are produced. The student can illustrate
for himself the broad basis of this difference by blowing into a
glass of lemonade, first through a thin hollow grass and then
through a dandelion stalk, and noting the pitch of the two
bubbling sounds. Again, he can listen to the sound of fine
bubbles as they break in a freshly poured-out glass of cham-
pagne or any other " fizzy " drink. Crepitations are obviously
discontinuous sounds ; they are particularly heard during inspiration, when the air current is stronger, though the coarser
varieties may be heard during expiration also. Coughing, with
its deep inspiration and forcible expiration, greatly increases
their audibility. *Fine crepitations* are tiny crackling noises
determined by the separation by the incoming air of two sticky
wet surfaces, either in the finer bronchioles or in the alveoli ;
this causes the making and breaking of very small air bubbles.
They are heard, therefore, at the end of inspiration ; and, as a
certain degree of force may be necessary to separate the two
surfaces, it may take a deep inspiration or a cough to elicit
them. The student can get some idea of what they are like by
moistening the side of his first finger with saliva and rubbing
his thumb to and fro along it with a fairly firm pressure ; at
a particular stage of " tackiness," when the surfaces are
neither too wet nor too dry, he will hear soft, fine crackling
noises. He should listen first, of course, to the rubbing together of the dry finger and thumb, so as not to be misled by
any mere dry friction sounds due to simple roughness of the
skin surfaces. Usually, as might be expected from the nature
of their origin, crepitations are multiple—several together and
in succession. Sometimes, as in acute œdema of the lung,
there may be whole showers of the medium variety.

As with other sounds, adjacent consolidation of the lung transmits them loudly. Again, the presence of a cavity may alter the timbre of crepitations by reason of its effect as a resonating chamber ; they then become, in the old term, *consonating*. These cannot be adequately described in words ; the student must become familiar with them at the bedside. A pneumothorax also can act as a resonating chamber, giving an amphoric or metallic timbre to the ordinary crepitations, which become *metallic tinkling crepitations*. These consonating crepitations are not necessarily produced in the cavity or the pneumothorax itself ; they can occur in the lung parenchyma near by and be resonated by the cavity.

Pleural friction rub—Normally the smooth glistening pleural surfaces pass over each other easily and without a sound. If the pleura is inflamed, roughened and covered with sticky fibrinous exudate, a rubbing sound is produced ; coarse, " leathery " and rasping if the roughening is considerable, softer and fainter if the inflammation is not so marked. The rub is usually heard at the same time in the inspiratory and expiratory phase, so that it has its own particular rhythm for the particular patient. It ceases when the patient holds his breath, and a bout of coughing does not alter its rhythm, its site or its intensity. Pressure of the bell of the stethoscope upon the chest wall increases the sound, probably by increasing the friction between the two pleural surfaces at the point of origin. In acute inflammation it can only occur when there is sticky pleural exudate, without enough fluid exudate to separate the two pleural layers and so prevent their rubbing one against the other ; it is apt, therefore, to be a very fleeting phenomenon, and, in consequence, the student must not be surprised to find that he seldom gets a chance to hear a pleural rub. By the time that any fluid effusion has been absorbed, the sticky fibrinous deposit will either have been absorbed or organised, so he is unlikely to get a second opportunity of hearing a friction rub on that particular patient's return journey to health. On the other hand, when the pleural surfaces are chronically roughened, yet can still move over each other, a very coarse creaking, painless and persistent rub can be felt, and may be audible even without a stethoscope.

The movement of the visceral pleura over the parietal pleura is greatest over the lower part of the lungs, least over the apices ; hence pleural friction is seldom heard at the apices, even with a deep breath, and it is best heard at the bases or in the axillary regions. Where the friction is marked it may be felt by the doctor's hand, and sometimes even the patient is aware of it. The softer friction rubs are sometimes mistaken for crepitations, but coughing does not alter them, whereas increased pressure on the bell of the stethoscope makes them more audible. A pleural friction rub at the edge of the cardiac area may simulate a true pericardial friction ; it will disappear, however, when the patient holds his breath.

Succussion splash (Hippocratic succussion)—This classical but not very common sign was first observed and described by Hippocrates, who mistakenly thought it a sign of empyema. It occurs in hydropneumothorax, but all cases of hydropneumothorax do not give it (see also Chap. XXVII). It is best elicited by shaking the patient by the shoulders and listening with the ear against the chest ; occasionally it may not be heard when the patient is standing or sitting, but may then be brought out when he is lying in bed.* As the pneumothorax acts as a resonating chamber the splash has a characteristic amphoric or metallic quality. A former Guy's physician named Henry Marshall Hughes, who in 1845 wrote a little book on the practice of auscultation, explained it by a simple and homely illustration. A cask containing beer full to the bung does not produce a sound when it is shaken. With a cask containing air and beer, a distinct noise is heard when it is agitated. So with air and fluid in the pleural cavity. " It is unnecessary to describe it further. It is like the noise produced by shaking fluid in a cask. It can scarcely be mistaken."

Post-tussive suction is a very rare phenomenon. It can only occur when there is a cavity with walls so lacking in rigidity that a bout of coughing can compress it and empty it almost entirely of its contained air. The re-entry of air during the inspiration which follows the coughing fills the cavity again. As the air is aspirated into the expanding cavity a sucking sound is heard ; it can only be an inspiratory murmur and does not take on a cavernous timbre because the cavity is not acting as a resonating chamber.

The bell sound (*bruit d'airain*)—See Chapter XXVII, p. 429.

* To attempt to elicit succussion splash while the patient is acutely ill may be positively harmful.

The student has " to observe physical signs, and think in lesions " : to associate and correlate the symptoms and signs which he finds in any particular patient, in order that they may lead him to a correct diagnosis. Each sign forms part of the necessary diagnostic data ; but, as Josef Skoda wrote in 1839, " the findings of percussion and auscultation depend never upon the disease itself but always upon the changes produced in the organs." A combination of signs may indicate, for example, consolidation of part of the lung ; the cause of the consolidation may be pneumonia, or infarction, or, rarely, neoplastic infiltration.

Moreover, any single physical sign may be open to more than one interpretation. An appearance of fulness on one side of the chest, for example, may be due, among other things, to pleural effusion or to pneumothorax. Other physical signs help to narrow down the possibilities ; in the example given above, the percussion note will distinguish between an accumulation, on the one hand, of fluid (dulness), and on the other, of air (tympany). Again, consolidation and pulmonary collapse both show dulness to percussion ; in the former, however, there is no appreciable displacement of the mediastinum, and the breath sounds are bronchial : while in the latter, there may be marked displacement of the mediastinum, and breath sounds are absent.

The association and correlation of physical signs make it possible to describe " typical signs " of consolidation, of collapse, of pleural effusion, of pneumothorax, and of fibrosis and thickened pleura. It is a useful intellectual exercise for the student to make from time to time his own lists of these typical signs (under the accepted headings of " inspection, palpation, percussion, auscultation "), and to note, for example, how fibrosis differs from collapse, or effusion from pneumothorax. Thus, *consolidation* is characterised by diminished expansion on the affected side : increased vocal fremitus : greatly impaired resonance or dulness (not " stony ") percussion : increased vocal resonance and whispered pectoriloquy : and bronchial breath sounds. Unless there is exudate in bronchi or alveoli, râles will not be heard. *Fibrosis* causes shrinkage of the lung and traction on the neighbouring organs. The chest wall over the lesion is retracted, and movement is diminished. The heart and trachea are dragged towards the side of the lesion.

The percussion note is impaired, usually because of associated pleural thickening. Breath sounds are present, though diminished owing to the poor respiratory excursion.

In later chapters the student will find, presented in detail, the signs associated with the physical changes caused by various diseases; when he comes to read them he will be well advised to refer back constantly to these early fundamental chapters on physical signs.

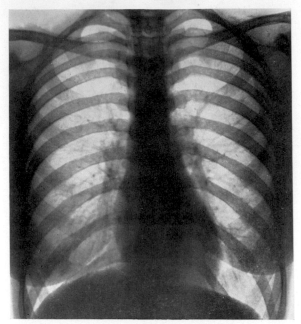

PLATE 1—The normal chest.   Anterior view.

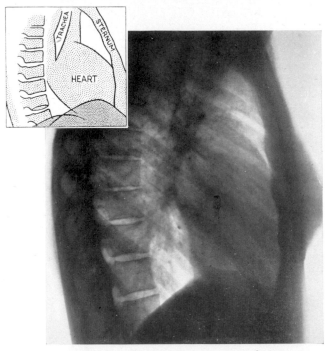

PLATE 2—The normal chest.   Lateral view.

[*To face page* 89.

CHAPTER VI

RADIOLOGY

RADIOLOGY of the chest is a matter for the expert. Nevertheless the student should be aware of the X-ray appearances of the normal chest so that he can compare them with the abnormal. He will then be able to take an intelligent interest in the radiological investigation of the patients under his care, and to make an attempt to integrate this type of investigation with the clinical picture and perhaps the post-mortem findings. The ideal way of educating him in the value of radiology is to ensure that as far as possible he follows his own patients to the X-ray department, learns from the radiologist the meaning of the films taken or of the findings when the patient is screened, and listens to the discussions between the radiologist and physician, which should be the rule in a teaching hospital.

If possible the radiograph is taken with the patient erect and with the tube six feet away from the film, with which the patient is in close contact ; the rays are then approximately parallel, so that there is a minimum of distortion, and the employment of the standard distance makes it possible to compare serial films under standard technical conditions. Obviously pictures can be taken in an enormous number of positions, but for useful information in chest disease two are essential—the **postero-anterior** (or " **anterior** ") view (Plate I), where the patient is standing facing the film (sometimes the antero-posterior view is also helpful), and the **lateral** (Plate II). For special purposes the right and left anterior oblique and the left posterior oblique positions are also used.

With the classic *postero-anterior* (or " *anterior* ") film one can gauge whether the patient is strictly in correct position by noting whether the inner ends of the clavicles are symmetrically placed in relation to the shadow of the vertebral column. If the patient is twisted out of the straight, the image will be distorted. The film gives a view of the whole thorax. The median shadow is made up by the vertebral column and the mediastinal organs, especially the heart and the aorta, pulmonary artery and the venæ cavæ. The right border of this shadow indicates the border of the right auricle (in its lower half), and the border of the superior vena cava (in its upper half). On the left border of the cardiovascular shadow there are three important bulges caused by (1) the aorta (" aortic knob "), (2) the pulmonary artery, and (3) the left ventricle. Above, and in the midline, is the translucency of the trachea. On each side of the median shadow are the clear areas of the two lungs, crossed by the shadows of the ribs. The costo-diaphragmatic sinuses (or costo-phrenic angles) are normally clear and well defined. The hilum shadow, caused mainly by the pulmonary vessels and not so dense as the median shadow, is seen at each side of the heart ; on the left it may be partly covered by the heart shadow. The diaphragm is clearly seen, the right side normally higher than the left. Sometimes the shadow of the scapula is seen overlapping the lung field, and in women the shadows of the breasts, with their clear-cut rounded lower borders, may somewhat inter- fere with the translucency of the lung bases.

The antero-posterior or " *posterior* " view is a little different in that the scapulæ are more sharply defined in the picture, and the shadow of heart and aorta is somewhat magnified, as in this position they are farther away from the film.

The supine view is a useful additional position in the in- vestigation of pleural effusions ; it is also the usual position adopted in the X-ray investigation of the chests of infants.

In any case in which the anterior or posterior view shows ab- normal intrathoracic shadows a *lateral view*, with the abnormal side next to the film, should be taken. The lateral view is often of very great help in assessing the site and extent of consolida- tion, cavitation, collapse, effusion or tumour, and in differentiating between an opacity due to consolidation or interlobar effusion.

The oblique positions are used to get a picture in which the shadows of the aorta, mediastinum, and hilum are moved away from that of the spine (right anterior oblique), or the œsophagus can be made to stand out clearly by a " barium swallow " (left posterior oblique or right anterior oblique positions).

Radiology may reveal, on the one hand, changes of the above-mentioned anatomical features ; or, on the other hand, abnormal shadows or translucencies. The student should pay attention to the following points :—

1. **The thoracic cage**—The film may show developmental abnormalities, fractures or growths of the ribs ; in the rare condition of coarctation of the aorta, vascular indentations or " notching " of the ribs may be seen. The ribs may be crowded together because of pulmonary collapse or shrinkage of the lung due to fibrosis. They become horizontal (instead of slanting) and the intercostal spaces are widened, in emphysema. There may be scoliosis or kyphosis, with consequent variations in the rib spacings.

2. **The trachea** may be displaced towards a collapsed upper lobe, or pulled over by fibrosis (when it may be curved or kinked), or it may be pushed over by a tumour, or by a large collection of air or fluid in the pleural cavity, or it may be compressed by a thyroid swelling.

3. **The diaphragm** is displaced downwards in emphysema. It may be displaced upwards by phrenic paralysis or in eventration (usually unilateral), or by abdominal swellings, including subphrenic abscess. It may be distorted by the pull of adhesions. Its excursion can be studied by screening. Its range of movement is a good indication of the expansion of the lungs except when breathing is costal in type ; this range is small in emphysema, and there may be unilateral lack of movement in conditions which reduce the normal expansion of the base of the lung. Phrenic paralysis and eventration are characterised by paradoxical or see-saw movement, the paralysed side moving upwards into the thorax during inspiration (from increased intra-abdominal pressure), while the intact side moves downwards in its normal way. The *costodiaphragmatic sinuses* become clear on inspiration ; if one sinus does not light up on inspiration there is some abnormality present, such as pleural thickening or effusion.

4. The position of the **mediastinum** is indicated by the shadow given by the heart as well as by the translucency of the trachea ; only experience will enable the student to discern easily when and to which side the heart shadow is displaced or the significance of abnormal mediastinal shadows (mediastinitis, mediastinal glands, aneurysm, tumours).

5. The **hilum** shadow may be abnormal in size or density ; here also the pathological significance of this can only be learned by experience.

6. **The lungs**—The lungs appear on the X-ray film as two

translucent areas faintly striated by " lung markings," which represent the shadows of blood vessels and radiate out from the hilum like a fan. The lung fields light up a little on inspiration and darken on expiration. In the absence of fluid a defect of illumination, therefore, denotes a defect of air entry, whereas excessive illumination indicates cavitation, cyst or emphysema (which may be generalised or local). Sometimes the interlobar fissures can be seen if there has been a thickening of the pleural membrane along them. They may be normally seen in a lateral view. Abnormal shadows are produced by airless lung tissue, which may result from collapse of the lung, inflammation of various types, and deposits of new growth or tubercle or pneumoconiosis.

7. **The pleura**—Shadows of pleural thickening may be seen. An appreciable amount of fluid, pus or blood in the pleural cavity gives a dense shadow ; if air is present in addition to fluid, the upper border of the fluid is always horizontal (best seen in the erect position) and surmounted by a clear zone of translucency due to the air. Pneumothorax is shown by a clear space not traversed by lung markings, between the thoracic wall and the sharp line of the visceral pleura which marks the surface of the collapsed lung.

These are but a few of the signposts which may help to guide the student partly on his way. More will be said about the relevant radiological investigations in the chapters dealing with the various diseases of the chest. Lipiodol radiography is discussed in Chapter IX.

Two recent technical advances are the *tomograph* and the *serioscope* ; by the former, films can be taken of the lungs at various depths, as though one were looking at serial sections ; by the latter the chest can also be examined layer by layer by the use of an ingenious stereoscopic device. They are of particular value in the demonstration and localisation of cavities, growths and foreign bodies.

Modern practice in diseases of the chest would be impossible without the help of the radiologist. It is, however, important for the student to realise that the evidence obtained from an X-ray examination is but one link in the diagnostic chain ; it must be confirmed by or correlated with clinical and pathological findings before the final and complete diagnosis is arrived at.

CHAPTER VII

COLLAPSE OF THE LUNG

"COLLAPSE of the lung" is a phrase which denotes merely a reduction in the volume of the lung, of a lobe or even of a sector of a lobe. It gives no indication of the underlying physiological or pathological factors. **Atelectasis** is not truly a collapse ; it is a term applied to the state of the lung or parts of the lung which have failed to expand when the new-born babe begins to breathe.

When the pleural membranes become separated by an accumulation of fluid, pus or blood, or by the entrance of air— whether accidentally as a result of trauma causing a communicating opening through the chest wall with the outer air, or deliberately by the induction of an artificial pneumothorax— the negative intrapleural pressure becomes less negative and the surface tension between the membranes non-existent. The loss of these two factors, which keep the lung expanded and the elastic tissue in tension, allows an elastic recoil of the lung, with consequent **relaxation collapse,** provided there are no pathological adhesions to prevent the lung collapsing. **Compression collapse** is a stage farther than relaxation collapse ; it is a positive rather than a passive state, being due to a degree of force exerted on the lung when the accumulation of air or fluid in the closed pleural space changes the normal negative to a positive pressure.

When a bronchus is occluded, either by pressure from without or by obstruction within the lumen, air is absorbed by the circulating blood from the lung alveoli supplied by this bronchus. The affected segment of lung collapses to a striking extent. This is **absorption collapse. Massive collapse of the lung** is the term sometimes used when the obstruction is of a main bronchus and has caused absorption collapse of the whole lung or of an entire lobe. It is more especially used to denote such a collapse which has developed with dramatic suddenness.

Restoration of the normal intrapleural negative pressure in the cases of relaxation or compression collapse, or removal of the obstruction to the bronchus in absorption collapse, thus allowing air to return to the alveoli, will result in re-expansion of the lung, provided always that infection and associated fibrotic changes have not already supervened in the collapsed part of the lung.

Bronchial obstruction can result from aspiration of foreign bodies, plugs of viscid sputum, blood clot (especially after operations on the nose and throat), and diphtheritic membrane, and very occasionally from an excess of lipiodol injected into the bronchial tree for diagnostic purposes. If the vocal cords are paralysed, food and other particulate matter is especially liable to be sucked into the lower air passages. Local interference with the mucociliary mechanism may result in the accumulation of secretions at a particular point in the bronchial tree, especially if at the same time the cough reflex is depressed. A new growth, benign or malignant, may block the bronchial lumen, but usually its development is slow and gradual, and the symptoms are therefore much less acute, and at first may not be noticed by the patient. Tuberculous bronchitis and cicatricial stenosis of the bronchus may also cause collapse of the lung. Pressure from without, as by tuberculous hilar glands in children, mediastinal swellings such as aneurysm of the aorta and new growths, and tumours of the lung pressing on the larger bronchi, may be sufficient to occlude a bronchus and produce pulmonary collapse. Occasionally a polyp or a pedunculated adenoma may cause intermittent occlusion, with consequent intermittent collapse and periodic changes in the signs and symptoms.

Obstructing plugs of viscid mucus or mucopus are liable to occur in whooping-cough, asthma, pulmonary tuberculosis, acute bronchitis and bronchopneumonia ; but very rarely in lobar pneumonia, for in spite of the thick tenacious sputum of the early stages of the disease the consolidation in and around the alveoli prevents aspiration whether of air or mucus into the affected lobe. In ordinary chronic bronchitis collapse of the lung is relatively uncommon, probably because the sputum is on the whole looser than in more acute inflammation, and coughing is not usually painful. Any condition, moreover, which produces increase in secretions combined with interference with the cough reflex may conduce to bronchial obstruction and pulmonary collapse. It is particularly liable to occur, therefore, after abdominal and thoracic operations and injuries.

According to the site of the occlusion in the bronchial tree, the collapse of the lung may be *total*, of the whole of the lung ; *lobar*, of a whole lobe ; *segmental*, of a main subdivision of a lobe ; and *lobular*, of a lobule (or *multilobular*, if scattered lobules of the lung are affected). It should be remembered that, other things being equal, the narrow bronchi of children are more easily occluded than the wider ones of the adult ; this goes far to explain the relative frequency of pulmonary collapse during whooping-cough, bronchopneumonia and asthma in childhood, and is an important factor in the development of bronchiectasis in early life. Moreover, it suggests that many of the supposed examples of " congenital pulmonary collapse " are probably acquired in early infancy.

THE MECHANISM OF THE COLLAPSE

When a large bronchus is suddenly blocked it takes a few hours for the air to be absorbed from the alveoli by the circulating blood and the lobe supplied by it to become deflated. When it is deflated it will tend to change in size from A to something like A¹ in Fig. 60, the right lower lobe being taken as an example (it does not in fact do so, because the collapsed lobe continues to be held in close apposition to the chest wall).

The rapid shrinkage of lung volume exerts a strong radiating traction force, as can be shown by the greatly increased negative pressure which develops in the potential intrapleural space. The loss of volume must be made good. The chest wall is drawn in, the ribs are

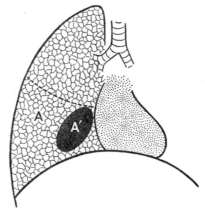

FIG. 60

On collapse of the right lower lobe the tendency to change in size might be from A to A¹, but as the collapsed lung is in fact held closely in apposition to the thoracic cage, the true picture is as seen in Fig. 62.

crowded together, and the intercostal spaces are sucked in. Owing to the rigidity of the chest wall, however, this

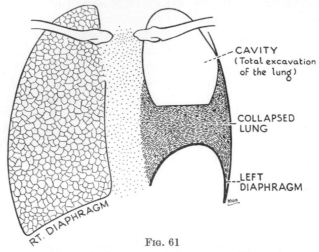

FIG. 61

Diagrammatical representation of an X-ray film of a patient with pulmonary tuberculosis of the left lung and cavities, in whom a phrenic paralysis has been established as part of the treatment. The lung is collapsed, with the result that the paralysed left side of the diaphragm is drawn unusually high into the thorax. For the significance of " total excavation of the lung," see p. 100.

contributes little to the restoration of equilibrium. The

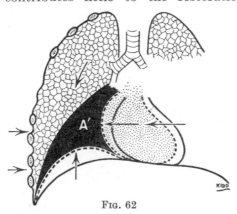

FIG. 62

To show collapse of the right lower lobe and the compensatory mechanisms brought into play—mediastinal displacement, ascent of the diaphragm, crowding of ribs and sucking-in of intercostal spaces, and compensatory emphysema of the rest of the lung.

dome of the diaphragm is raised, sometimes considerably (Fig. 61), and helps to reduce the drag. There is some compensatory emphysema of the rest of the homolateral lung. The main contribution, however, is made by the mediastinum, which because of its mobility is dragged over to the affected side. In consequence there is displacement of the apex beat of the heart

(Fig. 62). Similarly, collapse of the upper lobe causes a dragging over of the trachea. To compensate for this mediastinal shift the opposite lung also undergoes rapid compensatory emphysema.

The larger the bronchus occluded and the greater the amount of lung collapsed, the greater is the elastic traction. In the collapsed portion of lung the alveoli are airless and the vessels and bronchi are crowded together. The elastic traction on the bronchi in the collapsed zone causes them to dilate; the degree of dilatation is conditioned by the degree of traction and the distensibility of the bronchi. The larger bronchi with cartilaginous scaffolding dilate less easily

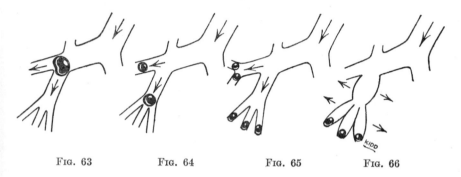

FIG. 63   FIG. 64   FIG. 65   FIG. 66

FIG. 63.—Occlusion of large bronchi by a soft plug.

FIG. 64.—The plug is sucked down, being split as it meets the spur of the bifurcation.

FIG. 65.—The pieces of plug are sucked farther down to smaller bronchi and arrested there.

FIG. 66.—Fusiform dilatation proximal to the obstructions, determined by the elastic traction forces.

than the medium or smaller ones; moreover, any bronchus whose wall is weakened by secondary infection will dilate more easily than if it were normal.

When the obstruction is due to a plug of mucus, mucopus or a piece of soft blood clot, the increased intrathoracic negative pressure tends to suck the material farther down the bronchial tree towards the periphery, the plug being split into smaller pieces as it meets the spurs of the bronchial bifurcations (Figs. 63 to 66). The alveoli which were originally collapsed must still remain airless, unless perchance the plug misses one or

7

more bronchial divisions as it moves on and is split up, so that

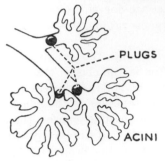

a free air-way is re-established to them. When the traction force is exerted mainly on the medium-sized bronchi the dilatations are *cylindrical* or *fusiform* ; but when the pieces of plug are sucked down as far as the finest bronchioles (which contain no cartilage and little muscle) the dilatations are likely to be *saccular* (Figs. 67 to 69).

Fig. 67

The plugs have been sucked down to the terminal bronchioles.

These dilatations which follow bronchial obstruction may occur quite independently of secondary infection ; though when secondary infection supervenes and destroys the elasticity of the bronchial walls, and later fibrosis

adds its own traction forces, the dilatations may become very large. Collapse of a whole lung, by producing a marked intrapleural negative pressure, may result in the sucking of pieces of friable plug into most of the peripheral bronchioles, determining so many saccular dilatations that the lung appears to be honeycombed with cysts.

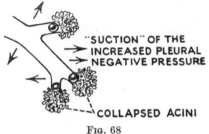

Fig. 68

Following the complete obstruction, air has been absorbed from the air-sacs.

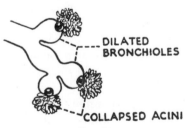

Fig. 69

The terminal bronchioles dilate into saccules.

When bronchial obstruction persists, the whole of the lung distal to it is in danger of secondary infection, by reason of the interference with the normal defences of the lung. This infection may take the form of a chronic low-grade peribronchial inflammation, characterised by round-celled infiltration, or of more acute lesions such as pneumonia, septic broncho-pneumonia, lung abscess or suppurative bronchiectasis.

As has already been said, so long as there is no complicating infection, removal of the obstruction allows re-aeration of the lung and restoration to normal of the calibre of the bronchi and of the position of the mediastinum. This can happen even when there is complicating infection, provided that the plug is removed (either by coughing or by the bronchoscopist) before permanent damage is done to the bronchial walls. Once infective changes have destroyed the elasticity of the bronchial walls or disintegrated the normal architecture of the lung by ulceration and fibrosis, recovery to normal becomes impossible, and sooner or later chronic pulmonary suppuration becomes almost inevitable (chronic lung abscess, or more commonly suppurative bronchiectasis). The distinction between simple and infected collapse of the lung is therefore of paramount clinical importance.

Once the dilated bronchial walls are seriously damaged they become abnormally tolerant of accumulating secretions. Mucopus collects in them without stimulating the normal response of coughing, and not until the secretions accumulate proximally to the area of tolerance do they start the cough reflex. This explains why infected bronchiectasis is characterised by periodic bouts of coughing which cause the evacuation of large quantities of sputum. Such copious expectoration is especially common after changes of position, as, for example, on rising from bed in the morning ; and the effectiveness of postural drainage in clearing the bronchial tubes depends to a great extent on producing a flow of secretions into a healthy portion of the bronchus of supply, with consequent stimulation of the normal cough reflex.

Secretions may spill over into an adjacent bronchus, occluding it and causing infected collapse of its corresponding alveoli ; or they may be discharged during a bout of coughing into other bronchi in the same or the opposite lung. Extension of collapse, with resulting bronchiectasis, from one part of the lung to another is always due to a fresh bronchial occlusion ; this happens frequently in patients with infected bronchiectasis or with chronic pulmonary tuberculosis.

In chronic pulmonary tuberculosis special factors come into play ; hilar adenitis, hæmorrhage, viscid sputum and tuberculous bronchitis may all cause bronchial occlusion and absorption collapse. Moreover, if there is a tuberculous cavity in the collapsed part of the lung (a plug of sputum from the cavity being often the cause of the collapse), the traction on the lung may suck part of the occluding plug back into the cavity, re-establishing a free air-way into it, but leaving the other bronchi still blocked and the lung collapsed. The cavity, which became smaller when the lung collapsed and the air was absorbed from it (it might even disappear), not only regains its original size but, owing to the excessive traction on its soft walls, more air is drawn into it. It expands still farther, therefore, until equilibrium of pressure is achieved (Figs. 70 to 74). Under certain circumstances it may dilate to a size nearly that of its own lobe, producing an apparent "total excavation of the lung," in which the greatly dilated cavity is surrounded by a thin zone of collapsed lung (Fig. 61, p. 96).

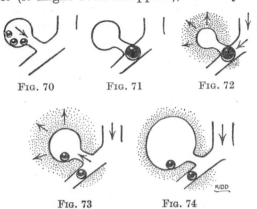

FIG. 70   FIG. 71   FIG. 72

FIG. 73   FIG. 74

FIG. 70.—Sputum in a cavity is evacuated.
FIG. 71.—A plug of sputum obstructs the bronchus supplying the cavity and the lung round it.
FIG. 72.—Absorption of air from the corresponding zone of lung; diminution in size of the cavity; traction forces act on the collapsed lung.
FIG. 73.—A piece of plug sucked back into cavity, re-establishing the air-way to it; rest of plug sucked farther down the bronchus; cavity increases in size.
FIG. 74.—Equilibrium of pressures established by entrance of air; cavity much larger than it was initially.

SYMPTOMS AND SIGNS

The effect on the patient of simple absorption collapse depends largely on the extent of lung involved but partly also on the rapidity of its development. If only one segment is affected, or if the occlusion develops gradually (as in bronchial carcinoma), the whole episode may be symptomless, though physical signs show what has happened. Total collapse may, however, be dramatic. In the typical case of acute extensive absorption collapse ("massive collapse of the lung") there may be an abrupt onset of dyspnœa and shock, so intense as to simulate pulmonary embolism or spontaneous pneumothorax. At other times the attack is like that of pneumonia or heart failure, or of a combination of both. The patient is ill and prostrated, breathing rapidly and showing cyanosis. He has paroxysms of cough, unproductive or accompanied by a little viscid expectoration. Pain, which may be severe, is referred either to the mediastinum or to the affected side of the chest. Except when there is some associated intrapleural disease to explain them, both pain and cough are probably due to the pull on the parietal pleura and the mediastinum associated with the excessively negative intrapleural pressure. The temperature ranges from 100° to 104° F., and the pulse rate is much quickened.

The physical signs are those of the displacement of the mediastinum, of the airless lung and of the compensatory over-distension of the healthy lung. The chest wall is retracted on the affected side, its intercostal spaces narrowed and depressed, its normal respiratory expansion absent. The heart and trachea are found to be pulled over to the collapsed side. Vocal fremitus is absent and the percussion note is markedly impaired —an impairment emphasised by comparison with the hyper-resonant note of the sound side. There is no air entry into the affected lung, so that the normal breath sounds are absent. If and when the occluding plug of mucus is later sucked from a larger into the peripheral bronchi, ausculation will reveal bronchial breathing and exaggerated voice sounds, for now the bronchi are patent as far as the peripheral occlusion and are surrounded by solid, airless collapsed lung. Here, again, the extent of the mediastinal displacement makes it clear that this is not the simple consolidation of lobar pneumonia.

If the obstruction remains and the collapse becomes chronic, some degree of permanent bronchial dilatation will almost certainly result. If it remains non-infected by pyogenic organisms, there may be some expectoration from simple bronchitis and also occasional attacks of hæmorrhage from granulations due to low-grade inflammation, or there may be no abnormal symptoms whatever. *Infected collapse*, when acute, presents the picture of pneumonia, with or without pleurisy, but physical signs and radiological appearances show the underlying collapse. *Infected chronic collapse* gives the symptoms of suppurative bronchiectasis with or without chronic lung abscess.

THE X-RAY APPEARANCES OF COLLAPSE OF THE LUNG

It is not always easy by ordinary clinical examination to recognise small degrees of mediastinal and diaphragmatic displacement. Radiograms of the chest can be of great help

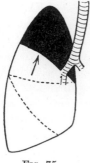

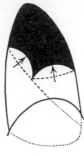

Fig. 75.—Diagrammatic representation of changes due to collapse of right upper lobe. Anterior view.

Fig. 76.—Collapse of right upper lobe. Lateral view.

FIG. 75   FIG. 76

because they show not only these changes but also the zone and extent of the collapse of the lung. A mental picture of the bronchial tree and of the areas of lung supplied by the

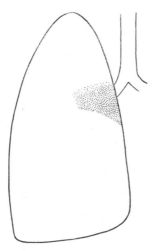
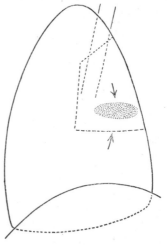

Postero-anterior view.   Lateral view.

FIG. 77

Collapse of antero-lateral segment of right upper lobe.

various bronchi is necessary for the proper interpretation of both physical signs and radiological findings. A study of Figs. 25, 26, 32 and 33 with Figs. 75 to 86 will help to correlate the various bronchi and the areas of lung collapse produced by their obstruction.

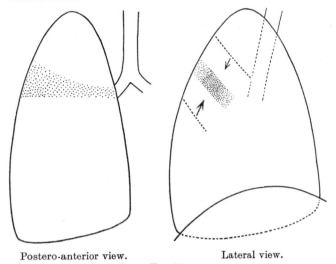

Postero-anterior view.   Lateral view.

FIG. 78

Collapse of postero-lateral segment, right upper lobe.

Right upper lobar collapse—The horizontal fissure is displaced steeply upwards, with a more or less concave lower

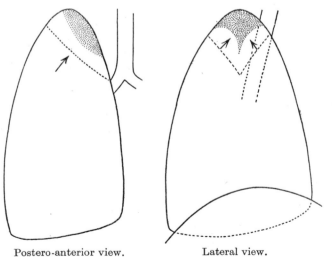

Postero-anterior view.   Lateral view.

FIG. 79

Collapse of apical segment, right upper lobe.

border to the collapsed lobe, and the trachea is pulled over to the affected side (Fig. 75). In the lateral view the lower and middle lobes are shown bulging into the collapsed lobe, so that

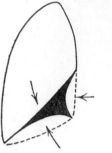

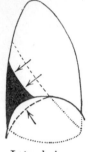

FIG. 80
Collapse of right lower lobe.

Anterior view.   Lateral view.

the border of the heavy shadowing due to the collapse takes on a " gull's wing " appearance (Fig. 76). In this limited and

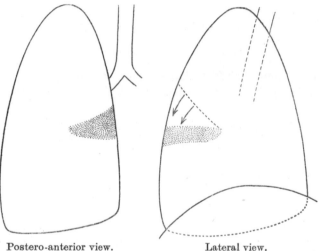

Postero-anterior view.   Lateral view.

FIG. 81
Collapse, "dorsal" lobe of right lower lobe.

The anterior view shows a somewhat ill-defined shadow based on the hilum. The lateral view is, however, characteristic; the segment collapses, to give a bend-like shadow, and the upper end of the interlobar fissure descends, to follow the collapse.

apical collapse the diaphragm is so little affected that there is no appreciable change in its position.

Examples of segmental collapse are illustrated in Figs. 77 to 79 and 81.

Right lower lobar collapse—In the anterior view the lobe collapses to give a triangular shadow (Fig. 80, see also Fig. 62), and in the lateral view (Fig. 80) the oblique fissure is drawn

FIG. 82

Collapse of right middle lobe.

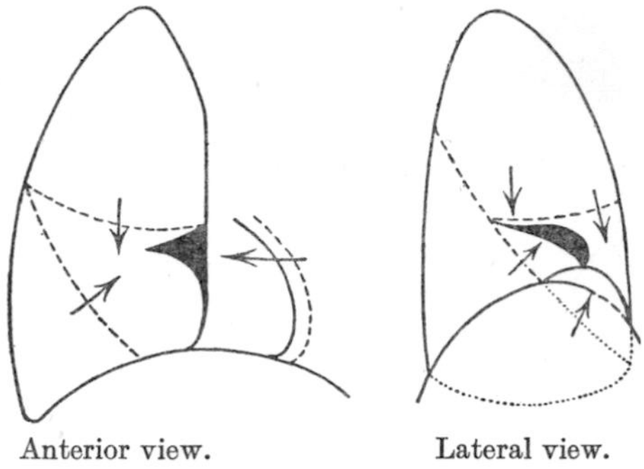

Anterior view.   Lateral view.

backwards and the posterior part of the diaphragm upwards. The upper lobe shows compensatory emphysema, especially in the costophrenic angle.

Right middle lobar collapse—The radiological appearances

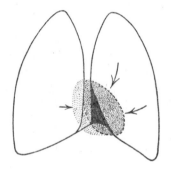

FIG. 83

Collapse of left lower lobe, which shows as a darker shadow inside the heart shadow.

(Fig. 82) make it clear that as the middle lobe collapses it recedes from the chest wall and is covered by the upper lobe, which thus intervenes to prevent the exhibition of any abnormal physical signs, save diminished movement.

Left lower lobe collapse gives somewhat similar appearances to that of the right lower lobe. In the anterior view the sharp interlobar line is situated inside the heart shadow (the right border of which is displaced towards the side of the collapse) (Fig. 83), and may be invisible in a radiogram of indifferent penetration.

Left upper lobe—The upper and middle lobes are fused

on the left side, so that the anatomical upper lobe consists of the " true upper lobe " and the lingular process which corre-

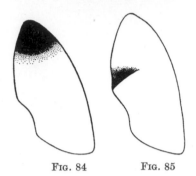

FIG. 84

Collapse of the left " upper " lobe. The absence of an interlobar fissure leaves the lower level of the collapse ill-defined in a radiogram.

FIG. 85

Collapse of the left " middle " lobe or lingular process. The absence of an interlobar fissure leaves the upper level of the collapse ill-defined in a radiogram.

FIG. 84   FIG. 85

sponds to the middle lobe on the right side. Collapse of the " true upper lobe " on the left side, therefore, does not show in the X-ray film a clear-cut lower border, because there is no horizontal fissure to demarcate it (Fig. 84).

Collapse of the " middle " lobe (lingular process) gives an

FIG. 86

Collapse of the anatomical left upper lobe, *i.e.*, " upper " and " middle " lobes.

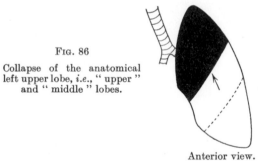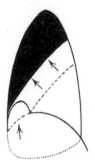

Anterior view.   Lateral view.

X-ray picture which is like that on the right side, but again it is less typical because of the lack of a well-outlined horizontal fissure (Fig. 85).

Collapse of the complete anatomical lobe (true upper lobe and lingular process combined) shows the well-defined outline of the upwardly displaced oblique fissure, as in Fig. 86.

Total collapse of a lung gives the radiological picture of a markedly displaced mediastinum together with compensatory emphysema of the opposite lung. The corresponding diaphragmatic outline in a right-sided collapse cannot be distinguished from the general shadow ; on the left side the gastric air bubble outlines the lower surface of the dome and shows that it has been drawn up into the thorax. The ribs on the affected side are crowded together and the intercostal spaces narrowed.

Bronchoscopy is of first importance in determining the nature and site of the occlusion in the larger bronchi.

Lipiodol bronchography (see Chap. IX) will also show the occlusion when the block involves one of the larger bronchi. In those cases in which the plug has already been sucked into more peripheral bronchi or bronchioles it is not the occlusion that is demonstrated but the resultant proximal bronchiectatic dilatations (see Figs. 66 and 69). In collapse due to plugs of sputum the condition is often, unfortunately, of long standing by the time diagnosis is made, and the bronchiectasis is well established. As has already been explained, the factors which determine whether the dilatations will be cylindrical (or fusiform) or saccular are, firstly, the yield of the bronchial walls, and, secondly, the radiating elastic and fibrotic tension on them. The less muscular and cartilaginous the bronchi the more they will yield. Bronchial walls damaged by infective destruction will yield much more than normal ones. The greater the amount of lung collapsed the stronger will be the distorting traction on the bronchial walls. The best conditions for the development of saccular bronchiectasis will therefore be total unilateral collapse of the lung, with occlusion of the terminal bronchi by innumerable pieces of " sputum-plug " sucked into them. In many cases of collapsed lobes with consequent bronchiectasis, the dilated spaces may be seen on an ordinary X-ray film (even without a bronchogram), honeycombing the collapsed lobe.

DIFFERENTIAL DIAGNOSIS

The crucial diagnostic features are the displacement of mediastinal structures towards the diseased side, and the absence of air entry. These together serve to distinguish collapse of the lung from lobar pneumonia, infarction, pleurisy with effusion and fibrosis of the lung on the same side, or from pneumothorax of the opposite side. It must be emphasised, however, that the collapse of a segment of a lobe may be symptomless, its discovery being made only on examination of an X-ray film.

The importance of the history cannot be over-emphasised. Collapse, unlike pneumonia and spontaneous pneumothorax, rarely develops with dramatic suddenness in a person who, until that moment, has been well. There is a preceding history of operation, probably on the nose, pharynx or abdomen ; or an anæsthetic has been given ; or there has been cough, sputum, repeated small hæmoptyses and pain, strongly suggestive of bronchial carcinoma ; or the patient has been suffering from whooping-cough, measles or bronchopneumonia. Sometimes the history is suggestive of a bronchiectasis over a number of years.

An abrupt onset of pain and dyspnœa with cough and dulness to percussion over the affected area may be due to pneumonia or to obstruction collapse. The clinical picture of a true lobar pneumonia is, however, characteristic, and although by reason of the airlessness of the alveoli the mediastinum may sometimes be displaced slightly to the side of the lesion, this displacement is never great. In pneumonia, also, the bronchi are patent (save in the rare instances of "massive pneumonia"), and the breath sounds are bronchial, in contrast to the complete lack of air entry which is a feature of bronchial obstruction.

In those cases where collapse is suspected from the character of the signs or where the first intimation is the shadow seen in the X-ray film, it is the geographical precision of the X-ray shadow which enables the exclusion of other causes possibly responsible for the clinical picture.

Once collapse is seen or suspected, the first step is the exact localisation of it by anterior and lateral X-ray films (and, in certain patients, by further films after instillation of lipiodol). The second step is bronchoscopy. By this latter method (with, if need be, biopsy of any abnormal intrabronchial structure which may be discovered) it may be possible to see the occluding plug of mucus or an obstructing tumour. It may also be possible to aspirate the plug of mucopus, or to remove the intrabronchial protruding tumour mass, so allowing air to re-enter and re-expand the lung.

TREATMENT

There are three principles to guide treatment : (1) to prevent the collapse occurring, if possible ; (2) to dislodge the offending obstruction when it does occur ; and (3) to deal with the secondary results of occlusion, including any infection. An inhaled foreign body must therefore be removed as soon as possible ; an occluding bronchial neoplasm must be dealt with as best one can (see Chap. X). Occlusion by a plug of sputum or mucopus following operation or trauma demands more detailed discussion. Ill-conceived and excessive medication before operation may conduce to the accumulation of thick and tenacious sputum and inhibit the valuable defensive mechanism of cough after it. In the days of almost universal ether anæsthesia, large amounts of secretion were produced, and atropine given pre-operatively inhibited the serous part of the secretion more than the mucous, so tending to make the secretion viscid. When nowadays gas and oxygen combined with a basal narcotic are so often used, there seems to be little call for atropine. Any source of infection in the mouth or upper respiratory tract may add to the dangers of accumulating secretion, and operation should be avoided in the presence of such active infection. Smoking should be forbidden for some weeks before any anæsthetic, as it irritates the upper respiratory tract. Breathing exercises for a week or so before abdominal operation may be of great value. After operation, especially on the abdomen, the patient is likely to suppress his cough because it hurts him. Firm bandaging of the abdomen will help him to cough with less apprehension, and small doses of morphia just sufficient to take the edge off the pain will allow him to cough more freely. With age and asthenia the risks of a poor cough reflex increase, and extra care must therefore be taken against the factors which conduce to collapse. *Carbon dioxide* inhalations early after the anæsthetic are helpful ; they cause hyperventilation by increasing the respiratory movement and therefore act mechanically against the tendency to stagnation of secretions in the dependent bronchi. The gas can be administered through a nasal catheter or B.L.B. mask, in a 7 per cent. concentration mixed with oxygen, or the same concentration can be given in an oxygen tent. At a pinch, a rebreathing anæsthetic bag may be used, with the addition of carbon dioxide from a " Sparklet " capsule, if available. After operations in which pulmonary collapse is especially to be feared, humidification of the air (as by a steam tent) helps to keep the secretions fluid, so that they are more easily coughed up.

If bronchial block from a plug of mucus does develop, with its consequent absorption collapse, anything which may tend to liquefy the secretions and assist effective cough should be given, iodides and alkalis for the former and antispasmodics (ephedrine, for example) for the latter. By themselves they are usually not enough, even when combined with CO_2 inhalation. *Percussion postural drainage* is simple and surprisingly helpful if the patient is fit enough to endure it. He is placed in a position where the affected lung is uppermost ; retained secretions beyond the block gravitate downwards, stimulate normal mucous membrane and cause coughing, which is often sufficient to expel the occluding plug, especially if percussion with the palm of the hand is made over the collapsed lobe. This manœuvre is best done with the patient on a special postural bed ; unfortunately, ill patients with serious abdominal or thoracic wounds are not easy subjects for the discomfort of this somewhat acrobatic posture, or for pummelling of the chest. Nevertheless, this may be a case where serious ills call for desperate remedies.

Bronchoscopic removal of an offending plug is theoretically the appropriate and most direct treatment, but in practice it is not always successful. Routine early bronchoscopy can hardly be adopted, because so many patients recover with the measures already described. Where there is clear evidence of bronchial block and absorption collapse, however, these simpler measures must not be persisted in if, after trial for forty-eight hours, they have failed. Unhappily, by the time bronchoscopy is undertaken the sputum may already have been sucked into the peripheral bronchi and so out of reach. When the plug or plugs can be removed they are often impossible to aspirate by suction, and are so tenacious that they must be removed by forceps ; there must be no half-measures, and the search for them must be thorough and expert.

In extensive collapse, with acute and dangerous symptoms due to the high negative intrapleural pressure, dramatic relief, especially of the pain and dyspnœa, can often be obtained by a temporary *artificial pneumothorax*. Air is introduced into the pleural cavity in an amount sufficient to restore the intrapleural pressure to normal (− 7 cm. of water) ; it compensates for the altered pressure equilibrium due to the pulmonary collapse, abolishes the pain due to drag on the mediastinum, reduces the suction-traction of the chest wall upon the collapsed lung and so diminishes the development of bronchiectatic dilatation, and gives the patient back his power of coughing. If, therefore, the intrapleural pressure is so highly negative as to cause distressing symptoms (it may " rise " to as much as − 40 cm. of water instead of the normal − 7 cm.), pneumothorax should be induced without any waste of time. It will not only relieve the acute symptoms and help coughing, especially if the other measures to liquefy the sputum and aid the cough are not neglected ; but by diminishing the intrapulmonary tension it will, as has been said, make less likely the migration of the sputum into the small bronchi and bronchioles, from which it is most difficult to dislodge them.

In practice it is not always easy to diagnose collapse of the lung nor to decide what is the actual precipitating cause when it is recognised. Where the crucial physical signs and the X-ray films make the diagnosis certain, or even likely, the doctor must realise that the problem has become one where the help of special investigations and treatment is needed. After operation especially, it is not enough to be content with labelling a patient as " chesty " and expecting him to recover with the aid of a kaolin poultice and a " Mistura Expectorans." Many do in fact recover, Nature being kinder than perhaps the doctor deserves, but some will be in danger of developing bronchiectasis later, with or without chronic pulmonary suppuration. Early recognition and early treatment of pulmonary collapse is the patient's right and the doctor's duty.

CHAPTER VIII

FOREIGN BODIES IN THE AIR PASSAGES

FOREIGN bodies of all sorts may be accidentally inhaled into the air passages. Children and lunatics are obviously much more prone to this accident than are well co-ordinated adults in full possession of their faculties.

WHAT HAPPENS WHEN A FOREIGN BODY IS INHALED

In the course of careless or rapid eating something may " go down the wrong way," or something in the mouth (a pin, a piece of bone, a toy, even a denture) may slip into the larynx when the patient unexpectedly coughs or sneezes, or laughs or even talks. Children are apt to " prove all things " by putting pins, nails, toys, paper clips or any other interesting plaything into their mouths. The accident may happen to an adult while he is under an anæsthetic, or during the extraction of a tooth.

The inhaled object is usually sucked into the larynx during a deep inspiration. Most commonly it is impacted there, if only momentarily. Straightway there is violent resentment of the intrusion, and the larynx goes into spasm. The patient chokes and coughs and feels that he is suffocating, dyspnœa is intense and inspiration becomes prolonged and wheezing. His face becomes blue and a cold sweat breaks out over his body. There is usually pain and a subjective sensation that a foreign body is in the throat. A large object which causes complete or almost complete obstruction in the larynx or trachea brings about asphyxia and death in a few minutes. On the other hand, the foreign body may pass on and the initial symptoms subside. A small body such as a pin may even be inhaled and lodge in a bronchus without producing symptoms.

If the foreign body remains impacted in and partially

112

obstructing *the larynx,* in addition to the dyspnœa and pain, hoarseness or aphonia and difficulty in swallowing are also present. A croupy cough develops, which is made worse by the subsequent œdematous laryngitis. Unless the object is bulky, or, being pointed, is impacted, it usually falls into the trachea, helped by the strong inspiratory suction which pulls it through the glottic opening. Passing *into the trachea,* it may for a time move freely up and down when the patient coughs. Every time it is coughed against the under surface of the glottis it provokes a paroxysm of laryngeal spasm and aphonia ; the noise of the impact may be heard as an " audible slap," and is heard most easily in the open mouth during coughing. Its impact against the sides of the trachea may be felt as a " palpable thud " if the fingers are placed on the outside of the trachea. As it brushes less forcibly against the tracheal wall it may cause a fluttering sound, " tracheal flutter." When the cough forces it against the glottis so as temporarily to shut off the expiratory stream of air, phonation ceases suddenly and dramatically. Usually dyspnœa is marked, not only because of the foreign body but also because of the associated traumatic, subglottic œdema. The croupy cough, continuous or in paroxysms, may mislead the doctor into thinking that he is dealing with laryngeal diphtheria or whooping-cough. With the stethoscope held close to the open mouth a more or less intense, high-pitched " asthmatoid wheeze " may be heard, occurring with inspiration or expiration or both, according to the physical conditions present. Until there is secondary tracheo-bronchitis there are no special changes in the normal physical signs over the lungs, save that if obstruction in the trachea is considerable it intensifies the " glottic " factor in the normal breath sounds so that it is more easily heard, and the breath sounds are bronchovesicular in character.

A foreign body usually travels as far down the air passages as it can get ; it stays in the trachea only because it is too large to go farther, or because its shape or sharpness cause it to become impacted there. Otherwise it is sucked down and is more likely to enter the right bronchus than the left ; and if it goes farther, the dorsal branches of the bronchial tree rather than the ventral. Rarely a foreign body may move about from one bronchus to another or from one lung to the

other as a result of coughing and so bring about bizarre variations in the physical signs.

With the passage of a foreign body from the larynx or
trachea *into a bronchus* the symptoms are as a rule greatly
relieved, for not only is the bronchial mucous membrane less
sensitive but also the effects of obstruction are restricted to
the portion of lung supplied by the obstructed bronchus. At
the same time, however, certain characteristic " bronchial
effects " develop from the presence of the foreign body there ;
they depend on the degree of obstruction and on the intensity
of the inflammatory reaction. The size and shape of the
object largely determines where it will lodge and how much
obstruction it will cause ; its nature determines the degree of
immediate inflammatory reaction and the secondary suppurative changes which may follow. Thus a metallic object such as
a pin may cause negligible obstruction and very little inflammatory reaction, at least for a considerable time, whereas a
grossly infected tooth quickly produces an intense inflammation
with suppuration. Similarly, organic material such as a nut,
a bean or a grain of corn is apt to cause an acute inflammation
of the larynx, trachea and bronchi ; the inflammation is a
reaction to irritating fatty acids present in such vegetable
matter, and is characterised by intense œdema and thick,
tenacious pus. The younger the patient the more dangerous
it is, and unless the inhaled nut or grain is removed, death is
likely to follow rapidly. Moreover, as the material absorbs
moisture and swells, it may progressively block the lumen of
the air passage in which it lodges.

A foreign body lodging in a bronchus may occlude it either
completely or partially.

1. **Complete obstruction of the bronchus**—Collapse of the
portion of lung supplied by that bronchus follows obstruction,
with the danger of inflammatory and suppurative changes distal
to the obstruction (see Chap. VII). Thus bronchopneumonia,
bronchiectasis, lung abscess and empyema may sooner or later
complicate the picture.

2. **Air may pass in but not out (" ball-valve obstruction ")**—
With a solid and not necessarily smooth foreign body, air may
pass beyond it during inspiration when the suction of the
inspiratory muscles is strong and the bronchus dilates.
During expiration, which is a much weaker muscular process,

the bronchial mucous membrane remains closely wrapped round the sides of the foreign body and air cannot be forced out past it (Figs. 87 and 88).

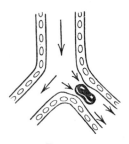

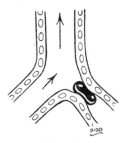

FIG. 87

Air passing beyond a foreign body during inspiration.

FIG. 88

Complete obstruction during expiration, so that air cannot pass out.

As a result, the obstructed part of the lung becomes over-distended with the air which cannot escape during expiration, a condition known as *obstructive emphysema*. The over-distended lung moves little if at all, the percussion note over it is hyper-resonant or tympanitic, the voice sounds are absent, and breath sounds are not heard save on the rarely captured occasions when an inspiratory quota of air is still able to penetrate into the affected part of the lung before it is distended to full capacity. Clinically the condition may be mistaken for pneumothorax. Occasionally, indeed, the contained air bursts its way into the pleural cavity through a weakened portion of the lung surface, causing a spontaneous pneumothorax : very rarely air escapes into the mediastinum. An X-ray picture of the chest shows the greater transparency of the affected side owing to the excess of air in it ; the distended lung displaces the heart and mediastinum towards the sound side and depresses the diaphragm on its own side, restricting its normal excursion. By compensation the movement on the sound side is increased, and this is seen on the X-ray screen, especially in the diaphragmatic excursion ; because of this the contrast in transparency of the two lungs is most easily seen at the end of expiration. In full inspiration the increased compensatory expansion of the sound lung will so fill it with air that there is little difference between the translucencies of the two lungs.

3. **Partial obstruction of the bronchus**—Here the symptoms and signs vary according to the degree of the obstruction, and any associated inflammatory changes in the lung beyond it. With any appreciable amount of obstruction, inflammation and suppuration are very likely to occur. Even with mild degrees of obstruction the affected side shows deficient expansion ; the other signs are those of accompanying bronchitis, of œdema of the lung, of bronchopneumonia, or of lung suppuration.

To sum up, it is clear that the symptoms and signs of inhalation of a foreign body depend on a series of factors. There are the variations in the foreign body itself. A pin, for example, will cause no appreciable obstruction and relatively little local irritation, though it may be responsible for periodic recurring hæmoptyses, and in the intervals no signs or symptoms. A round piece of nut, on the other hand, may obstruct a large bronchus and at the same time produce an intense inflammatory reaction. There is the irritation and inflammation caused by the foreign body, including swelling of the mucous membrane, which may be severe enough in itself to occlude a bronchus. There is the position at which the object has been arrested. There is the amount of retained exudate and the conditions of emphysema or collapse present in the lung at any particular time, either distal to the foreign body or in other parts of the lungs. There are the complications due to exudate being sucked into the sound lung, past a partial occlusion. Finally, and on rare occasions only, there is the shifting of the object elsewhere from its original position.

DIAGNOSIS

The original episode is often dramatic enough, with its sudden bout of coughing, choking and dyspnœa, coupled with the disappearance of the foreign body itself. Yet it is surprising to find how often the accident escapes recognition ; Chevalier Jackson has found over a large series of cases that in approximately one out of every seven the foreign body was overlooked for periods varying from a month to thirty-six years. There are several reasons for this. A child may be too young to tell of the accident ; an adult may have been unconscious, anæsthetised or drunk, or not quite sure of what has happened.

Often after the initial attack of choking the object passes into a bronchus, and if it is metallic and not large the distressing symptoms are greatly relieved for the time being, often for months. Occasionally, even, the foreign body is inhaled straight into a distal bronchus without setting up any reflex in its passage.

The *symptomless interval* may reassure both patient and doctor ; the patient may feel that he was mistaken, the doctor may be inclined to brush aside the suspicions of alarmed parents, especially if he can find no very obvious pathological signs in the chest. Sometimes, indeed, neglectful or unaware of the original attack of choking, he may tell the patient or his parents to " go home and forget about it." All too often, because of the " symptomless interval," they do ; so that when, weeks or months later, cough and fever develop, they are put down to " influenza " or pneumonia. But the illness does not subside as it should. An X-ray picture is taken, and a diagnosis of " unresolved pneumonia " may further delay the institution of proper treatment. Even if there is obvious collapse of the lung, bronchiectasis, abscess or empyema, the original cause may still be overlooked ; on rare occasions, indeed, it is discovered only when the surgeon or pathologist comes to examine in more detail the specimen of bronchiectatic lobe, removed years after the original episode.

The **differential diagnosis,** therefore, may be difficult if a history of the accident has not been obtained. As has already been said, in the acute stage laryngeal or tracheal diphtheria may be erroneously diagnosed ; later the condition must be differentiated from true bronchial asthma, and from other types of inflammatory or suppurative conditions in the lungs, including empyema. As might be expected also, the chronic cough with febrile attacks may lead to a diagnosis of tuberculosis ; but tubercle bacilli are never found in the sputum, and the physical signs are almost always entirely basal, an uncommon finding in tuberculosis. Pressure on the bronchi from without, by mediastinal swellings such as enlarged glands or aneurysm, may at times give a clinical picture somewhat like that of an inhaled foreign body ; here, again, the history will help, and in cases of doubt X-ray examination of the chest usually solves the problem. If a foreign body is suspected and is not seen in an ordinary anterior film the probability must be borne in mind that it may be situated behind the heart, or it may be obscured by the diaphragm, or by mediastinal or lung changes consequent on the presence of the foreign body. It may be necessary, therefore, for the radiologist to take a series of films from various angles and of varying penetrations. A poor X-ray film which fails to reveal an opaque body when it is there is a catastrophe. Inhaled vegetable bodies, non-opaque to X-rays, usually cause acute symptoms ; the X-ray picture does not show the foreign body, but it does indicate any changes which may be present in the lungs as a result of its inhalation. Obstructive emphysema can be recognised by the skilled radiologist and is very suggestive of an inhaled foreign body ; so can collapse of the lung distal to an occluded bronchus, though here there are several other possible causes of obstruction. The position of a foreign body causing appreci-able obstruction can usually be accurately determined by its effects, provided the student knows the anatomical distribution of the bronchial tree.

The diagnosis of an inhaled metallic foreign body is usually easy ; the non-opaque foreign body, in most cases of a vegetable nature, often presents difficulties, and careful questioning to elicit the circumstances of the original accident may go far to clinch the diagnosis. If there is reasonable likelihood of a non-opaque foreign body in the air passages the patient should always have the benefit of any doubt there may be, and direct inspection of the bronchi by a first-class bronchoscopist is called for, particularly as these inhaled objects of a vegetable nature are dangerous to life.

PROGNOSIS

Wishful thinking and the hope that a foreign body may be coughed up is badly misplaced ; in only about 3 per cent. of cases does this occur. The younger the patient the more dangerous is any inhaled organic material ; with inorganic, metallic objects the outlook is much better, though here, too, there is ultimate danger of serious suppuration in the lung. Grossly infected objects, such as a carious tooth, are extremely dangerous to life unless they are quickly removed. Even in long-standing secondary suppuration of the lung, removal of the foreign body may result in a remarkable degree of recovery.

TREATMENT

Obviously an inhaled foreign body must be removed as soon as possible, and by an expert. It is no task for the " occasional bronchoscopist." For whether it be a lost coin or a lost peanut he must search diligently until he finds it, and its removal may call for the highest skill and persistence. Delay, even when the patient is desperately ill, has no justification. Planned bronchoscopy is the only way ; there is no hope in inverting the patient and shaking him on the off-chance that the object may drop out like a coin from a money-box. Indeed, to do so is dangerous, for it may unexpectedly move, become impacted in the glottis and suffocate the patient. There is one exception to primary bronchoscopic removal ; in the later stages, when an empyema has formed as the result of secondary suppuration, it is usually better to drain the empyema first and remove the foreign body later. It should always be remembered that in young patients subglottic œdema may supervene after bronchoscopy, so that a temporary tracheotomy may become necessary ; the doctor must therefore not be caught unawares by this complication.

PROPHYLAXIS

It is clear that most instances of inhaled foreign body need not occur. Pins and tacks should not be put in the mouth, and mothers should be warned that if they do so, not only do they run risks themselves but they set a bad example to children, who are nothing if not imitative. Doctors and dentists must exercise particular care when engaged on manipulations about the nose and throat. Small children should not have access to easily inhaled objects ; they should not be given nut toffee or nut chocolate nor should they be allowed to eat nuts unless they are crushed fine. It only needs a sudden, unexpected, deep inspiration for the accident to happen.

CHAPTER IX

BRONCHIECTASIS

BRONCHIECTASIS is a mechanical state, at least in its earlier phase, before infective changes have supervened. It is a condition in which there is dilatation and distortion of the larger or smaller bronchi, or of the bronchioles ; usually there is an associated thickening of the lining mucosa, and some round-celled infiltration of the walls. The size of the bronchial tubes affected depends on the position of the obstruction responsible for the collapse of the lung, on the area of the lung involved in this collapse, and on the resulting traction forces. The causes and mechanism of bronchiectasis have been discussed in the chapter on Collapse of the Lung (Chap. VII).

True congenital bronchiectasis due to malformations during growth is rare ; that due to failure of the fœtal lung to expand properly after birth is usually associated with lung collapse, and is probably caused by occlusion of bronchi by amniotic fluid or mucus. Simple failure to expand, not due to actual blocking of the bronchi, would show a diffuse distribution at the edges of both lungs, rather than over a single lobe. The bronchi of infants and young children are narrow ; for this reason they are easily blocked by tenacious secretion, such as is produced especially in measles, whooping-cough and bronchopneumonia.

When the causative factor is non-infective and the lung is previously healthy, symptoms of the bronchiectatic changes may be few or absent. The supervention of an inflammation will cause hyperæmia and congestion, and subsequently a certain amount of peribronchial thickening and fibrosis in the collapsed lung. The effect of this is a tendency to hæmorrhage, and the development of or increase in catarrhal symptoms and signs. If, however, secondary septic infection becomes established the results are serious, for ulcerative destruction of the bronchial walls follows ; they become weakened and much more easily distensible, while abscess cavities involving both bronchi and lung parenchyma may develop. When the original bronchial occlusion is caused by septic material, particularly when organisms of putrid infection are concerned, it must often happen that even though the occluding plug is dislodged, and finally coughed up, the bronchial walls have already been so damaged and softened that they remain permanently dilated and deformed. They become more so as the resulting fibrous tissue gradually contracts. It is thus clear that the whole clinical picture, the treatment and the prognosis are from the outset more serious if the primary occlusion is infected ; or that it becomes more serious once progressive infection has supervened on a simple block.

PATHOLOGY

The pathological appearances of bronchiectatic lobes before the development of secondary pyogenic infection are of heavy, airless and collapsed lung, with the dilated tubes running through it. In the long-standing non-septic cases, round-celled infiltration of the bronchial walls and surrounding fibrosis of greater or less degree indicate chronic low-grade inflammatory change. The epithelial lining of the tubes may persist for many years after the development of the dilatation, and save for the instances of bronchiectasis caused by the inhalation of grossly infected material, the conversion into ulcerated abscess cavities is a comparatively late manifestation. Then the dilated tubes become filled with copious purulent secretion, the epithelial lining (including the cilia) is destroyed and replaced by septic granulations, the walls are devoid of cartilage and elastic tissue ; there is much fibrosis round the abscess cavities and the pleura may be thickened and adherent over the affected lobe. In the non-infected stage the other parts of the lung may be emphysematous, but once infection is established there may be a " spill over " of the pus into adjacent bronchi which, in turn, gives rise to areas of bronchitis or of bronchopneumonia.

Chronic bronchiectasis with low-grade inflammation may be likened to pyelectasis with recurring pyelitis ; at any time the inflammation may " flare up " into an acute exacerbation, so that the clinical history may be punctuated by attacks of pneumonia or pleurisy, nearly always on the same side and in or near the originally affected part of the lung.

THE NATURAL HISTORY OF THE DISEASE

The origin of the changes which lead to the development of bronchiectasis can, as a rule, only be recognised when tracing back the past history. If there has been a recognisable collapse after inhalation of a foreign body ; if immediately after operation on the nose or throat, or at any rate within two or three days, cough and sputum develops, with or without pain in the chest ; if a child is suffering from whooping-cough or measles, and recovery is exceptionally slow, then the possibility that the existing lesions will lead to bronchiectasis may and should be suspected.

A typical story is of whooping-cough or measles in childhood from which recovery was slow. The child was ill for many weeks, or there were known complications such as " pneumonia." At last, however, the condition settled down and the patient apparently recovered completely ; or perhaps it left him " chesty," with a troublesome cough each winter, due to a mild complicating bronchitis ; or it may be that as many as five or six attacks of pneumonia or pleurisy on one particular side disturbed the years of childhood and adolescence. In some patients the only striking symptom may have been the coughing up of blood at recurrent intervals, possibly in considerable quantities ; in between these attacks the patient might apparently be quite well.

The length of time between the onset of the dilatations and the development of recognisable symptoms varies greatly. It depends on the degree of collapse of the lung, on the extent and character of the involvement of the lung tissues and on the type of infection, if any. On the one hand, after inhalation of a foreign body such as a small piece of metal, it may be several years before the patient is aware that a slowly progressive cough may have serious significance. On the other hand, when it is realised that, within nine or ten days of an acute influenzal bronchopneumonia, extensive fibroblastic proliferation of the lung may be found, it is understandable how quickly pulmonary destruction and distortion can not only be developed but also become permanently established, so that recovery from the acute infection leaves behind permanent damage.

Radiograms may give one increased grounds to suspect the nature of the lesion, but it is only by the introduction of lipiodol into the bronchial tubes that the exact disposition and extent of the dilatations can be seen by means of anterior and lateral X-ray films.

It is a far graver story when septic infection supervenes. As has been already described, suppurative changes occur, the bronchial walls are weakened and finally abscess cavities form. Purulent secretion accumulates in the dilated bronchi and in any cavities which may be present. The sensitiveness of the diseased bronchi is blunted, so that they do not resent the presence of the accumulated secretion. When, however, some of the secretion reaches an area of healthy mucosa, whether because of change of position on arising from bed in the morning, or of an attempt at physical examination of the chest, the normal cough reflex is set in action and a violent bout of coughing results. A large quantity of the accumulated secretion is then expelled, after which the patient feels more comfortable, less " toxic " and able to breathe more easily. Unfortunately, even violent coughing may not empty the dilated bronchi, because their anatomical position makes this impossible unless the patient adopts the appropriate position for draining them.

With these advanced changes, there develops the typical clinical picture of suppurative bronchiectasis—chronic cough, copious expectoration, general toxæmia, clubbing of the fingers, dyspnœa and maybe frequent attacks of hæmoptysis. To this may be added local extension of infection, giving rise to pleurisy, or to an empyema localised and encysted by the accompanying fibrosis, to bronchopneumonia in adjacent parts of the lung, and even to pericarditis. The infection may be distal in its spread by means of septic emboli ; the most frequent manifestation of this is metastatic abscess of the brain. If the patient does not succumb to some of these infective complications, right heart failure or amyloid disease will eventually cause his death.

The secretions may stagnate in the bronchi and drainage become interfered with by mucosal swelling. This will give rise to all the symptoms of a closed pulmonary abscess—high fever, rigors, rapid loss of weight and profound constitutional, toxic manifestations.   If secondary infection by anærobic organisms occurs, it determines a fœtor of the sputum and the breath which is distressing alike to the patient and to those who come into contact with him.   This fœtor has a curious, unpleasant musty sweetness, which in olden days was likened to " the scent of apple blossom mingled with a kind of *arrière-goût* of fæces."

Apart from diminution of the expansion of the thorax on the side of a unilateral bronchiectasis, the student must not expect to find specific **physical signs** other than those of the associated or complicating lesions—of bronchitis, for example, or of collapse, of fibrosis and of compensatory emphysema or of lung abscess.   Occasionally an abscess of the brain may present itself in a patient who has never complained of serious chest trouble.   Seeing that bronchiectasis in the upper lobes is rare, save when it complicates pulmonary tuberculosis, the physical signs are mostly confined to the lower parts of the lungs.

DIAGNOSIS

It is already clear that persistent cough and expectoration, or recurrent respiratory illnesses with some degree of fever, may lead the doctor to suspect tuberculosis.   In children this is all the more likely because the child may fail to gain weight and growth in the normal way.   But tubercle bacilli are never found in the sputum, save where the bronchiectasis is but a secondary complication of an already established tuberculosis of the lungs.   In patients without gross secondary infection, periodic attacks of hæmoptysis will also suggest tuberculosis, but here again tubercle bacilli are absent, and an X-ray film of the chest does not show any tuberculous infiltration of the lungs.   As has been said, it may instead show collapse of a lobe, or honeycomb cavities, or even (unless a lipiodol broncho-gram is done) nothing grossly abnormal.   In older patients differential diagnosis from simple chronic bronchitis may be necessary.   If the bronchiectasis is not infected this may be difficult on clinical grounds alone, and often can only be made by the presence or absence of dilated bronchi in broncho-grams, but if there is secondary infection, then copious ex-pectoration initiated by changes of position, hæmoptysis, fœtid sputum or breath, and clubbing of the fingers indicate something more than mere bronchitis.

A **lipiodol bronchogram** clinches the diagnosis, and if properly done marks out the extent of the disease. The introduction of lipiodol into the bronchial tree is a specialised procedure and necessitates facilities for radiographing the chest immediately afterwards. The principle consists in anæsthetising the upper air-ways, and introducing the oil so that it will efficiently delineate the various bronchial branches. Only one side of the chest should be injected at a time. It is as well to make sure beforehand that the patient is not sensitive to iodine, which is a constituent of the oil. The aim is to outline the bronchi of the various lobes ; the amount of oil necessary for this depends on whether the bronchial tree is fairly normal, whether there is collapse of one or more lobes or whether the capacity of the bronchi is much increased by reason of dilatation. The normal lung tree can be filled by about 15 to 20 c.c. of lipiodol ; less is needed if there is collapse, more if there is marked bronchiectasis. If the patient has much expectoration, a preliminary course of postural emptying of the bronchi is called for. X-ray screening of the patient will tell the operator how successful is the filling and how much lipiodol is needed.

For the introduction of the oil a No. 5 gum-elastic catheter is convenient, inserted into the trachea through the nose. One side of the nose, the throat and the larynx are successively anæsthetised and the catheter is then introduced through the nose and pushed gently down during inspiration until it slips through the larynx into the trachea. Then 1 c.c. of 2 per cent. cocaine or novocaine solution is injected through the catheter in order to anæsthetise the tracheal mucous membrane. To fill the lower lobe bronchi, 5 c.c. of the lipiodol, warmed to body-heat, is injected with the patient sitting and leaning forwards and over towards the side to be filled (for the anterior basal bronchi) and another 5 c.c. with him leaning backwards and sideways (for the posterior basal bronchi). These injections should fill also the middle basal, the dorsal and the middle lobe bronchi. The patient should now be screened, and if the filling is satisfactory films should be taken. He then lies down and another 5 c.c. is injected to fill the upper lobe branches ; for this he will need to lie sideways, at first half on his back and then half on his front, in order that the oil will flow into the posterior and anterior divisions. The adequacy of the filling can again be controlled by screening, and films taken. If the lipiodol bronchograms are successful the anterior and lateral views combine to give an excellent shadow picture of the size, character and distribution of the bronchial tree.

This method is the surest, but there is a simpler procedure which can be used if filling of the upper lobe is not essential. An ordinary Record syringe fitted with a curved delivery cannula is used, and the lipiodol is dropped into the anæsthetised trachea over the base of the tongue, which is held drawn out. Neither of these methods is suitable for young children ; for them injection of the oil through the cricothyroid membrane with a special trocar and cannula may have to be done under general anæsthesia. It can be used also for adults with local anæsthesia. In infected cases the method may be dangerous by reason of secondary infection of the puncture wound when the patient coughs up foul sputum.

Usually the lipiodol is coughed up in the course of a few days, though sometimes a portion of it remains in the lung for a long time. The persistence of the lipiodol is usually seen when the bronchi are normal and the oil extends into the alveoli. It then produces scattered X-ray shadows, which may obscure those of underlying disease in a later film. It is unwise to inject lipiodol when the vital capacity is reduced to less than 50 per cent., or when there is active phthisis, or when the patient is suffering from thyrotoxicosis.

PROGNOSIS AND TREATMENT

The natural history of any disease determines to a large extent the indications for its treatment. Until the last few years the frequency of the non-infected variety of bronchiectasis was hardly realised. While patients with non-infected bronchiectasis may remain comparatively well and free from noticeable symptoms, the onset of secondary pyogenic infection changes the disease into one which will almost surely be progressive and fatal. Then, even at best, the patient enters upon the path of chronic invalidism. The child suffers tiresome respiratory infections, especially in the winter, which interfere seriously with the even course of his schooling ; his growth is stunted and the accompanying toxæmia fatigues him. Child or adult may suffer embarrassing accidents from the typical productive cough, seeing that exertion or even laughter may bring about violent bouts of coughing and copious expectoration. Work, play and social life become, therefore, difficult and hazardous. If breath and sputum become fœtid, the sufferer is a misery to himself and an offence to his fellows, however tolerant they may wish to be. The young woman realises that she cannot look forward to marriage and the young man that he is kept literally at arm's length by even the kindest of his friends.*

Cure of the disease can only be obtained by total extirpation of the diseased part of the lung. Any other form of treatment is but palliative ; but to state this is to raise immediately a series of questions, some of which are most difficult to answer. Though uncomplicated bronchiectasis is not in itself dangerous, what are the chances of infection supervening sooner or later ? Again, what are the chances of recovery after so serious an operation as extirpation of one or more lobes of a lung, and what likelihood is there afterwards of the ability to live and work normally ? In other words, is the cure perhaps worse than the disease ?

Given a patient with non-infected bronchiectasis, it is impossible to assess with any accuracy either the expectation of life or the likelihood of infection supervening within a

* In that somewhat Rabelaisian novel *Clochemerle*, by Gabriel Chevalier (Secker and Warburg), the following picture is drawn of Ernest Tafardel, small-town schoolmaster, town clerk and consequently right-hand man to Barthélemy Piéchut, the mayor :—

"The schoolmaster's fine maxims were spoiled by the quality of his breath, with the result that the people of Clochemerle fought shy of his wise utterances, which were wafted towards his hearers at too close quarters. . . . The haste with which the inhabitants of Clochemerle would flee from him, and above all their eagerness to cut short every confidential conversation or impassioned dispute, was attributed by him to ignorance and base materialism on their part. When people simply gave way to him and fled without further argument, Tafardel suspected them of despising him. Thus his feeling of persecution rested upon a misunderstanding. Nevertheless it caused him real suffering, for being naturally prolix, as a well-informed man he would have liked to make a display of his learning. He concluded from this isolation of his that the race of mountain wine-growers had, as the result of fifteen centuries of religious and feudal oppression, grown addle-pated. . . .

"But the mayor was a clever fellow, who knew how to turn everything and everybody to good account. Like the good politician he was, Piéchut turned to his own advantage his secretary's pestiferous exhalations. If in some troublesome matter he wished to obtain the approval of certain municipal councillors of the opposition, the notary Girodot, or the wine-growers Lamolire and Maniguant, he pretended to be indisposed and sent Tafardel, with his papers and his odorous eloquence, to their respective houses. To close the schoolmaster's mouth, they gave their consent."

specified period ; there is no doubt that a sword of Damocles hangs always over him, and any respiratory infection, apparently trivial or clearly serious, may be the one which will alter the whole course of the disease and start the patient on the downward road. Now that lipiodol bronchograms have made possible the diagnosis of bronchiectatic dilatation at a much earlier stage than formerly, especially before the onset of secondary infection, it remains to be seen whether the future history of these patients will modify the hitherto accepted grave outlook on the disease. At present it is clear that not many patients who are known to have developed bronchiectasis before the age of 10 survive beyond the age of 40 : but lipiodol was not available for diagnosis thirty years ago. As might be expected, certain of the saccular types are more dangerous than the cylindrical, for sacculation in any but the more peripheral bronchioles develops only when the bronchial walls have been badly weakened by infection. As for the operative risk, it is very high in the septic cases, but surprisingly low in children and young people who are carefully selected for operation before serious infective changes have developed. Moreover, in the majority of these *picked* patients—the actual figure is something of the order of 70 per cent.—the postoperative capacity for life and work is excellent.

Sound and balanced judgment for or against operation is therefore not always easy. A patient with non-infected bronchiectasis may be in reasonably good health, save for rare attacks of hæmoptysis or of some mild and passing respiratory illness. He may perhaps avoid serious secondary infection for the rest of his life ; on the other hand, secondary pyogenic infection may at any time supervene. Again, the older the patient the greater the risk of operation, so that the longer he avoids secondary infection the more risk he runs from later operation, if it is undertaken. To balance the various factors fairly would be much easier if the degree of risk of secondary infection which menaces a patient with non-infected bronchiectasis were known ; but full information on this point is unlikely for many years to come. What is known at present is that in the postmortem room it is very rare for examples of " clean " bronchiectasis to be unexpectedly discovered in patients who have died from other diseases ; in other words, in the teaching hospitals nearly all cases of bronchiectasis are discovered by the physician, and a latent, symptomless bronchiectasis very seldom persists harmlessly throughout the normal span of life.

In practical medicine our knowledge is incomplete, but such as it is we must use it. As in the law courts, we have often to make a decision on the grounds of " reasonable likelihood." Here the odds appear to be well in favour of the likelihood that if bronchiectasis is established in childhood, serious secondary infection can be expected by the time the patient has come to early middle age. Often it appears much earlier. Before the age of 21 years, operation at the hands of the expert chest surgeon is reasonably safe, provided that septic infection does not complicate the disease. It is best, however, to operate while the child is growing, for the necessary anatomical and physiological adjustments and compensations follow much more easily than later on when growth has ceased. On all counts, therefore, and especially in view of the long-term threat both to health and to life itself, operative extirpation of the diseased portion of the lung, at the stage before infection has supervened, would appear to be the right fulfilment of the responsibility we have to our patient. In other words, at any time after the age of 8 years established bronchiectasis should, if possible, be operated on as soon as diagnosed. It is no task, however, for the " occasional chest surgeon." Every device of preparation, skill and technique needs to be mustered to ensure a safe issue out of this affliction.

To advise a serious operation for a patient who has few or no alarming symptoms is a heavy responsibility. Nevertheless, the doctor ought to put before the patient or his parents the various factors involved and the likely future ; and he can leave it to the parents to decide what they wish to be done. If they decide against operation he should advise them of the wisdom of a further reviewing of the case from time to time and especially before the patient has come to the age when the operative risk appreciably increases. Most important of all, he must warn them that at the first signs of secondary infection, and before suppuration and toxæmia make operation dangerous, the whole situation *must* be reconsidered.

Even the presence of bilateral bronchiectasis does not always forbid operation. In children, provided that the disease is not too far advanced, it is occasionally feasible first to remove one lobe : and then, at a later date, when the compensa-

9

tory adjustments have been established, to remove the diseased lobe on the other side.

Before any operation, nasal sinus infection should be treated if it is present ; and if perchance there is any complicating pulmonary infection, an adequate course of postural drainage of the lung should be instituted. Often, because of persistent spilling over of infective material from the bronchiectatic zone, there is secondary bronchitis in other parts of the lungs. This does not necessarily contraindicate operation, though it calls for a postponement of it. By means of postural drainage and general tonic treatment, many such patients can eventually be made fit for operation. In many instances, preliminary treatment by sulphonamides and by penicillin (the systemic route is the best) will reduce infection to such an extent as to make operation feasible. When, on the other hand, chronic changes throughout the lungs have become established and the respiratory reserve seriously and permanently diminished, operation is no longer feasible.

It is particularly important to exclude tuberculosis of the lungs, bearing in mind that bronchiectasis may have arisen from bronchial occlusion by tenacious tuberculous sputum or by caseous material, or by pressure from without by a tuberculous gland. The third commonest cause of death after lobectomy is tuberculosis ; it was present but undiagnosed, active from the start, or " lit up " by the operative trauma. The family and personal history must therefore be carefully explored ; and persistent examinations, including culture, of the sputum for tubercle bacilli must be undertaken. It is better to examine the sputum a dozen or twenty times and to proceed to guinea-pig inoculation in case of doubt than to be in a hurry and carelessly operate on a tuberculous lung.

The operation is best not done on children in the winter or early spring, when respiratory infections are prevalent ; this does not hold for adults with established secondary infection. Lipiodol bronchograms will show the extent of disease in the lung—it is bad, for example, to extirpate the lower lobe of the left lung only, through lack of recognition of bronchiectasis in the left " middle lobe " (lingular process). The actual details of operation are a matter for the expert thoracic surgeon.

Medical treatment can only be palliative. It must often, however, be undertaken because surgical treatment has been refused or is inadvisable. It consists in building up the general resistance, in avoiding respiratory infections if possible, and in ensuring proper drainage of the infected tubes and cavities. Fresh air, a well-regulated life in a dry and healthy district, with as little exposure as possible to sudden changes of temperature, to cold winds and to fog, and general tonics, with iron if necessary, will probably do more good than any drugs directed to the bronchial mucous membrane. Vaccines, made from the organisms present in the sputum, are often used, but clearly they can be of little value when there is established septic infection. Periodic courses of penicillin may do something to reduce secondary infection and toxæmia.

Postural drainage, if properly carried out and persisted in, can be a great help, on the one hand, for improving the patient's general condition before an operation : and, on the other hand, for controlling the outpouring of the secretions and reducing toxæmia in a patient unsuitable for operation. The cardinal importance of using the position best suited for draining the affected area has already been emphasised earlier in this chapter. A study of Figs. 25 and 26, and 32 to 33 will indicate which positions are effective in allowing the secretions in the various bronchi to drain into the trachea ; they should be able to flow downwards towards the hilum. It is clear, for example, that to drain the posterior basal bronchus the patient must lie on his face with the head and chest directed downwards at an angle of about 45 degrees from the vertical ; and that the posture which best drains the " dorsal " lobe bronchus is almost the antithesis of that for the middle lobe bronchus. While postural drainage is made convenient and easy by the use of a specially adjustable Nelson bed, the patient can practise it in his own home with no more complicated apparatus than a bed or a chair and a few pillows ; the important point being that he should be instructed in the position which he has to assume if he is to obtain proper drainage of the affected bronchus. The method should be practised in the early morning and at night, and preceded by copious warm alkaline drinks ; when the patient is in position he should be encouraged to cough and get rid of the accumulated secretions. At first, ten minutes on the postural bed will be all that he can endure ; later, he will find that the period can be extended to half an hour, with benefit. In hospital, " percussion drainage " (vigorous percussion over the affected portion of lung, with the patient in the appropriate posture for bronchial drainage) is even more effective.

When the sputum is fœtid, postural drainage holds out as much promise of relief as most other forms of treatment, little as it is. Locally applied intratracheal injections of drugs such as menthol or guaiacol are not worth the inconvenience of the manipulation. More for the patient's comfort of body and mind than for any marked therapeutic effect, inhalations of creosote or menthol vapour can be prescribed, either with steam or through an inhalation respirator ; or creosote can be given by mouth in a mixture such as the following :—

$$
\begin{array}{lll}
\text{Creosoti} & . \quad . \quad . \quad . \quad . \quad . & \text{\reflectbox{R}xv} \\
\left.\begin{array}{l}\text{Tr. chlorof. Co} \\ \text{Glycerine}\end{array}\right\} & . \quad . \quad . \quad . & \text{āā} \quad \text{ʒi}
\end{array}
$$

a teaspoonful in milk three times a day. The patient may also find that a few drops of eucalyptus oil on his handkerchief gives him confidence and comfort. Otherwise symptoms are to be treated as they arise.

There is one group of patients, however, for whom medical treatment may be curative. From time to time the physician is confronted with a child who has had, say, an attack of measles and developed a very mild and localised form of bronchiectasis. The occluding plugs have been removed by coughing, but owing to a small degree of associated inflammation and infiltration of the bronchial walls a slight bronchial dilatation persists, but with no destruction of the mucosa. The child is subject to colds, is perhaps labelled a " catarrhal child," and is regarded as having a somewhat " delicate chest." Many of these children outgrow their disability, however, if they are made to live an outdoor life, and are carefully nursed through intercurrent colds or " influenzal " attacks. Doubtless the infiltration of the bronchial walls slowly subsides, resulting fibrosis is negligible, and for all practical purposes the bronchi regain their normal healthiness. Unfavourable conditions or neglect, on the other hand, will leave the patient open to recurrent infections and the eventual development of established bronchiectasis, such as has been described ; early care and supervision, however, may allow recovery and avoid the necessity for operation.

Prophylaxis—It is clear that the avoidance of prolonged bronchial obstruction by plugs of secretion in the respiratory illnesses of children, or after operation, is of paramount importance. This danger in persistent nasal sinus infection, in measles, whooping-cough or bronchopneumonia and in the " chestiness " which may follow operations and anæsthetics, should always present itself to the mind of the doctor, and any suspicion of such occlusion, with its resultant pulmonary collapse, should be a call for radiological and bronchoscopic investigation and treatment as already described in Chapter VII. It should be remembered that if an *infected* obstructing plug or foreign body is removed early, before serious damage has been done to the bronchial walls and the lung parenchyma, complete recovery is possible, including the avoidance of permanent bronchiectatic changes.

CHAPTER X

BRONCHIAL CARCINOMA AND OTHER INTRATHORACIC TUMOURS

ONLY in recent years has it been appreciated that primary cancer of the lung is so common that its incidence is only less than that of cancer of the gastro-intestinal tract. There are some intrathoracic tumours, on the other hand, which occur but rarely. The subject of intrathoracic tumours embraces a diversity of growths originating from the chest wall, the pleura, the lungs and bronchi, and mediastinal structures, and even tumours encroaching from without into the thorax. The differential diagnosis of many of them can often be made only at operation. For some types it is possible only to give general principles which will act as a guide. In the case of bronchopulmonary growths, early recognition is of such vital importance that they will be discussed in much fuller detail.

CARCINOMA OF THE BRONCHUS

Carcinoma of the bronchus is by far the commonest intrathoracic new growth. It affects males much more often than females, particularly in the fifth decade (40 to 50 years); an appreciable number occur, however, between the ages of 30 and 40 years, and instances have been recorded in patients as young as 16 years. There are no convincingly proved causal factors, apart perhaps from the radioactive dust encountered by those "pathological curiosities," the Schneeberg cobalt workers and the Joachimstal miners. The vast majority of cancers of the lung—some would say all—originate in a bronchus, nine out of every ten of them in the main bronchi or at the beginning of the secondary bronchi, and the odd ones, more or less peripherally placed, in smaller bronchi in the substance of the lung. These latter, when situated at the apex, produce a special group of symptoms and signs by reason of their anatomical relationships. Nearly all these bronchial carcinomata begin, then, in the mucosa of the larger bronchi at the root of the lung ; the growth soon spreads to the neighbouring lymphatic nodes in the mediastinum, and extends directly and by the lymphatics, in the opposite direction, to bronchioles and lung alveoli, while metastases are carried by the blood stream to distant parts of the body. Macroscopically the tumour may appear, therefore, as mainly a hilar mass, or as a diffuse infiltrating growth, or even as miliary tumours. As will be seen later, sometimes the clinical picture is predominantly one of lung abscess.

The bronchial mucous membrane is derived from the primitive hypopharynx, which also produces the squamous epithelium of the mouth and œsophagus ; it consists of a basal cell layer of small oval or rounded cells and of a superficial layer of ciliated columnar epithelium, with a variable number of ordinary columnar cells in between. From these cells the three common histological types of the neoplasm are derived — the anaplastic, undifferentiated " oat - celled " carcinoma (previously regarded as a mediastinal lymphosarcoma) : the columnar-celled : and the squamous-celled carcinoma, arising by metaplasia of either columnar epithelium, or (and this is more likely) of the more primitive oval cell of the basal layer. Many of these growths, however, are noteworthy for their pleomorphism, so that it is possible to find a mixture of these various types of cell in the same tumour. There is not enough clinical difference between the histological types to afford clear-cut indications for prognosis or treatment ; all that can be said is that the squamous-celled type tends to grow more slowly than the others, and to metastasise later, while the oat-celled type is the most malignant.

The most useful classification of these growths is that based on their site. If the tumour is near the hilum, in one of the larger bronchi, cough and hæmoptysis are early symptoms, bronchoscopy will show the bronchial portion of the growth, invasion of the mediastinal glands occurs in the earlier stages, and the nearness of the growth to vital structures increases the difficulties of surgical removal. If, on the other hand, the tumour is peripheral, it may cause few or no local symptoms until either the pleura is involved or metastases occur ; it cannot be seen through the bronchoscope, but if diagnosed without undue delay it offers better chances of successful surgical removal.

Symptoms and signs—The clinical picture varies so much from patient to patient that it is worth while considering how a bronchial carcinoma may develop, and what symptoms and signs it is able to produce. An early neoplasm growing in the bronchial wall (Fig. 89) will act as a foreign body, and the attempts to expel it result in *cough*, short, hard, unpro-

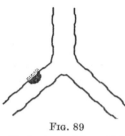

FIG. 89
Early stage of bronchial neoplasm.

ductive at first, maybe spasmodic. Perhaps a little mucoid sputum is soon brought up in response to the irritation. As the nodule increases in size it may ulcerate and bleed. This gives rise to *hæmoptysis* in the form either of a few gobbets of blood, or (if there happens to be an associated inflammatory reaction) as streaks of blood in muco-purulent sputum. A copious hæmoptysis is uncommon.

Imagine the growth to have increased still more in size until it produces *an appreciable but as yet incomplete blocking of the bronchus*. Since the lumen of the normal main bronchus is about as wide as a narrow finger, and the lobar divisions smaller still, the intrabronchial portion of the growth need not become very large before it embarrasses the proper ventilation of the corresponding lobe or lobes of the lung. The patient may become conscious of an inability to expand his lungs to the full extent, especially on exertion. Owing to this interference with ventilation of the affected lobe the blood flowing through it is imperfectly oxygenated. This blood joins the fully oxygenated blood from the normal parts of the lungs, with consequent depreciation of the full oxygenated quality of the systemic blood stream. This may cause, even at a comparatively early stage of the disease, some degree of *cyanosis*. The cyanosis is due to the amount of reduced hæmoglobin in the systemic circulating blood ; the dyspnœa results from the partial bronchial block, which interferes with the ventilation of a lung or of a lobe : this in its turn causes an imperfectly oxygenated blood supply to the heart, myocardial subfunctioning and consequent pulmonary congestion.

It may now be possible to hear a *wheeze* over the narrowed

bronchus, significant because it is unilateral and *localised*; sometimes the patient notices and localises it himself.

The partial obstruction of the bronchus impedes free drainage of secretions. This, together with the interruption of the normal defensive ciliary " staircase " movement over the area of the growth, renders the imperfectly aerated part of the lung particularly susceptible to infection. As a result there are *pyrexial attacks,* often referred to as influenzal, or giving the picture of a pneumonia, an abscess or pleurisy.

Further increase in the intrabronchial growth causes *complete blocking of the bronchus* (Fig. 90) and *absorption collapse* of the lung distal to the obstruction (see also Chap. VII). There is no entry of air during inspiration, and as the air in the alveoli becomes absorbed, there is considerable reduction in the volume of the lobe. The mediastinum is drawn over to the affected side, and the ribs fall in slightly. Owing to the comparatively slow growth of the obstructing nodule the develop-

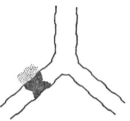

FIG. 90

Complete bronchial obstruction by neoplasm.

ment of the symptoms of collapse of the lung is much less dramatic than in acute obstruction, such as is produced, for example, by an inhaled foreign body. Often, indeed, they develop insidiously, though occasionally the mediastinal dislocation is rapid enough to cause discomfort and distress. A growth no larger than a cherry stone can block even a main bronchus completely, and may attain this size long before there are serious constitutional symptoms. It is possible for such a patient to have a cough, some dyspnœa on exertion and possibly occasional blood in the sputum, yet not to be seriously incapacitated ; on examination, however, one side of the chest is found to expand poorly, and there is dulness to percussion and complete absence of breath sounds over the affected lung. The physical signs are therefore out of all proportion to the symptoms. This marked difference between symptoms and signs is in striking contrast to the usual clinical picture in patients with simple abscess or with tuberculosis of the lung.

When the obstruction is of one of the main or secondary bronchi the collapse will be lobar or segmental. In certain of these latter examples, as, for instance, a block of the antero-lateral bronchus, the signs will, at first examination, appear to be bizarre ; because while there is dulness to percussion and silence to auscultation over the upper part of the chest in front, posteriorly there is a normal percussion note and the breath sounds are unaltered (Fig. 91).

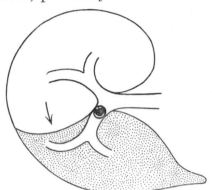

FIG. 91

Diagrammatic representation of cross-section of upper lobe, showing block of the antero-lateral bronchus and resulting collapse of the corresponding segment.

Occasionally the bronchial block is progressive from one bronchus to another, causing successive segmental lung collapse.

With the complete collapse of the lobe or lobes involved, the earlier cyanosis may improve, for the circulation through the collapsed and unaerated portion of the lung is so reduced that there is now not enough imperfectly oxygenated blood going to the right side of the heart to dilute the fully oxygenated blood from the rest of the lung.

As in partial, so in complete blocking of the bronchus, infection of the lung, with or without suppuration, is extremely likely to develop distal to the block—pneumonias of various types, infected bronchiectasis or lung abscess ; and as a complication of these, pleurisy, pleurisy with effusion, empyema or pyopneumothorax. These give rise to *irregular fever and toxæmia*. The combination of infection with deficient aeration of the lung may result in *clubbing of the fingers*, which quite often appears surprisingly early. Occasionally the patient's illness may present itself as an apparently mild or severe septicæmia.

Meanwhile, and even before it has obstructed a bronchus, the growth is spreading outside into the lung substance, and may extend to the glands and other tissues of the mediastinum. It then shows some of the many invasive manifestations of **mediastinal tumour,** as, for example :—

    (i) *Involvement of the phrenic nerve,* with consequent paralysis and elevation of the diaphragm. This is particularly likely to occur on the right side, for there the nerve courses through a small mass of glands lying below the inferior branch of the pulmonary vein. Such paralysis is therefore a valuable indication of glandular involvement, stamping the case as one in which surgical intervention is not feasible. Very rarely, in the early stages of implication, there is intractable hiccough from irritation of the phrenic nerve.

(ii) *Involvement of the left recurrent laryngeal nerve*, with fixation of the vocal cord. Very occasionally a patient with bronchial carcinoma may first seek advice from the laryngologist, because of hoarseness or aphonia.

(iii) *Pressure on the œsophagus*— This is not common, and is more likely to occur with a primary carcinoma of the left main bronchus, either by direct extension of the growth, or by enlargement of the glands just below the bifurcation of the trachea (Fig. 92).

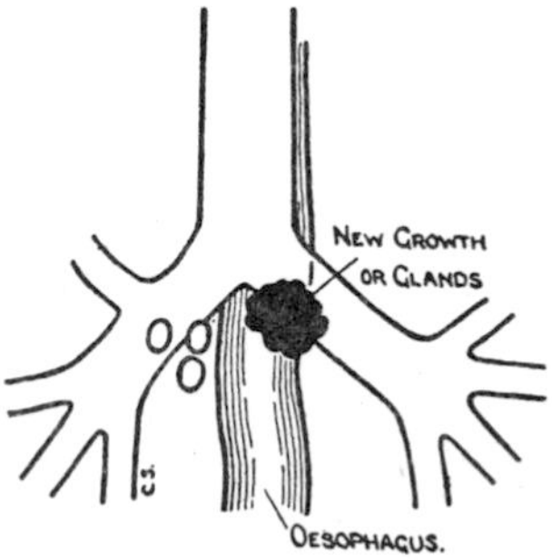

FIG. 92

To show pressure on œsophagus by new growth of left bronchus or by secondary glands in that situation.

(iv) *Involvement of the sympathetic*. (See the later section on Apical Bronchial Carcinoma.)

(v) *Pressure on the superior vena cava*, with venous engorgement of the head and neck, does not usually occur until a late stage of the disease.

(vi) *Direct invasion of the pericardium and heart* results in cardiac embarrassment and failure, or in pericardial effusion, and is again a late manifestation, occurring in perhaps 10 per cent. of patients.

(vii) *Pressure on azygos veins*, with dilatation of the superficial veins over the thorax.

(viii) *Invasion of the thoracic duct*, with chylous effusion.

(ix) *Involvement of the vagus nerve*, with gastric symptoms due to pyloric spasm, or cardiac arrhythmias.

The growth may extend from the mediastinum into the lymph nodes of the neck or of the axilla, or it may follow the line of glands along the aorta into the abdomen (where it sometimes invades directly the suprarenal glands, and so causes Addison's disease) and even into the pelvis, where invasion of the hypogastric nerves may confuse the doctor by causing retention of urine.

If the growth starts in a smaller bronchus nearer the periphery of the lung, there is likely to be early spread reversely along the lymphatics to the pleura, with pleurisy and finally *pleural effusion,* which may be serofibrinous, but more often is *hæmorrhagic.** Sometimes the pleural surface is seen to be studded with nodules of growth. Even if the carcinoma is near to the hilum, it is likely to extend into the substance of the lung, and occasionally a difficult clinical problem is raised by a growth which does not obstruct a bronchus until some considerable time after it has spread in fan shape along the lymphatics towards the periphery of the lung, producing a chronic indurative lesion, with the radiological appearances of what is sometimes called an " unresolved pneumonia." But this " pneumonia " does not resolve—a sinister persistence in any person at or beyond middle age. If perchance this invasion of the growth is punctuated by small nodules of cancer cells along its pathways, the X-ray picture may be like that of certain cases of lung tuberculosis.

Quite apart from infective or suppurative changes distal to a blocked bronchus, the intrapulmonary portion of the growth may at any time begin to necrose. This in itself can cause irregular fever, cough with copious sputum, night sweats and clubbing of the fingers ; while the X-ray film shows cavitation in the intrapulmonary mass. Occasionally this cavitation is obviously ragged, in contrast to the smoother cavitation due to a lung abscess which results from secondary infection of the collapsed portion of lung distal to an occluding bronchial mass.

Secondary metastases may occur anywhere (Fig. 93), and sometimes a metastatic deposit in an obvious place such as skin, spine, long bones or skull is the first indication of the disease. A secondary malignant deposit without an obvious primary growth should always make one think of the lungs ; I have seen secondaries in the skin in a lusty, symptomless farmer in whom an X-ray of the chest revealed a hilar shadow

---

* Sometimes malignant cells can be found in the pleural fluid. If the effusion is due to lymphatic blockage at the hilar " bottle-neck," malignant cells will not be found.

no larger than a penny. Similarly, a cerebral tumour frequently proves to be a metastasis from a bronchial carcinoma ; so much so that it should be a rule always to have X-ray films

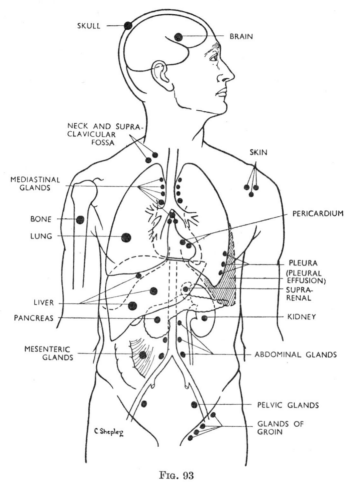

Fig. 93

Metastatic sites of bronchial carcinoma. (*After Christopher.*)

taken of the chest of any patient suffering from cerebral tumour. The malignant cells are carried by branches of the pulmonary vein to the left side of the heart, and thence by way of the carotid arteries to the brain.

Finally, the more general manifestations of loss of weight, fatigue, anæmia and cachexia are to be noted. Loss of weight is often a fairly early symptom and is steadily progressive ; more rarely, however, it only becomes obvious late in the disease, and then its progress is very rapid.

This schematic review emphasises the protean nature of the signs and symptoms of the disease. Any of these manifestations may, in fact, present themselves when the patient first seeks the advice of his doctor ; but in view of the preponderance of bronchial carcinoma in the larger bronchi it is clear that persistent cough and hæmoptysis are the most likely "early symptoms," to be followed by dyspnœa and infection of the lung expressed either as an "influenzal attack," pneumonia or pleurisy. When the growth starts more deeply in the lung symptoms are likely to be few or absent for some time, though here again hæmoptysis may occur, as also may pain from pleurisy. The earliest *signs* noticed will usually be those of collapse of a lobe or of a lung due to obstruction of a large bronchus, or of pleurisy with effusion, from lymphatic block or from a tumour near to the pleura. If, therefore, the diagnosis is to be made at a stage when any hope of effective treatment is still possible, it is futile to wait for the development of unequivocal physical signs. Even at the best the scales are still weighted against early diagnosis ; it is not encouraging to note the duration of symptoms before the patient seeks advice or the diagnosis is made. In a series of my own patients this was, on average, about six months. The insidious onset of the disease and the failure to realise that carcinoma of the lung is a comparatively common disease, are probably responsible for this delay. If, however, earlier diagnosis is to become more frequent the doctor must be more constantly suspicious, bearing in mind these guiding principles :—

(i) Applying the words of Osler, when speaking of pulmonary tuberculosis, half the diagnosis of bronchial carcinoma is to be on the look out for it, especially in any illness referable to the lungs which begins at or after middle age.

(ii) Persistent cough at any age should call for proper investigation, especially if it is accompanied by even slight hæmoptysis. In patients at the "cancer age," hæmoptysis occurring for the first time should be regarded as due to bronchial carcinoma until the contrary is proved.

(iii) In a patient of middle age who has not previously suffered from chest trouble, "influenza," atypical pneumonia or pleurisy which does not subside normally and satisfac-torily may be due to bronchial carcinoma. In an elderly person pleurisy with effusion and empyema without a clear primary cause may be complications of this disease. Lung abscess at this age must always be regarded with caution and suspicion.

(iv) In a patient of middle age, cough accompanied by a troublesome dyspnœa which is not adequately explained by the physical signs in lungs or heart, and which is new and recent, should lead one to think of the possibility of bronchial new growth. In the same way the onset of asthmatic wheezing at this age is not always due to simple asthma.

Whenever there is reason for suspicion an X-ray film of the chest must be taken, both in the anterior and lateral views. The sputum should be examined to see whether or not tubercle bacilli are present, and when the X-ray film suggests bronchial carcinoma, an expert clinical pathologist, using Dudgeon and Wrigley's wet film method,* has a fair chance of finding malignant cells. Whenever malignant disease of a bronchus is considered a possibility, bronchoscopy should be done, and especially if the X-ray film is seemingly normal in a middle-aged patient with hæmoptysis. If the growth is seen with the bronchoscope, a portion should be removed for section. In growths near the hilum, bronchoscopy is much more important than a lipiodol bronchogram, which is more helpful in detecting bronchial obstructions beyond the vision of the bronchoscope, though lipiodol may also reveal an obstruction in the larger bronchi.

The **diagnosis,** then, is usually clinched by special investiga-tions after suspicion has been aroused by the clinical history and physical findings. The radiologist as he screens the chest may find evidence of poor aeration of a lobe even before there is complete occlusion of the bronchus. The anterior and lateral films help to define the bronchus affected and the area of lung involved, as well as to give information about the mediastinum and maybe pleural involvement. Tomography may show the actual narrowing of the bronchus ; the lipiodol bronchogram will also mark the occlusion, though, as has been indicated

---

* *Journal of Laryngology and Otology,* 1935, **50,** 752. J. Bamforth (*Thorax,* 1946, **1,** 118) reports an encouraging percentage of successes. Another method is to centrifugalise the sputum, embed the packed deposit in a paraffin block and then cut sections—the *artificial block method.*

above, it is not so important, save for the peripheral tumours, as bronchoscopy, by which the bronchial portion of growth may be seen *in situ* and a piece removed for section. Examination of the sputum and pleural fluid, if any, may reveal malignant cells. If there is still uncertainty, inspection by the thoracoscope may give enough information to allow of a decision whether it is worth while proceeding to an exploratory thoracotomy, though usually thoracotomy will be necessary for a complete view.

The **differential diagnosis** will depend in practice on how the case presents itself. The problem may appear to the examiner as one of hæmoptysis ; of various infective processes either in the lung and pleura, or as a difficult " pyrexia of uncertain origin " ; of a mediastinal tumour, or of secondary and more distant manifestations, as, for example, cerebral tumour or enlargement of the liver.

The important thing is to become " carcinoma conscious." Just as when the doctor sees a patient with hæmoptysis, he considers the possibility of tuberculosis or bronchiectasis, so also must he think of carcinoma, especially if the patient is over 30 years of age. The same applies to patients who clinically and radiologically show the presence of a lung abscess. More particularly is this so when the preceding history is not typical, and there is no obvious antecedent history of infection. The abscess may be secondary to bronchial occlusion, or the growth itself may have undergone necrosis. A breaking-down growth resembling an abscess is more often seen when the tumour originates in one of the lesser bronchi, and is therefore situated in the more central or peripheral lung field. Differentiation in these cases may be extremely difficult. The history of the illness may be a guide. Moreover, if on examination of the X-ray films the abscess cavity is ragged, or is not central in the zone of shadowing, suspicion of carcinoma must be entertained. Recognition of a carcinomatous abscess is particularly necessary, because the opening of a carcinomatous abscess destroys any chance of radical removal of the growth.

TREATMENT

Until a few years ago carcinoma of the lung was regarded as an incurable disease. Radium and deep X-ray therapy had been hopefully tried, but found ineffective, though the latter may at times be helpful in controlling the pain associated with invasion of the pleura. It is true that the pathology of the disease does not encourage confident hopes of cure ; those growths which are likely to be diagnosed reasonably early are in the larger bronchi, near the hilum, when mediastinal invasion is liable to be equally early. The remaining 10 per cent., those situated peripherally, are liable for a long time to present few or no symptoms, so that early diagnosis is not easy. Both patient and chest surgeon are fortunate, therefore, if they meet before it is too late for successful surgical extirpation of the growth.

Nevertheless, thoracic surgery has recently made such progress that extirpation of the whole lung has become a possible and justifiable operation. Unfortunately, up to the present, surgery is in advance of diagnosis. With the increase in appreciation that carcinoma of the lung is often curable if operated upon early—say, within three months of the onset of symptoms : with the knowledge of what are the minimal signs which should make the diagnosis of carcinoma suspected : with the immediate transfer of such a patient to a chest centre where the more precise and specialised investigations can be made, a progressively increasing number of patients will be successfully treated for the disease.

In many instances there is bound to be uncertainty as to whether the growth is amenable to operation or not. For these, thoracotomy is indicated. If radical removal is impossible, the chest wall is closed ; but if extirpation is feasible, the operation is undertaken forthwith.

Contraindications to operation, making even thoracotomy superfluous, are an extension of the growth in a main bronchus to within less than an inch from the bifurcation of the trachea : signs of mediastinal invasion, such as right phrenic paralysis, paralysis of a vocal cord, fixation of the trachea or of the main bronchus : pleural effusion whether serofibrinous or hæmorrhagic : obvious secondary dissemination, such as metastases in the skin, skull, liver or elsewhere : and associated chronic bronchitis and emphysema, cardiovascular disease or cachexia.

Exploratory thoracotomy is not more serious—probably less so—than exploratory laparotomy. A hilar growth, when

10

it is found suitable for removal, calls for a skilled "dissection removal" of the whole lung ; a peripheral growth may demand this, or may need removal only of the affected lobe. The collected experience of lung surgery is not yet large enough to justify any final conclusions about the value and long-term success of operation, though individual successes are on record, In any event this body of knowledge can never become established unless the surgeon is given a fair chance to exercise his skill before the patient's doom is sealed by the progress of the disease.

If surgical removal of the growth is not possible, implantation of radon seeds can do nothing to check its progress ; an adequate dose of radon seeds cannot possibly be introduced through a bronchoscope. The temporary improvement which has sometimes been recorded as due to this form of treatment is almost certainly the result of the actual manipulation of inserting radon seeds into the bronchial portion of the growth. The mechanical trauma, combined perhaps with a small local effect of the radon, may re-establish an air-way, and allow drainage of the distal part of the lung. The only other line of specific treatment is by deep X-rays. Unfortunately, an adequate dose entails extensive irradiation which must of necessity damage and burn healthy lung, especially as the maximum dose must be given over a short period of time ; nevertheless, by simultaneous irradiation of the roots of the lungs and the mediastinum it is sometimes possible to arrest for a time the spread of the disease. It never cures a proven case of bronchial carcinoma ; after an interval the disease progresses again with great rapidity. Failure is due to recurrence of the growth in the damaged part of the irradiated lung, or to the fact that the patient cannot stand the drastic treatment. Sometimes X-ray treatment completely destroys a growth, converting it into a liquefied collection of necrotic material ; the patient is then in grave jeopardy of death from secondary bronchopneumonia.

Otherwise treatment consists of dealing with symptoms as they arise and of making the patient as comfortable as possible. A sedative linctus may help to relieve a troublesome cough, but sooner or later opiates will be needed for pain. When necessary they should be given without stint. Dyspnœa due to a pleural effusion should be relieved by the withdrawal of the fluid ; yet the fluid is almost certain to reaccumulate quickly. For empyema secondary to infection of the lung distal to a bronchial carcinoma, open drainage should be avoided, since the wound will not heal satisfactorily; frequent evacuation of the pus by needle and syringe is all that can properly be done.

APICAL BRONCHIAL CARCINOMA

In 1924 and again in 1932 Pancoast reported a small series of cases of tumour in the region between the root of the neck and the apex of the lung, to which he gave the name of " superior pulmonary sulcus tumour." By reason of the involvement of the brachial plexus and the sympathetic cervical chain a special clinical syndrome develops, comprising motor and sensory disturbances in the shoulder and arm of the affected side, atrophy of the muscles of the hand, and Horner's syndrome—ptosis of the eyelid, enophthalmos, unilateral miosis and anidrosis of the face and neck. Any lesion of the parietal pleura at the root of the neck may involve the brachial plexus and the sympathetic chain, so that apical tuberculosis has been found to produce the particular neurological picture. If the lesion is due to malignant growth, it may also bring about destruction of bony structures near by, such as the upper three ribs posteriorly, and the transverse processes and bodies of the corresponding vertebræ. Thus carcinoma of the thymus, intrathoracic sympathoblastoma and malignant metastases in this situation can all produce the syndrome. Almost all the cases of this syndrome are, however, instances of peripheral bronchial carcinoma, and the terms " Pancoast's tumour " or " superior pulmonary sulcus tumour " should now be discarded in favour of names which indicate the actual pathological condition. Most of them will therefore be cases of " apical bronchial carcinoma."

SECONDARY TUMOURS

Metastatic tumours of the lung and mediastinum are common enough, arising either by transmission along the lymphatics, as in breast cancer, or via the blood stream, as in primary sarcoma of bone, melanoma, chorionepithelioma, hypernephroma and the like. The nodular deposits may be large or small, so that the X-ray picture may show the lung invaded by fairly large, well-defined nodular shadows, or there may sometimes be a diffuse infiltration in which the tiny nodules give an appearance which may be mistaken for miliary tuberculosis. The treatment of a patient with secondary growths in the lung is purely palliative.

BENIGN INTRATHORACIC TUMOURS

These are less common than the malignant ones—indeed, they are rare. In the lung parenchyma, chondroma, fibroma and myoma can occur. In the bronchi both simple intra-bronchial polyp (consisting of hyperplastic mucous membrane) and fibroma have been reported. The most common benign intrabronchial tumour is the **bronchial adenoma**, which arises in the main or secondary bronchi, probably from the bronchial mucous glands. It is usually pedunculated, and being very vascular, bleeds easily. Sometimes in its growth it forces a way between the bronchial cartilages and expands again outside the bronchus, thus producing a " dumb-bell tumour." Micro-scopically it is not always easy to differentiate from bronchial carcinoma ; both radon and deep X-ray treatment will cause a small adenoma to disappear, and it is most likely that patients reported as cured of their carcinoma many years after deep irradiation were, in fact, suffering from benign bronchial adenoma. Cough and recurrent hæmoptysis are the only symptoms at first. When the adenoma blocks the bronchus the usual secondary changes in the distal part of the lung supervene. By this time the clinical history is usually a long one, far too long for carcinoma ; the patient may therefore be regarded as a case of " unresolved pneumonia," bronchi-ectasis, pulmonary tuberculosis with a " negative sputum," or chronic empyema. He may even die from the suppurative changes secondary to a condition which is curable. The history of recurrent hæmoptysis, together with radiological evidence of collapse of one or more lobes of the lung, should suggest that blocking of the bronchus is present, and call for broncho-scopy. The tumour can usually be removed through a broncho-scope by means of forceps, and the application afterwards of a radon container to the site of the lesion ensures that any pieces of growth left behind are destroyed.

TUMOURS OF THE PLEURA

Primary tumours of the pleura are rare, secondary meta-static deposits fairly common. The only important primary neoplasm is the so-called endothelioma or mesothelioma ; it is a diffuse infiltrating tumour which causes marked thickening of the pleura, together with pleural effusion which may be serous at first, but usually becomes hæmorrhagic later. The clinical picture is thus one of chronic pleurisy with effusion, the fluid reaccumulating rapidly after tapping the chest. Some pathologists think that this tumour is not primary at all, but secondary to a primary tumour either of a peripheral bronchus or elsewhere in the body, so small that it can be missed even at autopsy.

The fluid withdrawn from the pleural cavity is clear and straw-coloured, or it may be blood-stained. With clear fluid the differential diagnosis from tuberculous effusion may be difficult. In malignant disease of the pleura it is uncommon to find tumour cells in the effusion, though large, vacuolated "endothelial" cells may be seen. The rapid reaccumulation of the fluid after aspiration is very suggestive of neoplasm. In such patients air replacement of the effusion will allow study of the underlying lung and the pleural cavity by radiology and by the thoracoscope.

MEDIASTINAL TUMOURS

Retrosternal goitre is localised to the superior mediastinum and produces its symptoms when, sooner or later, it becomes impacted in the upper thoracic outlet. In consequence, there is pressure upon the trachea, the great vessels, the œsophagus and rarely the nerves. Pressure on the trachea is the most common ; the clinical picture is therefore one of severe "asthmatic" attacks and troublesome, sometimes almost suffocating, dyspnœa. Less often there is difficulty in swallow-ing, or the signs of venous obstruction, such as prominent veins over the upper thorax and œdema of the head and neck. X-ray films show a typical picture, and the goitre can be re-moved surgically by approach from the neck.

Thymic tumours are rare.

In the posterior (and occasionally in the anterior) media-

stinum, a tumour of a thoracic nerve sheath may occur
(**neurinoma**) ; sometimes it arises in the region of the intervertebral foramen, and takes the form of a dumb-bell tumour,
with prolongations into the spinal theca and into the
mediastinum. **Ganglioneuroma** is a growth arising from
sympathetic ganglion cells. They occur in the young as
well as the adult, and are easily removed without special
danger to the patient, provided that they have not produced mechanical damage to important structures, or that,
following pressure on a bronchus, secondary infection of the
lung has not supervened. Early rather than late removal
is therefore indicated, at a time when there may indeed be
no specific symptoms, and when the condition has been discovered by routine radiograms of the chest for some other
reason.

Dermoid cysts and **teratomata** are usually situated in the
anterior mediastinum. They may perforate a bronchus, so
that the patient coughs up cheesy material and pieces of hair ;
very rarely they may push their way through the hilum and
fan out through the breach into the interior of the lung. They
tend to become malignant. X-ray films show the tumour to
be in the anterior mediastinum ; the shadow may be of varying density with, at times, typically dense patches of calcification. Their removal is more dangerous because of their
connection with the root of the lungs. Once secondary septic
changes have occurred, the risk to life is greatly increased ;
operation should, therefore, not be delayed once the diagnosis
is made.

Lymphosarcoma can occur as part of a generalised lympho-
sarcomatosis, but it must be remembered that most of the cases
of what used to be called " mediastinal lymphosarcoma " are
in fact primary bronchial carcinomata with secondary invasion of the mediastinum. Both lymphosarcoma and the
enlarged glands of mediastinal **reticulosis (Hodgkin's disease)**
are radio-sensitive. X-ray therapy is therefore of great value
not only in treatment, but also in the differential diagnosis
of these conditions from carcinomatous spread into the mediastinum.

Seeing that the word " tumour " primarily signifies a
swelling or lump, **aneurysm of the aorta** must be added to
this list of mediastinal tumours. It is almost always due to

syphilis, and a positive Wassermann reaction in the blood is therefore a point in favour of the diagnosis, especially if it is accompanied by an obvious expansile swelling. The final differentiation from other mediastinal swellings frequently depends on the radiological appearances and especially on the discovery of a clearly defined, pulsating shadow, seen during screening of the chest.

HYDATID DISEASE OF THE LUNGS

By far the commonest site for the development of hydatid cysts is the liver ; next in frequency come the lungs. The disease is more common in Australia, Iceland and the Argentine than in Great Britain, though in certain regions here (parts of Wales, for example) an appreciable number of cases occur.

Man is only one of various animals which act as intermediate hosts for the parasite, *tænia echinococcus*. The mature form of the worm inhabits the intestine of the dog ; it is about 3 to 6 mm. in length, forms three or four segments only and possesses a head which is armed with four suckers and two rows of hooks. Its eggs are excreted in the dog's fæces and gain entrance into the human intestine with the ingestion of water or food (lettuce or watercress, for example) which they have contaminated, or from fingers which have fondled the soiled coats of infected sheep-dogs.

The ingested egg then hatches, and the resulting embryo bores through the intestinal wall and is carried by the portal blood stream to the liver, where it may lodge and grow ; sometimes, however, it is carried onwards to the right chambers of the heart, and thence to the lungs. Less frequently still, it may reach the left side of the heart and the systemic circulation.

Wherever it lodges, as it grows it surrounds itself with a thin, pearly, chitinous membrane ; outside this a dense capsule of fibrous tissue forms as the result of tissue reaction to its irritating presence. The central part of the developing embryo opens out to become a cystic space filled with a crystal-clear fluid rich in salts and protein. The cyst wall is therefore thinned-out embryonic tissue ; from it arise small bud-like projections which grow out into the central space. These buds will eventually form the heads of new worms ; some of them, however, will form *daughter cysts*, which produce buds in their turn.   In the lungs, however, the formation of daughter cysts is rare.

The buds, whether in main or daughter cysts, soon become invaginated, with the result that the future head of the parasite, with its suckers and crown of hooklets, is turned outside in. The student can visualise this by imagining a series of suckers and hooklets on the end of the finger of a rubber glove, and then picturing their position when the finger has been invaginated.

The ingestion by the dog of cyst-contaminated tissue of any animal who is an intermediate host results in the liberation of the living buds ; the heads become evaginated, and suckers and hooks fasten themselves to the dog's intestinal mucosa, while the worm grows to maturity.   If, however, the inter-mediate host lives on, so depriving the worm of its chance of maturity, the embryos may eventually die and the cystic fluid become absorbed.   As a result the cyst collapses to some extent, the chitinous membrane persists as a wavy remnant, and following the eventual deposition of calcium, the inspis-sated cyst contents come to resemble white mortar.   The whole is encapsulated in a solid ring of fibrous tissue.   If some of the inspissated material is microscoped, a few detached hooklets may be found here and there.

The protein of the cyst fluid is foreign to the human body, acting as an antigen which determines allergic manifestations such as eosinophilia or attacks of urticaria, and also specific humoral reactions which can be revealed by complement-fixation tests.   When in an already sensitised patient massive and rapid absorption of the protein takes place, as by the rupture of a cyst into the pleural cavity, the resulting ana-phylaxis may be fatal.

Hydatid cysts in the human lung remain latent until they produce symptoms which depend on their site and size : irritation of the pleura, causing pain, or of the diaphragm, causing cough ; pressure on a bronchus, causing cough, scanty mucus and hæmoptysis ; rupture into a bronchus, which may cause death by drowning of the lungs, or by suffocation from impaction of the cyst wall in the glottis : if the patient sur-vives these hazards the cyst cavity soon becomes infected, with suppuration of the contents ; or rupture may occur into the pleural cavity, with an anaphylactic reaction and the development of secondary effusion. Only when the contents of the ruptured intrapulmonary cyst include daughter cysts will pleural hydatids occur.

The physical signs also depend on the site and size of the cysts. Cysts near the periphery of the lung may give signs resembling those of encysted fluid, and there is danger of mistaking them for interlobar effusion or, possibly, encysted empyema. The danger arises from putting in a needle in order to draw off fluid for diagnostic or therapeutic purposes. Cyst fluid escapes along the track of the needle, or the cyst may be torn and pour its contents into the pleural cavity, with the risk of severe anaphylaxis. A similar danger has to be guarded against during the course of surgical removal of a hydatid cyst of the lung.

Hydatid cysts in the lung may be single or multiple. Occasionally a cyst of the liver perforates the diaphragm into the pleural cavity or even into the parenchyma of the lung.

Diagnosis is usually made by radiology, the typical shadow of the cyst being seen—rounded in the central and basal parts of the lung, pear-shaped in the apical situation. The diagnosis finds support from a known history of exposure to the worm, from an appreciable eosinophilia and from positive reactions to specific tests such as the complement-fixation test and the Casoni intradermal test. If there has been spontaneous rupture into a bronchus, sputum or pleural fluid may contain hooklets, buds or portions of the cyst wall.

Early operation is called for, except where operation would be unjustifiably hazardous. There are, for example, deeply situated parabronchial and hilar cysts, small and non-infected, for which expectant treatment may be adopted. Such patients need periodic supervision, however, for an enlarging cyst may eventually rupture into a bronchus or into the pleural cavity and cause death or grave illness.

A NOTE ON ADVISING SURGICAL INTERVENTION

The surgery of the thorax is not yet as firmly established as that of many other regions of the body. Thoracic surgeons are still pioneers, blazing trails through difficult country, making roads on which those who come after may tread securely. In the taming of unexplored country, an adventurous readiness to press forward needs to be complemented by the more deliberate and judicial qualities necessary for consolidation. The physician, on his part, is naturally hesitant in counselling operation so long as the risk to life remains great and the end results not certain. In almost desperate circumstances the doctor has sometimes a most difficult decision to make. He must not play with his patient's life, on the one hand, by risking it without just cause, to satisfy his own curiosity or desire for experience ; on the other, *by denying his patient a possible chance of recovery, even if it is a slender one.* The following paragraph from Thorkild Rovsing's preface to his *Clinical Lectures on Abdominal Surgery* (1914) is to the point :—

" The practitioner's responsibility is of a twofold nature. All practitioners properly feel the responsibility of advising patients to undergo operation, and they all feel this because the fears and many scruples of the patient react on their minds. On the one hand, the practitioner is far less sensible of responsibility if he refrains from advising surgical assistance in cases of certainty or doubt, simply because no one would saddle him in either case with the responsibility. No one, that is to say, save his own conscience. This responsibility is, in consequence, often overlooked and forgotten, more is the pity ; because, as a matter of fact, it is a greater and more serious responsibility than that incurred by advising surgical counsel. For in the latter case if interference be not necessary, the fact will be opportunely recognised by the experienced surgeon whose help has been sought, and thus no misfortune occurs ; while, on the other hand, neglect of a timely call for such surgical help, when needed, often results in loss of life. . . . It should always be every good physician's pride, above all things, to preserve the feeling of this responsibility steadily alight and awake in his conscience, and the more so because in the world's eye he can so easily avoid it."

CHAPTER XI

UPPER RESPIRATORY INFECTION—THE COMMON COLD

FEBRILE catarrhs affecting the upper respiratory tract are all apt to be loosely called " influenza " or " influenzal cold." Sometimes the doctor deliberately uses the term in order to persuade his patient to go to bed ; often the sufferer feels that his illness is more important as " a dose of 'flu " than as " a common cold." A certain amount of confusion is thus imported into this group of illnesses, and it is made worse by the absence of a clear-cut differentiation based on the clinical picture.

The **common cold** (" febrile catarrh ") is an acute catarrhal inflammation, usually beginning as an infection in the nose, and apt to spread to the nasal sinuses, Eustachian tubes, pharynx, larynx and maybe trachea and bronchi. It is now proved that the immediate agent is a filterable virus ; very quickly, however, there is secondary invasion by organisms which are indigenous in the nose and throat of ordinary healthy individuals—various strains of pneumococcus, streptococcus, staphylococcus, micrococcus catarrhalis and Pfeiffer's influenza bacillus being the most common. Spread of the disease is by droplet infection either from people already suffering from it or from carriers ; it is easily passed on in crowded gatherings and confined spaces. A sneeze can disseminate infection over a wide area. Given the infective " seed," the " soil " is undoubtedly made readier for its reception by such factors as chilling of the body, getting wet through, hyperæmia of the pharynx as by irritant dusts or fumes in the air, congestion of the mucosa by lack of proper ventilation and overheated, stuffy rooms, allergic reactions in the nose, and the presence in nose and throat of obstructive defects or foci of chronic infection.

It must be emphasised, however, that none of these contributory causes will produce a common cold if the infective agent is not present. This has been demonstrated time and again ; as, for example, in the records of Antarctic expeditions when the men remain free from infection, though exposed to the cold of blizzards with, possibly, semi-starvation, or to close confinement in poorly ventilated quarters : yet on the arrival of the relief ship and the introduction of infection brought from civilisation, febrile catarrh (or " coryza ") rages. Every person, having for a long time lost immunity, becomes a prey to the virus.

PATHOLOGY

The disease is seasonal, occurring most commonly at the back end of the year (late September or October), again in January and February, and again in April. With the coming of autumn and its chilly evenings, windows and doors are closed and people herd indoors in unventilated rooms. The virus passes through its preliminary hosts and increases in virulence at a time when the majority of people have lost their immunity. In September or October, therefore, the first epidemic starts, and a large percentage of those susceptible are 'attacked. By November they have recovered and acquired an immunity which for this disease lasts only a few weeks or months. By January, immunity has passed or is passing, with the result that January or February sees the second epidemic. There follows another period of immunity for the larger number of those attacked. Once more it passes away, so that by about April there is a third epidemic, usually cut short by the warm spring sunshine, which tempts people to ventilate their houses once again, and to disperse more often into the open air.

The characteristic lesion is a catarrhal inflammation of any part of the upper respiratory tract, including the nasal sinuses. It frequently starts in a recognisably localised spot, spreads along the submucosal lymphatics and causes a marked engorgement of the mucous membrane, which is red, swollen and covered by mucoserous exudate. The lymph glands draining the area are often enlarged and tender ; an inflamed gland behind the neck of the jaw may involve the auriculo-temporal nerve, so that the patient complains of earache. The pharyngeal follicles may stand out as tiny glistening masses against

the red inflamed mucous membrane of the throat, and the
tonsils also may be inflamed and swollen. Later, as the body
masters the infection, the exudate becomes mucopurulent.
The toxic products absorbed from the raw and inflamed
mucous membrane and its underlying tissues cause the generalised toxic manifestations of the illness.

SYMPTOMS

The incubation period after exposure to infection is from
one to three days. The patient becomes conscious of a localised burning or discomfort at the site of invasion—a " hot
spot," usually at the back of the nose or throat. The discomfort spreads slowly but relentlessly, and the mucous membrane of the nose, nasal sinuses and pharynx becomes red and
swollen. The nose becomes blocked, and if the sinuses are
involved there is a diffuse, dull ache in the face and head.
The inflamed mucosa exudes a watery, serous exudate, which
soaks many a handkerchief and is apt to excoriate the upper
lip ; the sufferer, however, gets no relief from sniffing and
nose-blowing. Inspiration of cold air hurts the nasal passages
and makes the headache worse. Extension of inflammation
to the Eustachian tubes causes temporary deafness, the tongue
becomes dry and furred, the throat feels swollen, there is loss
of the sense of taste, and it hurts to swallow. The inflammation may descend to the larynx and cause hoarseness ; and
to the trachea, with the resulting racking, unproductive
cough of tracheitis and a feeling of painful rawness under
the sternum.

The general constitutional symptoms depend on the severity
of the infection. The temperature may rise to about 100° to
102° F., though with a mild infection it may remain approximately normal. The patient feels uncomfortable, shivery
and depressed, with moderate aches and pains all over his
body, and if he continues with the routine of normal business
during the illness, the muscles become stiff and easily fatigued.
Digestive upsets, such as diarrhœa, retching, nausea and marked
constipation may complicate the picture.

It has been said that if the patient goes to bed and adopts
a particular form of treatment, he will recover in about seven
days, whereas if he adopts one of the other forms of treatment

recovery will take about a week.* The danger usually lies in trying to carry on normally, for not only does the sufferer hand on his infection to others but he runs a much greater risk of complications such as pyogenic nasal sinus infection, severe bronchitis, or bronchopneumonia. If the cold takes its normal course, however, congestion and swelling of the mucosa gradually subside, the secretions become mucopurulent and less uncomfortable, and the temperature falls to normal. For some days afterwards the patient feels weak and debilitated ; this is a stage when if he is not careful a relapse may easily occur.

DIAGNOSIS

Certain specific diseases like measles, whooping - cough, enteric fever, scarlet fever or diphtheria may begin with a febrile catarrh, but the course of the illness soon establishes the true diagnosis. Local irritants, drugs such as iodides, allergic reactions and vasomotor attacks may cause intense hyperæmia of the mucous membranes, and the diagnosis from a mild or abortive cold may not at first be easy. Happily, in these cases, with the patient's quick recovery the differential diagnosis soon becomes mainly of academic interest. True influenza, with its complications, is clinically allied to febrile catarrh and cannot always be clearly differentiated from it ; it will be discussed later (Chap. XII).

TREATMENT

An acute cold causes the sufferer intense discomfort and undermines him both physically and mentally. Quiet, comfort and warmth are desired. For this reason at least, still more to prevent the risk of complications, and most essentially of all, to avoid jeopardising his fellows, the patient should go to bed and stay there until he is better. There is no specific treatment, although individuals may boast how they can unfailingly abort a common cold by adopting their own particular measures. The wise thing is to recognise that the illness will take its course, and to make the patient as comfortable as possible meanwhile, treating symptoms as they arise.

* When lay people taunt doctors by asking them why they cannot find a cure for the common cold, it is because they resent giving the time necessary for cure. Even the most civilised persons hanker after magic at times.

He should have a hot bath, and then go to a warm bed, with a hot bottle to warm his feet or comfort any particular aching part of his body. The room should be warmed so that he is not breathing cold, irritating air. He should have plenty of hot drinks, sugared to taste, and if he feels like it he can have light and tempting food. A nightcap of hot whisky and water to sip, and a powder containing 5 gr. of aspirin and 5 gr. of Dover's powder will probably give him a comfortable night. In the daytime a mixture containing 15 gr. of sod. salicyl. with 15 gr. of sod. bicarb., t.d.s. will do much to relieve his generalised aches and pains ; if they are severe, this powder

R

Codein   .   .   .   .   .   . $\frac{1}{8}$ gr.

Acetyl salicylic acid ⎱   .   .   āā.   5 gr.
Phenacetin   ⎰

given four times a day, will be more effective.

The stuffy running nose is a source of great discomfort, compelling him to breathe through the mouth. Frequent steam inhalations (a teaspoonful of Friar's balsam or of oil of pine in a pint of boiling water) are comforting and better than oily instillations into the nose. The rubbing of the chest and neck, back and front, with camphorated oil is most helpful, for in addition to the local effect the patient breathes the slowly vaporising camphor. Instillations of watery solutions into the nose should never be used in the acute stage ; they may carry heavy infection into the sinuses. If the throat is sore, hot drinks retained in the mouth for a short time and then swallowed help as much as formal gargling ; even a hot antiseptic gargle can only act by washing away the superficial exudate, and as a local, very temporary application of heat. A hot bottle applied to the neck, or a warmed muffler wrapped round it, will help ; the old granny's primitive comforter of a woollen stocking filled with hot baked potatoes had its points. If the pharynx feels raw, warm linseed tea is comforting, coating it with a covering of smooth mucilage so that swallowing is not so painful. If there is laryngitis, the patient should not talk ; if tracheitis, the tearing, painful cough will probably not yield save to a linctus containing codein or heroin—for example, 20 minims each of syr. codeinæ, syr. tolutanæ and tr. opii camphorata, not more often than three-hourly. As sweating is likely to take place under this course of treatment, periodic sponging of the body and the wearing of woollen pyjamas are indicated.

After the pyrexia has subsided the patient should remain in bed for a day or two after a moderate cold, and for at least three days after a severe cold. Then he may get up gradually and move about the house, but he should not go out of doors for some days longer, especially if the weather is bad. A severe cold calls for a convalescent holiday, though most people, including doctors who should know better, have to get back to their work as soon as they can, and often do poor work in consequence. In the long run, less actual time and efficiency is wasted by getting thoroughly fit before returning to full activity. At this stage the best tonic is a holiday. Some form of vitamin product containing vitamins A and D especially is also advisable.

PREVENTION

Most people suffering from a common cold show a wicked lack of a sense of social responsibility. " It is only a cold " forms the excuse for much spurious heroism or sheer stupidity ; with the result that they carry on snuffling at their job, barking and sneezing their infection in the tramcars, the train, the workshop, the office, the cinema—church is the only place about which they seem to have any scruples. Even medical students turn in to their wards, breathe and talk assiduously over their cases of congestive cardiac failure and give them their terminal infection. A self-interested, let alone an enlightened, public opinion would force these irresponsibles to stay at home and keep their troubles to themselves. Meanwhile, during respiratory epidemics wise men will try to keep away from crowds, confined spaces and infected individuals. Spraying the nose and throat and gargling with antiseptics are of little use. Prophylactic inoculation with vaccines containing the usual secondary invaders is claimed by many to be of great value ; but carefully controlled tests,* such as those carried out at the University of Minnesota, make it clear that vaccines are of

---

* " In Shakespear's time and for long after it, mummy was a favorite medicament. You took a pinch of the dust of a dead Egyptian in a pint of the hottest water you could bear to drink ; and it did you a great deal of good. This, you thought, proved what a sovereign healer mummy was. But if you had tried the control experiment of taking the hot water without the mummy, you might have found the effect exactly the same, and that any hot drink would have done as well." —GEORGE BERNARD SHAW (Preface to *The Doctor's Dilemma*, p. lxxii).

little or no value either for reducing the incidence of colds or as safeguards against the complications arising from them.

Those less fortunate people who, despite the infection, have to carry on with their work should remember that they owe an obligation not to spread the infection to others. During the acute stage they must avoid close contact with their neighbours, especially when talking to them. They ought not to travel in buses or trains, where they are certain to infect the atmosphere. When sneezing, the mouth and nose must be completely enveloped in a large handkerchief. Medical students, doctors and nurses must, without fail, wear masks if they have to enter a ward or visit a patient. Such a mask is made of two layers of linen or muslin, with a sheet of celluloid between them ; the wearer must keep in mind that celluloid is inflammable. Failing celluloid, a sheet of brown paper will suffice. This mask must cover the nose and mouth, with an ample margin.

If a patient is subject to repeated colds because of some chronic infective focus in the upper respiratory tract, surgical relief may be possible ; in children the removal of unhealthy tonsils and adenoids may help greatly.

Reasonable hygienic measures such as a good diet, proper clothing and dry shoes, with leather and not crêpe soles, and moderate exercises are in any case a healthy discipline ; but an excessive and faddy " hardening off," in the hope that it will increase resistance to colds, is uncalled for. The common cold is no respecter of persons, and it visits the lusty athlete as often as the ordinary man. A daily dose of mixed vitamins throughout the winter will increase general resistance.

CHAPTER XII

INFLUENZA

RECENT researches both in England and America have shown that true epidemic influenza is due to a filterable virus, of which there are two main strains (viruses A and B) ; that antibodies appear in the blood during convalescence from the disease, and persist for some time ; that immune serum can prevent experimental infection in ferrets and mice ; and that active immunity to the disease can be induced by subcutaneous inoculation of the virus in experimental animals. As yet, however, there is a considerable gap between these discoveries and their effective application to the treatment of human sufferers ; the disease is still in the stage of experimental attack.

It is endemic throughout the world. From time to time terrible pandemics have swept across continents and oceans like a plague, destroying in a few weeks more lives than are killed in years of modern warfare. It is a disease of remote antiquity ; Boyd notes that what might well be an epidemic of it is described in the *Iliad*, and Hilton Fagge recalls that it was supposed to have attacked Charlemagne's army when returning from Italy in A.D. 786. Since the year 1510 there have been at least eight great pandemics, and innumerable smaller, localised epidemics. The last influenzal pestilence of 1918-19, during the war, as well as the previous one of 1889-92, showed that the pandemic has three separate waves. In the first, great numbers of persons are affected, but the disease is mild. This wave lasts some three to six weeks, and quickly recedes. After a short interval a second wave breaks savagely, still engulfing large numbers, but this time much more severely ; and by reason of the high incidence of complications it is infinitely more fatal than the first. It recedes rather more slowly, maybe with a sharp period of recrudescence. Then it might seem that the worst is over ; but soon there is another wave, advancing more slowly, its peak not so sharp and its decline slower. This lasts some eight to ten weeks, and possibly because of the residual immunity in persons already attacked it does not fall upon so many, but the complications are still frequent and serious, and the death rate high. In the years following the pandemic, periodic localised epidemics of varying severity occur. In the U.S.A. the recrudescences of infection due to influenza virus A have a periodicity of 2–3 years, to influenza virus B 4–6 years. In Great Britain this regular rhythm is not quite so sharply defined.

The epidemiological features, therefore, are the explosive spread of the disease ; the exceedingly high incidence ; the relatively short duration of the individual waves ; and the localised, restricted epidemics in the interpandemic periods. The death rate in the great pandemics is staggering. It has been put as high as 200 to 400 per 1000 cases during the serious waves, and certainly that of 1918-19 killed far more victims than died in battle or of wounds during the whole war. Here are one or two examples of the explosive suddenness of the outbreak, as it hits the community and the individual. In a soldiers' camp in New Jersey there were 3 cases one day and 3000 the next. In a few hours a whole household might be laid low, and a man sipping his breakfast coffee and reading his newspaper might be stricken down and die before nightfall. " Sir Thomas Watson says that when he was first called to 2 cases on 3rd April 1833 the symptoms were just those which frequently mark the commencement of an attack of continued fever, and that he did not then know what was about to happen ; but in the course of that and the following day, all London was smitten by the disease." * The reasons for this rapid spread are that the incubation period is very short (about forty-eight hours), and almost everyone is susceptible to the disease. Sufferers, therefore, transmit it before they realise how ill they are, or before they can be isolated, and it is readily received by the susceptible majority. The infection is through contact, by droplet dissemination of the virus, directly or indirectly conveyed. It is interesting to note that during the 1914–18 war it was introduced into one area of England a few hours after a batch of infected American soldiers had been landed at a port after crossing the Atlantic.

* Hilton Fagge (1886), *The Principles and Practice of Medicine.*

MORBID ANATOMY

Since the discovery of the virus of influenza in 1933, only small epidemics have been available for the study of true influenza, and it is not yet certain how far the observed lesions are due to the influenzal infection, and how far to secondary infective organisms. A fair statement at present would be that influenza produces general toxæmia and inflammation of the mucous membranes of the upper respiratory tract ; the severer the attack the more likely is the inflammation to descend to the trachea and bronchi, and even to become hæmorrhagic. The ciliated epithelial cells of the trachea and bronchi are thus damaged and many of them are shed, a toxic manifestation in all probability. As a result, one of the key defences of the lungs, the mucociliary mechanism (see Chap. I) is seriously impaired, and descending secondary organisms are then free to do their worst. In the nasal sinuses, and in the middle ear also, acute purulent infection may become established ; and in the lungs, purulent bronchitis, bronchiolitis or pneumonia. Occasionally the intense toxæmia causes Zenker's degeneration of muscle ; intestinal paresis may reveal itself by startling abdominal distension and tympanites ; the liver may be damaged with resulting jaundice ; thrombophlebitis may occur ; and there may be purpura, with hæmorrhages into the skin, muscles and viscera.

SYMPTOMS AND SIGNS

The uncomplicated, pure influenzal illness as seen typically in the first pandemic wave is characterised by the sudden onset of fever (101° F. or more), headache, shivering, muscular pains and prostration. There are usually no prodromal symptoms. A healthy man is suddenly struck down while he is working ; he feels very ill, aches intolerably in muscles and limbs, and in addition to the symptoms mentioned above he may have photophobia and abdominal pain. His appetite is quickly lost, and he looks ill, with flushed face, suffused conjunctivæ and often quickened respiration. The throat is congested, but there is no exudate ; there may be a tickling cough. Catarrhal manifestations in the upper respiratory tract do not usually develop until a few days later. Examination of the blood in the early stages shows a leucopenia, with a relative lymphocytosis, and examination of the chest shows nothing abnormal, save perhaps a few scattered râles. The fever persists for about four days, is remittent in type and sometimes diphasic ; it is apt to be accompanied by heavy sweats. The sufferer feels progressively weaker and uncomfortable. Sometimes there is a sharp epistaxis at the onset, and in some outbreaks there may be mild or severe gastro-intestinal disturbances, such as vomiting, nausea and diarrhœa. In the severer cases it is common to find a slight febrile albuminuria.

If fever still persists after four days, either the illness is not influenza or else some secondary infective complication has supervened. This may be an acute sinusitis, an otitis media with or without mastoiditis, a purulent bronchitis or a pneumonia. The secondary invaders are organisms normally present in the nose and mouth, of which the most dangerous are H. influenzæ, pneumococcus, streptococcus hæmolyticus and staphylococcus aureus. With purulent bronchitis the complication manifests itself by a change in the character of the sputum about the third day, signs of frank bronchitis of the larger and medium bronchi and persistence of an irregular pyrexia for about a week.

Influenzal bronchopneumonia is particularly seen in the second and third pandemic waves, and is usually a mixed infection, with H. influenzæ often predominating. In the fulminating type there is an intense bronchiolitis and a broncho-pneumonia which is accompanied by hæmorrhagic œdema of the lungs. The patient's lungs fill rapidly with fluid, the toxæmia is profound, and he may die within a few hours of the onset of his illness, though more often he survives for twenty-four to forty-eight hours. As the fluid accumulates in the alveoli he finds breathing more and more difficult, and an increasing livid cyanosis shows that he is slowly suffocating. His distressing cough brings up a frothy, watery sputum which may be stained red or salmon pink with blood. Hopelessly ill, he may remain conscious and alert almost to the end, without appreciating how ill he is ; or he may pass into a muttering delirium, picking at the bedclothes, and never recover consciousness.

If the attack is not so grave, the bronchopneumonia may become obvious on about the second to the fourth day of the illness, and is revealed by an exacerbation of symptoms—a marked quickening of the respiratory rate, pain in the chest, an exhausting cough which may bring up a little tenacious mucus or blood-stained froth, and obvious cyanosis. At first, and until the bronchopneumonic patches become confluent, there may be few signs, but they may be significant. The bronchiolitis may prevent appreciable air entry into the affected portions of the lung and so the corresponding breath sounds are weak ; if some air does penetrate, fine crepitations characteristic of exudate in the finer tubes will occur. As in ordinary bronchopneumonia, patchy areas of collapse may later be cleared by a bout of coughing, so that the physical signs can vary from time to time. A large enough area of confluent bronchopneumonia gives the signs of lung con-solidation, with diminution of expansion, dulness to percus-sion, bronchophony and bronchial breath sounds ; this is not a common picture, however, and in any case does not appear until several days after the onset of the illness. With the development of the bronchopneumonia the sputum may change in appearance, becoming frankly purulent. Seeing that the infection is usually a mixed one, the inflammation often takes on the character of the most virulent organism : if it is predominantly streptococcal, a synpneumonic streptococcal empyema may develop, perhaps in association with small streptococcal abscesses ; if due to H. influenzæ the picture is likely to be one of intense bronchiolitis (so-called " capillary bronchitis ") and bronchopneumonia ; and if to staphylococcus aureus, multiple abscesses in the lung may typically occur in association with the septic pneumonia. Pure pneumococcal lobar pneumonia is uncommon. If the patient survives these hazards, there is always danger of a localised collapse of the lung with resulting bronchiectasis ; sometimes the occluding plugs of mucopus may give only a ball-valve obstruction, with resulting obstructive emphysema. An X-ray film of the chest showing patches of shadowing due to collapse, contrasting with over-aeration due to emphysema, does not, therefore, give an easily interpretable picture of the amount of lung put out of action by the illness. By the ninth or tenth day a marked fibroblastic reaction in the lungs may develop, to lay the foundations for a later fibrosis of the lungs, if the patient lives. Extension of infection to the pericardium, mediastinum or meninges by the blood stream or by direct spread may further complicate the clinical picture. Other possible developments have been mentioned in the discussion of morbid anatomy (p. 164).

Pneumonia may occur also as a somewhat later manifestation, beginning on the fourth to the tenth day, giving the appearance of a grave relapse. It varies in degree from the inevitably fatal, fulminating type to one from which a slow recovery is made.

The description of the cyanosis of influenzal bronchopneumonia as a " curious heliotrope," or by other vivid terms, tends to import a certain air of mystery to it. It is well, therefore, to examine this symptom in more detail (see also Chap. II). The cyanosis which may be observed in these patients depends on whether the oxygen deficiency, due to interference with the proper aeration of the blood in the œdematous alveoli, is accompanied or not by retention of carbon dioxide and by full or empty peripheral capillaries. With excess of carbon dioxide in the blood there is a deepening of respiration, dilatation of the capillaries and therefore a deep blue or purple cyanosis resulting from the excess of reduced hæmoglobin in the dilated peripheral vessels. With marked œdema of the alveoli—and this occurs not only in bronchopneumonia but also in phosgene and chlorine gas poisoning, miliary tuberculosis and other types of pulmonary œdema—the Hering-Breuer reflex comes into play much earlier than normally, and the breathing is therefore rapid and shallow. Moreover, seeing that the diffusibility (and solubility) of carbon dioxide is twenty times that of oxygen, carbon dioxide will pass out of the blood much more quickly than oxygen passes in. The result of these various factors is a progressive lack of oxygen in the tissues, together with a washing out of carbon dioxide. The result is an excess of reduced hæmoglobin in the collapsed peripheral vessels ; the skin and mucous membranes show a faint blue (" heliotrope," " mauve ") colour rather than the deep purple of reduced hæmoglobin in dilated capillaries. Meanwhile, the oxygen deficiency produces a paresis of the medullary centres, so that the respiration becomes progressively shallower, the pulse more frequent and thready, the peripheral circulation more and more inefficient. Obviously this latter type of cyanosis is more serious than the former, in that it indicates a much more advanced stage of respiratory and cardiac failure.

An even graver stage is the greyish lividity, with profound peripheral vascular paralysis ; the patient is now almost moribund, with cold, clammy skin bathed in beads of sweat. The student can draw upon even his own limited experience for the significance of these varying degrees of cyanosis ; he can remind himself of the contrast between the florid purple of the healthy patient under an anæsthetic, suffering from some temporary mechanical obstruction to respiration, and the lead-like greyness of a patient dying from pneumonia.

Convalescence from influenza is apt to be slow, and if the patient is allowed to get up too soon he may suddenly relapse. The myocardium almost certainly has been damaged by the toxæmia (in the pneumonic complications, by the anoxia also), so that post - influenzal bradycardia and other functional disturbances are common. It is wise, therefore, to watch carefully the cardiovascular response to effort. Other later complications are mental depression, polyneuritis and a transient post-influenzal psychosis.

DIAGNOSIS

In pandemics the diagnosis is easy. In interpandemic periods the differentiation between *mild* influenza and the common cold may be difficult ; the onset of influenza is usually very sudden, and the catarrhal symptoms more delayed than in the common cold. The severer forms of influenza are characterised by splitting headaches and intolerable aching in the limbs for which it is almost impossible to find ease— features not seen in the common cold. In the early stages of the illness the problem may present itself as the diagnosis of a " pyrexia of uncertain origin." The course of the disease soon resolves it, however ; an old Irish practitioner used to temporise on these occasions by saying solemnly to the anxious relatives, " He has an inflammation ; but whether it is the high inflammation or the low inflammation it is not yet possible to tell "—a mode of approach effective in its day and generation, but not so likely nowadays to satisfy a public which thinks itself instructed in modern scientific medicine by an up-to-the-minute popular press. Influenza with gastrointestinal symptoms may have to be distinguished from acute gastro-enteritis or food poisoning ; in the latter a subnormal temperature is often present.

PROGNOSIS

This is affected by the character of the existing epidemic or pandemic. In the great pandemics, not only are the very young, the aged and the weakly carried off, but even the strong die in their thousands. Simple, uncomplicated influenza such as is seen in the first pandemic wave is comparatively mild in nine out of ten cases. Pulmonary complications are, however, always serious, and cause most of the deaths ; they also determine a considerable incidence of bronchiectasis and lung fibrosis in the patients who survive their acute manifestations. Cyanosis, high fever, a respiratory rate of over 40 per minute and peripheral vascular failure are all of unfavourable import. Chronic alcoholics and patients with previous cardiac and pulmonary disease clearly meet the disease with a grave handicap. The death rate among pregnant women is high.

TREATMENT

There is no specific cure for the disease. The patient should be confined to bed from the onset of the illness and kept there until convalescence is well established. During the febrile period at least 5 pints of fluid should be given in the twenty-four hours in the form of hot drinks with glucose or of simple cold water. The rest of the treatment consists in making the patient comfortable, treating symptoms much along the lines of those for febrile catarrh (see Chap. XI). The danger of bronchiolitis and bronchopneumonia calls for care in giving sedatives which are likely to depress the cough reflex ; but if the exhausting cough of tracheitis is present, steam inhalations and a codein linctus are advisable. Hot alkaline drinks are particularly important if the sputum is tenacious and difficult to bring up. If pulmonary or other complications supervene, the appropriate measures must be adopted (see Chap. XVIII). Early treatment of the anoxia of influenzal bronchopneumonia by oxygen therapy (see Chap. XIII) is of capital importance. The necessity of an adequate convalescence has already been emphasised.

PREVENTION

Control of the spread of an epidemic by isolation of affected patients is not easy, owing to the rapid onset of the illness and the general susceptibility ; to have any chance of success it must be exceedingly rigid and absolute. The wearing of facial masks has many practical difficulties for the general public. In hospitals, on the other hand, during a pandemic it should be imperative for every visiting consultant, for students and for nurses to wear adequate masks (see also p. 161). While the epidemic is in progress, visitors should not be allowed except in special cases, and these too should be made to wear masks. Gargles, sprays and nasal douches have no proved effect in preventing infection. Vaccination with living or dead virus is theoretically possible, but practical application of the theory is not at present feasible, even though recent researches hold promise of future effective immunisation. By analogy with other virus diseases, the intramuscular injection of 5 c.c. of serum or 15 c.c. of whole blood from a convalescent patient might give a short period of immunity, but as yet there are no large-scale studies available to guide us on this point. Vaccination against secondary invaders might reduce the mortality, but could not influence the incidence of the disease ; here again, controlled studies on a big scale are not available.

CHAPTER XIII

OXYGEN THERAPY

THE exchange of gases in the lungs takes place by simple diffusion across the alveolar epithelium and the endothelium of the capillary walls which separate the air in the alveoli from the blood in the capillaries. It is conditioned by the partial pressures of the gases, by their solubility, and by the integrity of the separating "pulmonary membrane."

As a background to the practical problems which arise during oxygen therapy the student should remember certain facts and figures which are fundamental. *Alveolar air* contains approximately 14 per cent. of oxygen, at a tension (or partial pressure) of about 100 mm. Hg. In *arterial blood* the oxygen tension is somewhat lower, about 90 mm. The hæmoglobin content of blood is normally 15 gm. per 100 c.c., and when fully saturated each gram of hæmoglobin combines with 1·34 c.c. of oxygen ; the full oxygen-combining power of blood is therefore approximately 20 c.c. O_2 per 100 c.c. Arterial blood, however, is normally only 95 per cent. saturated, containing 19 c.c. O_2 per 100 c.c. ; in addition, 0·3 per cent. of oxygen is carried in solution in the plasma. The oxygen content and partial pressure of *mixed venous blood* depends on the activity of the body tissues, the percentage falling from 14 c.c. at rest to about 4 c.c. during violent exercise, which creates a greatly enhanced call on the part of the tissues for oxygen to replace that which is being rapidly used up in metabolic activity. The tension varies, therefore, from 40 mm. Hg to about 20 mm. Hg under these extremes of circumstance.

Although it takes only a second for circulating blood to traverse a lung capillary, this is ample time for oxygenation, as the combination of oxygen with hæmoglobin is achieved in less than $\frac{1}{100}$ sec. Hæmoglobin in the blood behaves in a different way from that of hæmoglobin in simple solution. The oxygen-hæmoglobin dissociation curve in the latter is a rectangular hyperbola ; in the blood the curve is S-shaped.

171

This modification is due to several factors—the high concentration of hæmoglobin in the red blood corpuscles, the
presence of CO_2 at a tension of 40 mm. Hg or more, the
presence of inorganic salts, and the body temperature of 37° C.
The important practical effects of this alteration in the curve
are that, normally, about 5 per cent. of oxygen is available
for use in the tissues : that at lower oxygen tension levels
much more oxygen is made available : and that with an
increase of CO_2 tension in the blood the hæmoglobin gives off
more oxygen at any given oxygen tension.

The flow of oxygen from the atmospheric air to the blood
is from the alveoli, through the respiratory epithelium, into
the blood plasma, and then through the limiting membrane
of the red blood corpuscles to combine with the hæmoglobin ;
its discharge to the tissues is from the hæmoglobin of red blood
corpuscles, into the blood plasma, and then through the capillary
walls into tissue fluids.   Seeing that the solution of gases in
a fluid depends upon their partial pressures, the inspiration of
a lowered oxygen percentage at a high barometric pressure
may result in the same amount of oxyhæmoglobin as would
be produced by a normal percentage of oxygen at a normal
pressure.   On the other hand, a normal oxygen percentage at
low pressure (such as obtains at high altitudes), or alternatively
a low oxygen percentage at a normal pressure (such as obtains
in mines, or wells, or submarines), both result in a reduction
of oxyhæmoglobin in the blood.

Anoxia (lack of oxygen in the body) may be caused in the
following ways :—

1. *By an insufficient partial pressure of oxygen in the inspired
air.* This occurs at high altitudes where, though the
oxygen percentage is the same as that at sea level, the
barometric pressure is less ; or in mines or tunnels,
especially when the air is vitiated by " black damp "
or " fire damp," the barometric pressure being approximately normal but the oxygen percentage considerably reduced.

In order to compensate for the lowered O_2 tension
in the blood the breathing is accelerated, with resulting washing out of CO_2 from the blood.   This
deficiency of CO_2, known as *acapnia*, affects the
hæmoglobin-oxygen curve in the sense that the

amount of oxygen carried by the hæmoglobin, already insufficient in amount, is in addition less readily available to the blood and tissues.

2. *By obstruction of the air passages, as by a foreign body or bronchiolitis*, which denies the inspired air access to the respiratory epithelium.

3. *By interference with the passage of O_2 from the alveoli to the pulmonary blood stream.* This is well seen in œdema of the lung and in other conditions where the alveoli are filled with exudate ; and in emphysema where there is a great reduction in the respiratory surface through which O_2 is absorbed.

4. *By alterations in the oxygen-carrying capacity of the blood*, either because the hæmoglobin is much reduced in amount (as in anæmia) or because it has been altered by poisons such as carbon monoxide, nitrites or chlorates.

5. *By failure of an adequate supply of circulating blood to the tissues, even though the blood is fully oxygenated.* This is seen in circulatory failure, in which the peripheral blood flow through the capillaries is so slow that a large part of the O_2 supply is delivered to the tissues under an inadequate partial pressure. The circulatory inefficiency may be general or local.

6. *By admixture of oxygenated with de-oxygenated blood,* with the result that the blood in the systemic circulation is deficient in oxygen. This may occur in certain types of congenital heart disease where there is a communication between the left and right sided chambers of the heart ; or where there is a zone of poorly aerated lung through which the blood continues to circulate.

7. *By poisoning or exhaustion of the respiratory centre,* either by toxins (of influenza or pneumonia, for example), depressants (morphia), or shock.

8. *By poisoning of the tissue protoplasm* (as by cyanides), whereby the tissues cannot use oxygen although the blood may be well supplied by it. The poison interferes with tissue oxidation ; it paralyses the " respiratory enzyme " described by Warburg and prevents it from oxidising cytochrome—the reaction which con-

stitutes the fundamental oxidising system of body cells. Narcotics may also reduce tissue oxidation.

The effects of anoxia on the body are especially serious upon the " noble organs "—the nervous system and the heart muscle. The anoxia which results from diseases of the lungs may determine clinical manifestations such as sleeplessness, nightmares, restlessness, delirium, coma and failure of the respiratory and circulatory centres ; the myocardium is also damaged, and eventually peripheral circulatory failure supervenes. The significance of cyanosis as a measure of anoxia has already been discussed (see p. 51).

ADMINISTRATION OF OXYGEN

The lungs, blood and tissues are unable to store oxygen. While anoxia persists, therefore, restoration of the oxygen saturation of the arterial blood to normal, demands continuous administration of oxygen. The amount of oxygen necessary to achieve this restoration can be controlled by means of blood-gas analysis ; this, however, is not feasible in clinical work. Other criteria must therefore be adopted. Happily, certain simple observations are sufficient ; the appropriate dosage is that which provides relief of the cyanosis,* restlessness and delirium, together with a fall in the pulse rate.

If large portions of the lung are poorly ventilated, with no circulatory flow through them, owing to the consolidation of extensive lobar pneumonia, to collapse of the lung, or to other conditions, oxygen therapy is unlikely to be so successful as in the early stages of diffuse alveolar exudation such as pulmonary œdema, bronchopneumonia or irritant gas poisoning. Nevertheless its usefulness can only be assessed in any individual case by trial and by observing its effect upon the patient. It is hardly applicable to conditions of chronic permanent oxygen lack—for example, chronic cardiac failure or emphysema—though it may have a vital place in tiding the patient over an acute complication.

The oxygen can be given by nasal catheter, by nasal tubes such as the Tudor Edwards' spectacle-frame carrier, by the B.L.B. mask or by an oxygen tent. It is entirely futile to administer it by a glass funnel held in front of the patient's

* In patients with profound anæmia cyanosis may be absent, though anoxia is present (see page 51).

nose and mouth ; this method is not only wasteful but it cannot possibly supply the amount of oxygen which is necessary. With the nasal catheter or nasal tubes there is a considerable waste of oxygen during expiration, a phase of respiration in which though the gas continues to flow from the cylinder it is not drawn into the lungs ; nevertheless it is possible to treble the normal O_2 concentration in the alveolar air (from 14 to approximately 40 per cent.) by delivering some 5 to 6 litres of oxygen per minute. This rate, however, is extremely uncomfortable, and impossible to tolerate for any length of time because of the forcible current of gas which dries and irritates the mucous membrane.

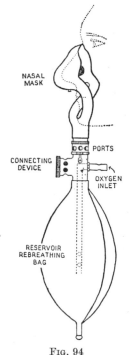

FIG. 94

The B.L.B. Mask

The glass spigot at the bottom of the reservoir bag can be removed at intervals in order to drain off excess moisture.

If a nasal catheter is used it should be of soft rubber (size No. 9), with three or four additional holes laterally placed. It is sterilised, lubricated with 1 per cent. cocaine ointment and inserted into the nostril to within $\frac{1}{2}$ in. of the back of the naso-pharynx ; the outer end is then bound down to the forehead with an efficient bandage, after it has been connected to the tube coming from the O_2 cylinder. This cylinder has attached to it a fine adjustment valve, and the oxygen is led through a flow-meter. The Tudor Edwards' spectacle - frame carrier, with small tubes leading into both nostrils, gives approximately the same oxygen concentrations but is more comfortable.

Oxygen tents are expensive, not readily available except in hospitals, and call for skilled personnel to supervise their use. A device as efficient, more practical, and comparatively simple to manipulate is the **B.L.B. mask.*** It has approximately double the efficiency of the nasal catheter or tubes, is not wasteful of oxygen, and is much more comfortable (Fig. 94).

The nasal mask must be adjusted to fit snugly ; the

* Boothby, Lovelace and Bulbulian, 1938.

rubber strap which holds it in position over the patient's face can be placed above or below the ears, whichever is more comfortable, and the malleable metal strips attached to the nose-piece can be bent into position so that it rests easily but firmly over the nose.

When the three air ports of the connecting device are closed the patient inspires entirely from the reservoir re-breathing bag, into which oxygen should flow at a rate which prevents it from collapsing completely at the end of inspiration. More air and less oxygen is breathed if one or more air ports are opened so that the patient breathes partly from the bag and partly from the atmosphere.

E.M.S. Memorandum No. 5 gives the following oxygen percentages obtainable in a healthy adult breathing through the nose :—

O_2 Flow. Litres per Minute.	Number of Holes Open.	Alveolar Air O_2. Per Cent.	CO_2 in Bag. Per Cent.
3	3	46	2·04
4	3	56	1·51
5	2	69	1·22
6	2	76	0·89
6	0	87	1·42
7	0	90	0·99
8	0	91	0·39

A flow meter, which can be of the simplest type, is always advisable, and if one or more air ports are open, is essential.

It is obvious that there must be no leakage when the mask is on the patient's face. A simple test of the apparatus is done as follows : the oxygen flow is adjusted approximately to the required amount and the mask fitted on the face. The patient breathes through the nose for a few minutes and then the mask is pressed on the face. If there are no leaks, the bag continues to distend and collapse exactly as before. If, however, the bag distends to a greater extent, oxygen has probably been escaping by the sides of the mask, which should then be readjusted by shortening the strap or moulding the metal strips of the nose-piece to give a better fit. It may sometimes be necessary to pack small strips of gauze under the edges of the mask, both to prevent leakage and ease the pressure on the skin. If the patient finds the straps or their metal buckle uncomfortable, they may be led over pieces of fairly thick gamgee tissue.

Nasal obstruction, sufficient to limit the efficiency of the mask, is uncommon.   Breathing through the mouth lowers the oxygen concentration, so that if the patient cannot breathe through the nose a special oro-nasal type of mask should be used, if it is available.   In practice, however, the " open mouth " is due either to dropping of the jaw in weak and desperately ill patients (when covering of the mouth by a folded handkerchief may be helpful), or to intolerance of the mask.   The latter is often seen in patients with severe cardiac failure, who in any case are found to respond poorly to oxygen therapy.   Intolerance may be particularly troublesome in an acute illness or chest wound when the patient is fighting for breath.   Much encouragement is often necessary to overcome a patient's fears of wearing the mask.   When this is accomplished it is best to close the three air ports for a time and allow a flow of 6 litres of oxygen per minute, to give a theoretical concentration of at least 80 per cent., in the hope that he will receive enough oxygen to relieve the breathing even if he is unable to breathe fully through the nose.

In patients with anoxia and cyanosis due to pulmonary lesions or to thoracic wounds, about 60 per cent. of oxygen in the alveolar air will as a rule relieve it, if oxygen inhalation is going to be successful.   This corresponds approximately to a flow of 4 litres per minute with two air ports open (see the table quoted).   Larger concentrations than this should not be administered for longer than thirty-six to forty-eight hours in view of the danger of oxygen poisoning.   The optimum concentration at any time must be decided for each individual patient according to his condition and to his response to treatment.

12

CHAPTER XIV

ACUTE BRONCHITIS

THE defences of the respiratory tract have already been described (Chap. I). If other defences fail, an inflammatory reaction to inhaled bacteria or other noxious material may occur anywhere in the tract from the nose and throat to the parenchyma of the lung itself. Established infection in the upper part of the respiratory tract puts the lower part of the tract in jeopardy, by reason of the danger of its spread downwards into the trachea, bronchi and lungs.

All upper respiratory tract infections—rhinitis, laryngitis, tracheitis, bronchitis—are essentially similar in their pathology. The resulting symptomatology, however, depends on the site, nature and extent of the infection ; and the farther it extends down the respiratory passages the greater is the general bodily disturbance. When the bronchioles are inflamed the lung parenchyma becomes involved, owing to local collapse of the lung units supplied by them and to subsequent extension of infection into them.

ACUTE TRACHEO-BRONCHITIS

Apart from such unusual causes as exposure to irritating gases such as bromine, chlorine, phosgene, mustard gas and nitrous fumes, acute inflammation of the bronchial mucous membrane is nearly always part of a tracheo-bronchitis which follows a catarrhal inflammation of the nose and throat. A cold in the head spreads downwards and " goes to the chest," or the bronchitis may be an important incident in the upper respiratory inflammation caused by certain other specific diseases, such as measles, influenza, whooping-cough, diphtheria and enteric fever. Respiratory epidemics prevalent in the long winter months and treacherous changes of weather which conduce to lowered resistance are always important factors in its occurrence. " Catarrhal " children, with unhealthy tonsils and adenoids, are particularly liable to attacks. The infection is, as a rule, a mixed one, by the usual secondary invaders ; pneumococcus, micrococcus catarrhalis, hæmophilus influenzæ, streptococcus and staphylococcus may be present and in varying numbers.

All too often the illness is the result of a neglected cold. It has already been pointed out how easily respiratory catarrhs are spread because of the failure to take sensible precautions ; a cold is often regarded as something trivial and an inadequate excuse for absence from work. The infection not only spreads through the community, but the patient himself is liable to develop complications from extension of the disease.

PATHOLOGY

Apart from the rare tuberculous variety, the essential pathology of acute bronchitis is very much the same, whatever the precipitating cause. The bronchial and tracheal mucous membranes are red and congested. In fatal cases the redness and swelling may be extreme, so that the mucous membrane looks velvety, and has been likened to the petal of a damask rose. The ciliated epithelium is damaged, often detached, and the submucosa is infiltrated with leucocytes. At first the mucous membrane is dry, later there is exudate, which at first is thin and mucoid, and then becomes mucopurulent. With the patient's recovery the mucous membrane recovers its normal appearance, but if the infection has been severe, with peribronchial infiltration, it may result in some thickening round the bronchi, with or without peribronchial fibrosis. In severe cases, with invasion of the medium and finer bronchi, the post-mortem appearances are very striking ; when the lung is cut across and squeezed, a bead of yellow mucopus appears at each bronchial orifice.

SYMPTOMS

The clinical picture of bronchitis varies greatly, according to the severity and extent of the infection. It may be a mild tracheo-bronchitis, with a little malaise but no pyrexia ; it may be more severe and may spread to the medium tubes ; or it may be the desperate illness of suffocative bronchiolitis, merging into bronchopneumonia. As might be deduced from the pathology, the salient symptoms in all cases are cough and expectoration. With widespread extension to the narrower tubes and consequent obstruction to the entrance of air into the alveoli, lobular collapse follows and marked dyspnœa and cyanosis become prominent.

A mild attack produces few general symptoms, with only slight malaise and no fever. In severer infections there may be pyrexia rising to about 101° F. The patient feels shivery and aches in body and limb. There may be tightness or a feeling of rawness under the sternum. *Cough* is never absent ; at first dry, it may be very distressing, especially if the tracheitis is marked. It is loud and barking, and often occurs in paroxysms so severe as to make the patient retch or even vomit. The rasping nature of the cough causes him to try to suppress it, usually in vain, and often it ends in a grunt or half-strangled cry of pain. In the less severe inflammations there may be a constant, vague, tickling sensation difficult to localise. Changes of temperature, as in passing from a warm room to the cold night air, may precipitate a bout of coughing which is intractable and very exhausting. The patient's discomfort is made worse if the infection spreads to the upper part of the œsophagus so that swallowing becomes painful as well. In this early stage there may be little, if any, *expectoration*—perhaps a little tenacious mucus, or maybe some thin, serous exudate, the bringing up of which in no way relieves the discomfort. Later, as the inflammation subsides and the exudate becomes mucopurulent, the cough becomes productive and much less painful ; thick mucopurulent sputum is brought up, and the patient feels infinitely more comfortable. His previous bouts of coughing may, however, have hurt the thoracic muscles, so that he still feels a painful stiffness in the sides or epigastrium. Sometimes, indeed, the violence of the paroxysms in the acute stage may even tear a few muscle fibres from their attachment to one of the rib margins, so causing an acute, very localised pain which may be mistaken for pleurisy (see p. 376).

If the inflammation extends to the smaller tubes, the fever and the general systemic effects are more serious. There is likelihood of widespread interference with the entry of air into the lungs, and an accumulation of exudate particularly at the bases. *Dyspnœa* and *cyanosis* are added to the picture, and if there is suffocative respiratory obstruction the veins of the neck are seen to be dilated and to throb. In children, with their smaller-calibred tubes, obstruction is more easily brought about than in adults, and the danger of frank broncho-pneumonia is much greater. They have to struggle hard for breath, and close observation reveals that each expiration is immediately followed by an inspiration, so that the respiratory pause occurs after inspiration instead of after expiration. The alæ nasi are working, and there is indrawing of the intercostal spaces. Involvement of the finest bronchioles, whether patchy or diffuse, cannot be distinguished clinically from broncho-pneumonia, and will be discussed under that heading.

PHYSICAL SIGNS

Bronchitis affects both lungs, and in itself does not cause any predominantly unilateral difference in expansion or any dulness to percussion. Unless complications are present the transmission of the voice is not altered, nor is bronchial breath-ing heard. Sometimes the vesicular murmur over some part of the lung is temporarily faint because of an obstructing plug of mucus or mucopus, but it returns after a bout of cough-ing which displaces the plug. The expiratory murmur may be much prolonged because the bronchial walls are swollen, infiltrated and narrowed, and so hinder the expulsion of air. Tenacious secretion in the larger tubes produces partial obstruc-tion, so that sonorous rhonchi are heard in both inspiration and expiration ; their site may change with coughing or they may disappear altogether from a particular part of the lung as a piece of sputum is displaced or coughed up. In the medium tubes the rhonchi will obviously be of higher pitch, are likely to be more easily heard during inspiration and may change in site after a bout of coughing. The smaller the calibre of the tubes the more sibilant the rhonchi ; and, as swelling of the mucous membrane is here apt to narrow the tubes very appreciably, the rhonchi are not so readily shifted by coughing. If the secretion is fluid, moist sounds (crepitations) occur instead of rhonchi, coarse in the larger tubes, fine in the smallest. Unless there is consolidation of the lung from a sufficiently large area of complicating bronchopneumonia the crepitations are not consonating, because the lung is still spongy (see Chap. V).

COURSE AND PROGNOSIS

Bronchitis is not a trivial illness, for there is always the risk of serious complications, especially in children and old people. It may last for only a few days, but usually it is two or three weeks before a patient fully recovers from even an uncomplicated acute attack. With proper care and treatment from the start the outlook is good. If the cough or fever persists longer than three weeks, it is possible that to the original bronchitis has been added some complication such as a localised, unresolved area of bronchopneumonia, or that it was itself but an incident in some underlying disease. Pulmonary tuberculosis is always to be borne in mind in these circumstances, and it is a sound rule to explore this possibility, by sputum and radiological examinations, whenever a cough persists longer than a month. Bronchitis confined to the upper lobes should invariably suggest the possibility of tuberculosis. The danger of absorption collapse of portions of the lung by reason of occluding plugs of mucus is always a real one, especially in bronchitis of the lesser-calibred tubes and whenever the secretions are liable to be tenacious, as in measles or whooping-cough. The consequences of collapse of the lung have been discussed in Chapter VII. Frequently repeated attacks of acute bronchitis are liable to end in the chronic form of the disease. Patients who succumb to an attack of acute bronchitis usually die within a fortnight of the onset of the disease, either from bronchopneumonia or cardiac failure. If they survive this period, their chance of recovery is usually good.

DIAGNOSIS

As a rule it is easy to say that a patient has bronchitis ; any difficulty there may be is in deciding whether it is part of some more serious disease. It is of primary importance always to bear in mind the necessity of determining whether the bronchitis is secondary to a common cold, or possibly to a specific fever, to pus in the nasal sinuses, or to chronic inflammation of the lung parenchyma, particularly tuberculosis. The other important task is to recognise the development of complications, especially bronchopneumonia.

TREATMENT

The general line of treatment is the same as that described for the common cold, adapted to the early congestive " dry " stage, the " moist " exudative period of recovery and the convalescence. Patients generally feel happier if they are propped up in bed with pillows rather than lying flat. For the dry stage, with painful cough and soreness in the chest, steam inhalations, rubbing of the chest with camphorated oil, copious hot drinks, including black currant or linseed tea, and a codein linctus are all helpful. Codein or heroin must be given carefully, however, and not for too long ; they should be used to take the edge off the pain and irritation, not to abolish the cough reflex. A useful mixture at this stage is an alkaline diaphoretic, for example :—

℞

Sod. citrat.	.	.	.	.	gr. xxx
Liq. ammon. acetat.		.	.	ʒi
Syr. tolu	.	.	.	.	♏ xxx
Aq. camph.	.	.	.	ad	ʒfs.

Four-hourly.

For children, ½ to 3 minims, according to age, of Vin. antimonialis may be added, the doses of the other ingredients being adjusted also. Sod. iodide, 5 gr., may be added to the mixture for adults if there is expectoration of sticky mucus ; this, together with hot alkaline drinks, will help to liquefy the sputum, so that expectoration is easier. An old-fashioned remedy which is very comforting at this stage is " hot chlorodyne " ; a dose of 10 minims of Tr. chloroformi et morphinæ (B.P. 1885) is put into a tumbler of very hot water which the patient slowly sips.

A **poultice** covering the whole of the chest up to 2 in. from the edge of the sternum on both sides (Fig. 95) gives great relief. It helps reflexly to reduce bronchial spasm, so preventing much discomfort and aiding respiration and expectoration. In the absence of a competent nurse the family doctor may himself have to poultice a patient, or alternatively to instruct a willing but untrained relative in the practical details.

The linseed poultice is the best type, though nowadays the making and applying of it is something of a lost art. The kaolin ("antiphlogistine") poultice is perhaps easier, so that it is liable, mistakenly, to be regarded as foolproof; but unless

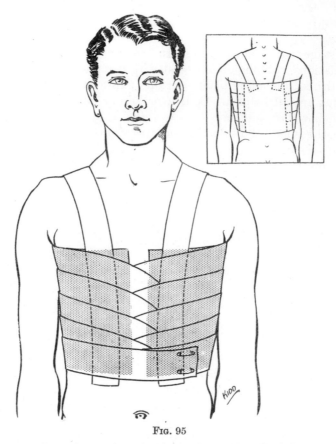

Fig. 95

The poultice is shown by the stippling. The tails of the bandage are criss-crossed, each tail being firmly tucked into its corresponding axilla, and overlapped by the next.

it is applied with proper attention to detail it can become exceedingly uncomfortable.

To make a *linseed poultice* a bowl and spoon are required to mix the linseed, and a spatula to spread it. The bowl and spoon should be heated, and the spatula placed in a jug of hot water. A little boiling water is poured into the bowl, and linseed meal is sprinkled into it with one hand while the other hand stirs with the spoon until the water is absorbed and the mixture is of a consistency which enables it to come away cleanly from the sides of the bowl. The linseed is then placed on a piece of muslin or old linen, previously cut to the right shape for encircling the chest ; it is spread evenly and quickly by means of the hot spatula up to within an inch of the border, thus allowing for a neat turnover. The linseed should be spread about $\frac{1}{8}$ to $\frac{1}{4}$ in. thick and then covered with a single layer of gauze. The poultice is next folded together, placed between hot plates and carried to the patient. It is then opened out—if properly made it will not stick together—tested with the back of the hand to see that it is not too hot, and applied to the chest, which has previously been lightly greased with vaseline. It is covered with a layer of jaconet, and then with a pad of brown wool and bandaged in place. The bandage should be a five-stranded, many-tailed one, made out of a 4-in. open-weave (not domette) bandage, and with the two shoulder-strap pieces to prevent it slipping downwards ; it is bound firmly to the chest and fixed by safety-pins so that when the patient moves, the poultice cannot flap away from the chest wall and so allow cold air to come between it and the skin. It must be renewed every four hours. When poulticing is discontinued the chest is covered for a time with a pad of cotton-wool, held comfortably in place by means of the many-tailed bandage.

To make a *kaolin poultice* the opened tin of kaolin compound is placed in a saucepan containing enough water to come not more than half-way up the tin, lest the water boil over the edge of the tin and spoil the compound. It is allowed to boil gently for about twenty minutes in order to heat the kaolin all through. A piece of lint is made ready, of suitable size to cover the chest. A spatula or carving knife to spread the kaolin is put into a jug of boiling water. The lint is put smooth side up on a table or spreading board, and when the kaolin is ready an adequate amount is turned on to the lint and spread rapidly, smoothly, and as thinly as possible. The edges of the lint are turned in neatly, the poultice is covered with a single layer of gauze and placed flat on a hot tray ; if it is folded it will stick together. Though the kaolin should be spread piping hot, the poultice must be carefully tested for heat by placing the back of the hand on it, in order to avoid burning the patient's skin. As soon as it is of bearable heat it is applied to the previously greased chest, covered with a pad of wool, and bandaged in place with a many-tailed bandage. An ordinary bandage is worse than useless, for it allows the poultice to come away from the front of the chest whenever the patient bends forwards, with a resulting draught of cold air and the eventual development of an unpleasant clamminess. If there is much dyspnœa the wool pad may make the poultice too heavy, and it should therefore be omitted. The kaolin poultice need be renewed only every twelve hours. After poulticing, the patient should be allowed to lie undisturbed until the time comes for renewal ; all examinations, washings or other attentions should therefore be concluded before the poultice is applied.

Sleep is especially important and may be difficult to ensure at the beginning of the illness when the cough is painful and unproductive. In addition to the methods already described for giving the patient comfort, 10 gr. of Dover's powder, with 5 gr. of aspirin if there is much aching in the limbs, should be administered before settling him off for the night. To those who are used to it the whisky nightcap should not be withheld. Elderly persons and children especially need sufficient nourishment in the form of glucose added to their hot drinks, warm diluted milk and one of the proprietary foods such as Benger's, according to the severity of the attack and the powers of digestion.

When the breathing is relieved and the cough becomes loose the diet can be gradually increased. Mucopurulent sputum begins to be coughed up ; it usually comes up easily, helped by hot alkaline drinks, unless there is associated bronchial spasm. This is often troublesome, and is a factor in the dyspnœa which distresses the patient. For moderate spasm the following nasty tasting but effective mixture may be given, followed by a hot drink, every four hours :—

R

Sod. iodid.	.	.	.	5 gr.
Tr. lobeliæ	.	.	.	$7\frac{1}{2}$ minims.
Aq. chloroform.	.	.	to	$\frac{1}{2}$ oz.

If the spasm is severe, ephedrine hydrochloride, $\frac{1}{4}$ gr. should be added to the mixture.

If the bronchitis spreads to the narrower bronchi and cyanosis develops, oxygen should be given without delay by the B.L.B. mask or Tudor Edwards' spectacle frame to the adult, or in some form of oxygen tent, if available, to the young child. The danger of bronchopneumonia is great ; this severe type of bronchitis, with pyrexia and marked constitutional disturbance, calls for chemotherapy similar to that given for frank pneumonia (see p. 223). Heart failure may develop, especially in the aged ; in addition to the oxygen, 1 c.c. of nikethamide (coramine) by hypodermic injection, every four or six hours according to need, is then advisable.

In patients who progress favourably from the onset, the temperature has fallen to normal and the expectoration has become thin and watery by the end of seven to ten days. The diet may now be further increased both in bulk and in variety. At night and on waking hot alkaline drinks and a dose of the original medicine will help to clear the bronchial tubes of any accumulated secretion. About four days after cough and expectoration have ceased the patient may be allowed up in his bedroom, provided that he feels up to it. A few days later he can be allowed into other rooms in the house, provided that they are warm. According to his progress and the state of the weather, he can gradually be allowed out of doors. An adequate convalescence is important, for relapse may occur, or an annoying residual cough remain. A complete change of air, preferably to an equable seaside climate, is an even better tonic than the most elegant preparation of iron and strychnine. This does not always apply to old people, however, who may not be able to endure comfortably a visit to the seaside. The treatment of bronchiolitis cannot be separated from that of bronchopneumonia and will be discussed later (Chap. XVIII).

CHAPTER XV

CHRONIC BRONCHITIS AND EMPHYSEMA

(a) CHRONIC BRONCHITIS

CHRONIC catarrhal inflammation of the bronchi is not often the result of acute attacks alone ; usually there are other factors, so that the important problem is to discover the primary condition which underlies it. There may be, for example, some infective focus in the upper respiratory tract which determines recurrent inflammations of greater or less severity—pus in the nasal sinuses, oral sepsis or infected tonsils and adenoids. The infected material is liable to drop into the trachea and bronchi, especially during sleep, and it may overcome the primary defences of the lung. The focus may be in the lung itself—infected bronchiectasis, fibrosis leading to the stagnation of secretions, or tuberculosis. Apparently typical senile bronchitis may on occasion show tubercle bacilli in the sputum, a point which underlines the necessity for bacteriological examination of the sputum in every case in which cough and expectoration continue for more than four weeks. Pressure on the bronchi from outside, as by a mediastinal growth or an aortic aneurysm, may determine a partial mechanical occlusion and consequent bronchitis. Compression of the trachea by a thyroid swelling may result in persistent bronchitis. In all these examples the chronic bronchitis is but an incident in a more important disease.

Chronic congestion of the lung from cardiac insufficiency is an important predisposing cause, perhaps because the poor oxygenation of the blood reduces the efficiency of the ciliary defence ; and there are certain general illnesses which favour catarrhal infection, such as rickets in children, and obesity, alcoholism, hyperpiesia and chronic renal disease in adults. Bronchitis is likely to be worse in winter—" winter cough " was the name given to it by the old physicians—by reason of the evil influence of damp, fog, treacherous weather and prevalent respiratory epidemics. Dusty occupations are bad for

188

the bronchitic, as is excessive smoking, especially when inhaling of the tobacco smoke is practised. Structural damage to the lung, of which emphysema is a common example, establishes with the bronchitis a particularly vicious circle.

PATHOLOGY

The appearances differ according to the stage of inflammation. The bronchial mucous membrane may be red, swollen, hypertrophic and granular, with an exudate of mucus or mucopus into the lumen ; or it may have become pale, smooth and atrophic, with little or no exudate. Round-celled infiltration of and around the walls, engorgement and fibrosis are present in varying degree. In the long-standing atrophic types the cylindrical epithelium becomes cubical or even squamous, the mucous glands atrophy and weakening and thinning of the walls result in a diffuse, mild dilatation. This can be recognised at autopsy by the fact that the scissors can be made to run along the small bronchi as far as the lung periphery instead of stopping well short of it, as in healthy lungs. With the increase of fibrosis, resistance to the blood flow through the pulmonary capillaries increases, and the end result is right-sided cardiac failure.

SYMPTOMS

The patient is, as he says, " chesty," with cough, expectoration and dyspnœa in varying degree according to the pathological lesions present. The *cough* may be constant or paroxysmal ; at first it may attack him only in the winter months, but later it may cling to him, though not so severely, during the summer as well. It is made worse by exposure to fogs and mists, keen winds and sudden changes of environmental temperature. Physical exertion may bring on an attack, especially if cardiac insufficiency is present also. The *expectoration* varies according to the condition of the bronchial walls and the state of infection. In the atrophic type there may be no sputum at all (hence Laennec's descriptive term, *bronchitis sicca*, dry bronchitis). On the other hand, it may be thin and mucoid or thick and mucopurulent. There is no pyrexia and no pain, except in the acute exacerbations. Often the patient appears quite well until he undertakes some exertion, when he becomes breathless and has a prolonged and distressing bout of coughing ; later in the disease the breathing becomes quick and may be wheezing, even when he is at rest. If there is associated disease such as fibrosis of the lung, emphysema or cardiac failure, its appropriate symptoms are added to the clinical picture.

PHYSICAL SIGNS

The signs are those of secretion in the larger and medium bronchi, with coarse or medium râles, usually moist (crepitations), but sometimes dry (rhonchi). In the purely atrophic bronchitis without expectoration, râles are not heard. Owing to the irregular thickening and increased rigidity of the tubes in the hypertrophic form the expiratory murmur is often found to be prolonged.

DIAGNOSIS

The presence of chronic bronchitis is easily recognised. It is more important to discover what is the underlying cause and what complications are present.

COURSE, COMPLICATIONS AND PROGNOSIS

The tendency is for the winter cough to become worse as the years go by, until it is more or less permanent throughout the year. Superimposed attacks of acute bronchitis may occur and leave the patient still more disabled. Peribronchial fibrosis is common, and the chronic cough and partially obstructed bronchi help the development of true emphysema (see Chap. XVI). Attacks of true bronchial asthma may be precipitated by the chronic inflammatory damage, though frequently what is called " asthma " in these patients is in fact the dyspnœa of cardiac insufficiency. The disease progresses, sometimes slowly, sometimes rapidly, until in the end right-sided cardiac failure dominates the picture. A fairly frequent result of the chronic cough in old people is the development of herniæ through the weak abdominal wall. If the bronchitis is but a minor part of more serious disease such as myocardial damage or bronchiectasis, the course and prognosis is obviously dependent on the main factor.

TREATMENT

There is a tendency among students and house physicians to dismiss these patients as " old chronics " and to lose interest in them ; any such dulling of humanity and responsibility must be resisted, the more so because when hospital is left behind for general practice, these patients " are always with us," needing hope which we can so rarely guarantee, and help which we can in some measure often give.

The principles of treatment are to remove the cause if possible, to prevent acute exacerbations and to try to arrest the progress of the chronic disease, and to give the patient as much comfort as possible. Unhealthy tonsils and adenoids, or rickets in children, nasal sinusitis and oral sepsis in adults, can usually be dealt with. The effects of inoperable bronchiectasis in the adult may be diminished by postural drainage and other appropriate treatment. Cardiac failure needs prolonged rest. It is worth remembering that in old people chronic renal disease may be due to an enlarged prostate, so that a rectal examination may occasionally be one of the most important preliminaries to the treatment of a chronic bronchitis.

A careful regime is essential. The sufferer should avoid all excesses—overheated, stuffy rooms, excessive and stuffy clothing, over-smoking, overfeeding, and too much alcohol. He should not go where there are likely to be respiratory infections, nor should he live in cold, damp and foggy places. The bronchitic is wise who builds his house upon the rock, not on clay or marshland or in a misty river valley. In fine weather it is good for him to take reasonable exercise well within his limitations. If he can afford to winter in a temperate climate (Bournemouth, Torquay, the Cornish Riviera and Colwyn Bay are suitable in England) he should do so.

It is obvious that a man's pocket determines to a large extent his chances of delaying the advance of the disease. If his circumstances force him to " keep at work until he drops," to live unsuitably so as to be near his means of livelihood, his chances are poor ; whereas if he is fortunate enough to be master of his economic fate he may survive reasonably long and in fair comfort. This is one of the diseases which brings home what Bernard Shaw has described as a " real woe " of the doctor—" the uselessness of honestly prescribing what most

of the patients really need : that is, not medicine, but money." *
These patients come to the out-patient departments of our
hospitals or to their panel doctors and leave an atmosphere
of gloom and frustration behind them, because the doctor
knows how little he can do for them in the absence of that
economic prescription.

The *diet* of the chronic bronchitic should be light and
digestible, and flatulence should be avoided because it may
embarrass the heart. He should avoid large meals, especially
at night. The obese patient is often greatly helped by a regime
which reduces the weight by gradual stages. Constipation is
often troublesome, for most of these sufferers have to live
restricted and sedentary lives, and it must be suitably treated.
During the winter regular doses of cod-liver oil or preparations
of vitamins A and D may do good. *Medicinal treatment* should
be as simple as possible, because the digestion of these people
is easily upset. A hot alkaline drink night and morning (as
much bicarbonate of soda as will lie on a sixpence, in a tumbler
of hot water) will help to clear the tubes of secretion. For
useless unproductive cough a codein linctus may be necessary.
If the sputum is brought up freely, nothing more is needed to
help it than periodic hot alkaline drinks ; if it is difficult to
get up there is probably associated bronchial spasm, and a
mixture containing sodium iodide and tincture of lobelia, with
ephedrine if need be, is called for in addition to the hot drinks.
It should not be continued for too long, as it may upset the
digestion. With the onset of cyanosis and cardiac insufficiency,
oxygen and cardiac stimulants are needed ; if there is congestive
failure, digitalis, together with venesection with the removal
of 10 oz. of blood, may relieve the burden on the heart for the
time being. For patients whose disease is not too far advanced,
special respiratory exercises may be useful (see p. 200). Emphysema nearly always complicates the picture and may call for
further therapeutic measures, which will be discussed in
Chapter XVI.

Plastic (Fibrinous) Bronchitis is a very rare condition, characterised by the
coughing up at intervals of a plug of sputum which when unrolled in water is found
to be a cast of part of the bronchial tree. It is mentioned here only because the
striking pictures of such casts in earlier textbooks may too readily fix the attention
of students or their examiners on an unimportant rarity.

---

* G. Bernard Shaw : Preface to *The Doctor's Dilemma*.

CHRONIC BRONCHITIS AND EMPHYSEMA — *Continued*

(*b*) EMPHYSEMA

THE word "emphysema," which means "inflation," is applied to a number of conditions which ætiologically have little in common. When any portion of the lung fails to expand because, for example, the alveoli are collapsed or are filled with exudate, the deficiency must be made good, partly and immediately by the sucking-in of the thoracic wall, and later, if the collapse is considerable, by fuller expansion of the remaining healthy portions of the lungs. In such cases the increase in the volume of the lungs plays by far the greater part, seeing that the chest wall is comparatively rigid. This extra expansion of the lung is a physiological response to the failure of other parts of the lung to function ; it is known as **compensatory emphysema.** It may be temporary, as in transient collapse of the lung or in bronchopneumonia ; or permanent, as in long-standing collapse or following lobectomy.

Interstitial emphysema denotes the escape of air from ruptured bronchi or alveoli into the interstitial tissues of the lung ; it may track towards the hilum and mediastinum, and occasionally may even reach the neck and the subcutaneous tissues there. It usually results from violent respiratory efforts, especially paroxysms of coughing such as may occur in whooping-cough or respiratory obstruction.

Surgical emphysema is caused by injuries which lacerate both layers of the pleura ; air escapes through the laceration of the lung, accumulates in the pleural space, forces its way through a tear in the parietal pleura and infiltrates the subcutaneous tissues. The extent of the subcutaneous emphysema depends on the amount of air which escapes from the torn lung.

Chronic atrophic vesicular emphysema is a senile condition in which, unassociated with mechanical strain, atrophy of alveolar walls and of lung tissue occurs as part of the decay of

old age. " They fade away like the grass . . . in the evening
it is dried up and withered." The lungs are thin and shrivelled
(" small-lunged emphysema "). The sufferers are old and frail,
with a sluggish circulation and feeble muscular power, both
of which forbid effort ; life's activity is slowing down to a
standstill, and for this reason there is commonly little exertion
to arouse distress of breathing. The symptoms are those of
generalised senile decay.

In sharp pathological and clinical contrast to these varieties
of emphysema is the disease which forms the main subject of
this chapter, **" hypertrophic " vesicular emphysema.** The
adjective " hypertrophic " is misleading, for, as will be seen,
it is a condition characterised by dilatation of the alveoli and
of the alveolar ducts, accompanied by *atrophy* of many of the
alveolar walls. They " give," partly because their walls are
atrophied, and partly because they have lost their elastic
support. Sir William Jenner's description of the condition as
" large-lunged emphysema " indicates the increase in volume
of the lungs (following the loss of elasticity) without confusing
the pathological issues ; unfortunately, however, the term
" hypertrophic " has become so much part of the nomenclature
that it is not easy now to discard it. It will therefore be used
in inverted commas, in order to remind the student not to take
it at its face value.

It has already been seen that when portions of the lung
collapse, following the absorption of air from the alveoli, the
resulting mechanical stresses tend to dilate the bronchi (see
Chap. VII). When, however, the bronchi are partially obstructed and the alveoli still open, mechanical strain makes
its impact predominantly on the thin-walled alveoli and their
ducts, so that they become distended. The strain may be
sudden and violent, producing **acute " hypertrophic " vesicular
emphysema** ; the respiratory efforts during suffocation are an
example. It may, on the other hand, be gradual and long-
continued (**chronic " hypertrophic " vesicular emphysema**).
The whole of the lungs may be involved (*generalised emphysema*),
or only parts of them (*localised emphysema*).

PATHOLOGY

Sir John Floyer, the Lichfield physician who in 1711 sent young Samuel Johnson to London to be touched by Queen Anne for the King's Evil, was perhaps the first Englishman to :write about vesicular emphysema. As with so many pulmonary diseases, however, Laennec was the first to recognise its clinical and pathological significance and to give the classical description, to which he devotes a whole chapter in his book on auscultation.

The old idea that the stresses which produce emphysema are expiratory broke down on the fact that in expiration most parts of the lung are closely supported by the thoracic wall, which thus prevents alveolar distension. It is now recognised that inspiratory stress, associated with partial bronchial obstruction, is the more likely ætiological factor. Inspiratory muscles are much more powerful than expiratory ; their action produces marked suction-traction on the lung. The entry of air in inspiration is therefore much more forcible than is its escape during expiration. For the same reason, partial occlusion of the air passages is far more easily overcome by inspiration than by expiration ; when the obstruction acts as a valve, the expiratory effort fails to expel any air, with the result that there is progressive distension of the alveoli. The mechanism of this valve-like action is similar to that described on p. 115 and illustrated in Figs. 87 and 88.

Acute emphysema may occur not only after the inhalation of a foreign body (see Chap. VIII) but also with violent respiratory effort, as in asphyxia, or in the acute paroxysms of asthma or in whooping-cough. Focal patches of it are also associated with bronchopneumonia, especially in children. When certain of the smaller bronchi are completely obstructed, compensatory emphysema balances patchy collapse of the lung ; but when the obstruction is partial, true vesicular emphysema follows. Chronic " hypertrophic " generalised vesicular emphysema usually results from chronic bronchitis, less commonly from chronic asthma ; continued hard manual labour may act as a gradual contributory factor, because during heavy lifting or straining the filling of the lungs produced by deep inspiration is prolonged by temporary closure of the glottis. The inspiratory phase of coughing has a similar effect.

The valvular obstruction, described above, results in over-inflation of the thin-walled alveoli (especially during the early stage of coughing, when there is a marked rise in intrapulmonary pressure). This presses out blood from the capillaries, and when it is long-continued, leads finally to capillary atrophy. The affected lung tissue is therefore pale. The diminution of the capillary bed imposes a strain on the right side of the heart, which is a considerable factor in the final development of cardiac failure. Degenerative changes take place in the walls of the alveoli, notably of the elastic fibres, causing a marked loss of pulmonary elasticity. Rupture of the septal walls of the alveoli may therefore readily occur (Fig. 107), especially if there is additional inspiratory strain, as in heavy bouts of coughing. In consequence, air sacs of considerable size are eventually formed (**emphysematous bullæ**). The rupture is most likely to occur in situations where there is most yield and least support for the lungs, namely, at the lung margins (especially the apices and the sternal and diaphragmatic margins). With the disappearance of many interalveolar septa, the total respiratory surface is lessened, the vital capacity and respiratory reserve reduced, and the residual and dead-space air increased. This is the result of a prolonged pathological process; by this time the changes in the terminal bronchioles which originally produced the valvular mechanism and over-inflation of the alveoli have largely subsided. The dilated alveoli or groups of alveoli which have lost their elastic support are not now actively over-distended (in the sense that an inflated rubber balloon is distended), but are like bags of tissue paper which are readily dilated, and readily collapse.

The loss of pulmonary elasticity causes a reduction of the intrapleural negative pressure from the normal – 7 cm. of water to one which gradually approaches zero as the disease progresses. Expiration is less complete, and the chest remains partially expanded. The more serious the disease, the more the chest tends to remain in the position of inspiration. Its shape at rest changes gradually to that of full normal inspiration. The accessory muscles have then to be used for ordinary breathing, though they are able to achieve only a limited additional expansion. The respiratory excursion of the chest is reduced from the normal $2\frac{1}{2}$ in. or so to a mere $\frac{1}{2}$ in. or less. The final result is a *barrel-shaped chest*,* with the dome of the diaphragm flattened ; the costal cartilages tend to calcify, perhaps because of their greatly reduced movement, though this explanation of the change is not generally accepted.

The result of all these factors is to make breathing mechanically difficult, especially on exertion, and to interfere seriously with the gas exchanges in the lungs. The blood is imperfectly supplied with oxygen ; the normal 95 per cent. saturation may fall to 85 per cent. or less, even at rest, and the deficit is greatly increased during exertion. At the same time there is an increase in the carbon dioxide of the blood. Apart from other factors the increase in the amount of residual air will itself diminish the normally effective diffusion of the respiratory gases. Furthermore, the emphysematous person finds it impossible to compensate for his disabilities by increasing the pulmonary ventilation. A healthy person who is made to breathe air enriched by 7 per cent. carbon dioxide develops a ventilation six or seven times that of normal ; the patient with advanced emphysema is lucky if he can double his normal figure.

SYMPTOMS AND SIGNS

Chronic " hypertrophic " generalised vesicular emphysema is associated so often with chronic bronchitis that the diagnosis " chronic bronchitis and emphysema " has become almost a medical cliché. The lack of normal pulmonary ventilation and the interference with oxygen exchange determines the two chief symptoms of *dyspnœa* and *cyanosis*. The onset is insidious, and the patient is at first not much troubled in his breathing unless he exerts himself. The slow development of the disease allows a certain degree of gradual compensation for the disabilities caused by it. At rest, therefore, he may not at first notice the moderate quickening of breathing ; effort, however, reveals the poverty of his respiratory reserve. As the disease progresses the breathlessness increases, respirations

* The anteroposterior diameter of the chest is increased, the sternum thrown forward ; costal angle obtuse ; costal cartilages prominent ; intercostal spaces widened ; dorsal kyphosis increased, back rounded, shoulders raised ; clavicles prominent ; the neck appears shorter than normal, because of the elevation of the thorax and shoulders.

even at rest being quick and shallow, and the contours of the chest gradually alter towards the " barrel-shape " characteristic of the full inspiratory position. Ears, lips and extremities become cyanotic, especially so during exertion or even with change to the recumbent posture, for the call of the tissues for sufficient oxygen cannot be met. An attempt is made to compensate for the deficient oxidation by means of an increase in the circulating red blood corpuscles (*polycythæmia*).

The heart has to pump its blood through a greatly diminished pulmonary capillary bed ; the result is an increase in the pulmonary blood pressure and dilatation and hypertrophy of the right ventricle. Moreover, as the elasticity of the lungs decreases and the distension increases there is great difficulty in expiration. The intrapleural pressure becomes less and less negative, and the venous pressure consequently increased.* This, together with the poor oxygenation of the heart muscle, adds to the strain not only on the right side of the heart but on the whole myocardium. Congestive cardiac failure, attacks of cardiac dyspnœa and left ventricular failure are all liable to supervene. A menacing vicious circle has become established ; the patient needs better pulmonary ventilation and a more adequate oxygen intake, yet he is less and less able to achieve them.

The physical signs are predominantly those of enlarged, voluminous lungs, which encroach far more than normally on the heart and liver. The percussion note is hyper-resonant ; the area of lung resonance is considerably increased, and the normal cardiac and hepatic superficial dulness diminished. Expansion is poor, the vibrations of the voice are less easily felt or heard, and the breath sounds are feeble. The heart sounds are soft and distant, owing to the myocardial damage and to the overlying air-cushion of distended lung. Either bronchitis or passive congestion is nearly always associated with the emphysema, and therefore the adventitious sounds due to bronchial or alveolar exudate are usually present.

A spirometer tracing reveals graphically the respiratory disability. If the patient is at rest and breathing as quietly as possible, the tracing may be normal save for a certain degree of rapidity of breathing. When, however, the emphy-

---

* The negative pressure in the thorax directly affects the pressure in the great veins, and indirectly in the whole venous system.

sematous patient is asked to take a deep breath, the tracing shows the attempted deep inspiratory excursion, and then the expiratory return towards the normal level. Unlike the normal individual, however, he cannot achieve a full return to the normal level at once ; the lung has been filled beyond its feeble expiratory capacity, its elasticity is impaired and it is only after a number of expiratory phases that the relative excess of air is driven out.

TREATMENT

The disease is, as a rule, slow but progressive, and its disabilities are increased by the usually associated bronchitis. Acute exacerbations of bronchitis are especially disabling. Once established, emphysema is incurable, for the damaged lungs cannot be repaired. The patient must therefore live within his limitations and adopt a careful regime directed against his bronchitis ; the student should remind himself of the details which have already been described in Chapter XV. It is especially important for him to avoid respiratory infections, for the respiratory reserve is already so impaired that otherwise trivial infections are dangerous. Even the most banal common cold cannot be neglected with impunity. If the patient suffers from true bronchial asthma, every measure which promises the possibility of abolishing or minimising attacks should be put in hand (see Chap. XXX).

The difficulty of expiration is sometimes lessened and the patient helped to breathe in comfort by the use of a tight abdominal binder ; this increases the intra-abdominal pressure, so raising the level of the diaphragm and giving it continuous support. This would seem to be an ingeniously logical method of treatment, and some patients are greatly benefited by it. Others, however, cannot tolerate it ; it may be (though there are no convincing observations on the point) that the ascent of the diaphragm under these conditions produces a " more positive " (that is, less negative) intrapleural pressure in such patients, which would tend still further to hamper the return of blood to the heart.

A moderate degree of bronchial spasm is often present in patients with chronic bronchitis and emphysema. This can be relieved by ephedrine, with appreciable diminution of the dyspnœa.

The deficiency of proper oxygenation of the tissues often makes the patient stupid, forgetful and irritable in the daytime and results in disturbed sleep at night. Inhalation of oxygen for fifteen to twenty minutes before bedtime may allow him to fall into natural, refreshing sleep, so improving the outlook for the morrow. Aminophylline (a combination of theophylline with ethylenediamine) often has the same effect as oxygen inhalation, by reason of its stimulating action upon the respiratory centre and the coronary and cerebral circulations. It may be more convenient to administer than oxygen. It should be given at night in the form of two 0·1 gm. " tabloids " (B. W. & Co.). Cardiac failure is treated in the appropriate way. With the hope of increasing the elasticity of the thoracic cage, excision of costal cartilages has been suggested ; but experience seems to indicate that either there is no place for surgery in the treatment of this disease or the wrong type of operation has hitherto been attempted.

Massage and remedial breathing exercises may sometimes help the patient, but much depends on the condition of his heart. Gentle abdominal massage may help to remedy the constipation due to enforced lack of exercise. The chief aim is to assist expiration and to mobilise the thorax. Patients with chronic bronchitis, slight emphysema and no cardiac symptoms are given exercises adapted to their age and strength. Following a natural inspiration, they attempt a full expiration, the masseuse helping by means of strong pressure vibrations as they breathe out. Other suitable manipulations are available, under expert guidance, including spinal frictions, applied especially to the upper thoracic regions ; they have the further advantage of helping to loosen mucous deposits in the bronchi. Physical treatment of this stage of the disease differs from that of ordinary chronic bronchitis only in that the masseuse has to go more slowly and carefully.

With marked emphysema and cardiac involvement much less can be done. Very gentle massage may do no harm, and careful chest vibrations may make the patient more comfortable. Later, if there is improvement, even expiratory exercises may be added, but they must not be forcible ; at all times the effect on the patient must be watched lest the treatment do more harm than good.

CHAPTER XVII

THE PNEUMONIAS (1)

THE word " pneumonia " has a long history, going back to Hippocrates' " peripneumonia," and signifying for the ancient authors an acute illness either with pain in the side or with severe dyspnœa. As the study of morbid anatomy and of physical diagnosis developed, the term acquired a more precise meaning. Morgagni added to it the concept of solidification of the lung ; Laennec described the pathological stages of the disease and showed how to diagnose them by auscultation ; and Rokitansky distinguished lobar from lobular or bronchopneumonia. The pneumococcus was discovered by Pasteur in 1880, and before long it was proved that lobar pneumonia was caused by this organism. Since then, inflammations of the lung due to other organisms have been more clearly defined. Even before the discovery of the pneumococcus, clinicians were well aware of the difference between the lobar pneumonia " which consists of a series of changes by which the spongy pulmonary tissue is rapidly converted into a solid mass, returning afterwards, in cases that recover, to its normal condition," and the other varieties of pneumonia. So the German physicians called the first variety " croupous pneumonia," on the grounds that the fibrinous exudation was similar to that which characterises croup.

In recent years some physicians who are more at home with the X-ray film-viewing box than the post-mortem room appear to be somewhat nonplussed by " atypical pneumonias," and particularly by inflammations of the lung which do not make the patient acutely ill. Recently these inflammations have been labelled " pneumonitis," but this defines nothing more than the puzzlement of a man who sees shadows which he does not understand, and cannot interpret in terms of pathology (see also Chap. XXI).

It might be considered by some to be better to drop the name " pneumonia " altogether, and call every inflammation

201

of the lung a " pneumonitis." Why, however, should we
drop it for an upstart term (the suffix *-itis* has achieved its
specific connotation of inflammation only in the last 150 years)
which offers no advantages ? There is a whole history of
pathological meaning in the word " pneumonia," and it is
still strong and alive enough to grow in wisdom and stature
as our knowledge of the pathological processes reaches out
towards completeness.

PNEUMOCOCCUS PNEUMONIAS

To our knowledge of the pathology of pneumonia, as of
so many other pulmonary conditions, Laennec made a master's
contribution, describing the three accepted stages of the inflammatory reaction. Experimental methods were, however,
necessary to amplify what could be learned at the bedside
and in the post-mortem room, and the credit of the first experiments whose results were comparable with the pathological
reaction seen in man belongs to Lamar and Meltzer (1912).
Blake and Cecil (1920) extended this work, using pneumococci
of very high virulence, and claimed that pneumococcal lobar
pneumonia is a cellulitis of the lung which spreads outwards
from the hilum. The experimental work of J. F. Gaskell
(1925) of Cambridge is outstanding, though it has not received
as much attention as it deserves, and his Bradshaw lecture
on the Pathology of Pneumonia (*Lancet*, 1927, ii, 951) is one
of those classical papers in Medicine which the student should
read for himself.

What happens in any infection must depend on " the seed
and the soil "—the invading power of the organism and the
resistance of the host. Standardising as far as possible the
latter factor, Gaskell found that if he introduced pneumococci
by insufflation into the bronchus of a lobe of a rabbit's lung,
the results depended upon the virulence of the organism used
and not on the number of organisms injected. The experiments
were carried out with a single strain of pneumococcus whose
virulence could be altered at will by suitable manipulations ;
the virulence was measured in terms of the minimal lethal dose
for a 20-gm. mouse. When the coccus was of low virulence,
the animal either suffered no pathological changes at all or
else they were of little importance. With a rather more virulent strain, a patchy bronchopneumonia was produced, with

hardly any change in the bronchi or bronchioles. Organisms of a somewhat higher virulence gave a larger area of more intense inflammation—a lobular or a segmental pneumonia, with changes in the corresponding bronchioles. If the strain was of higher virulence still, the invasion could not be localised until a whole lobe was involved right up the limiting pleura—lobar pneumonia, with smaller bronchi and bronchioles widely and secondarily involved and merged into the general consolidation. With organisms of the highest virulence, there was an intense septicæmic invasion of the blood stream, in spite of an obvious early attempt of the host to localise it in the lung. The lungs showed intense dilatation of the capillaries, hæmorrhages, and diffuse, patchy serous exudate throughout —a fulminating, septicæmic or " miliary " pneumonia which has sometimes been mistaken for the earliest stages of a typical lobar pneumonia.

The **pneumococcus** is a member of the viridans family of streptococci. Its distinguishing marks are that it is soluble in bile, it is highly pathogenic for the mouse, and it has a capsule. The capsule contains a *specific soluble substance* (S.S.S.) of high molecular weight and polysacch aridenature,* distinctive both in quantity and in molecular structure for each of the many types of pneumococci now known to exist. By certain methods the organism can be robbed of its capsule, and then its virulence disappears. Some thirty strains of pneumococci have been discovered. Types I, II and III, and the miscellaneous remainder which was included under the term Group IV have been further studied, and can be divided largely into " epidemic " and " potentially pathogenic " members. Thus Types I, II, V and VII, together with XIV and XXII which attack children more particularly, are " epidemic " ; Types III, VIII, XVIII, together with IV, VI, XIX and XXIII which are more often found in children, are " potentially pathogenic." Types I, II and V and VII are responsible for the majority of attacks of lobar pneumonia, and hence may be presumed to be of comparatively high virulence. Types I and II are seldom found in the mouth and throat of normal individuals, so that the finding of either of these strains in the sputum

---

* Vaccination with mixed polysaccharides of types I, II, V and VII has been found to be a useful prophylactic measure against epidemic pneumonia among Army recruits in training.

of a patient in the early stages of a febrile illness strongly suggests pneumonia as the cause. On the other hand, pneumococcal strains of Group IV are frequently found in the mouth and contain the less virulent strains ; when they become pathogenic they usually cause only lobular pneumonia. Infections caused by organisms which normally inhabit the mouth and upper respiratory tract—and these include not only pneumococci of Type III and Group IV, but also a mixed bacterial flora which may determine various types of bronchopneumonia (see Chap. XVIII)—may be called endogenous. Exogenous infections arise by direct contact with a patient suffering from pneumonia, or with a carrier, or from inhalation of the infected dust of rooms or wards where patients with pneumonia have been nursed.

THE PATHOLOGY OF PNEUMOCOCCAL INFLAMMATION OF THE LUNG

The accepted stages of congestion, red hepatisation, grey hepatisation and resolution are well known, and their detailed description can be read in textbooks of Pathology. This classical description applies, however, to a " typical " reaction, the result of a particular balance between the seed and the soil which produces a lobar pneumonia. Though it is a commonly observed picture, it tends to over-emphasise one particular degree of inflammatory reaction to the pneumococcus ; with the result that the significance of other degrees of inflammation is not properly appreciated. After all, the battlefield of the lung may be the scene of engagements which may vary from an insignificant and ineffective local sortie to a general advance which rapidly overwhelms every defence.

It is well, therefore, to go back to fundamentals, to see how the body and lungs react to pneumococcal invasion under the differing conditions which arise from variations in the virulence of the pneumococci and in the resistance of the host.

There are cases of blood-borne " metastatic " pneumonia secondary to pneumococcal peritonitis or other pneumococcal lesions ; but usually the pathway of infection is by inhalation. The primary defences fail to prevent the organisms passing down the trachea and bronchi. The first alveoli which they can meet and from which they cannot be ejected either by cough or ciliary action are those which open out directly from the main bronchi near the hilum and fill the interbronchial spaces there. Gaskell points out that terminal lung units (*i.e.*, a terminal bronchiole with its associated air spaces) occur not only at the end of terminal branchings, but are also given off throughout the bronchial tree, arising from the largest bronchi, usually in pairs, and connected to such a bronchus by only a very small short ciliated bronchiole (Fig. 96).

It is here, in the neighbour-hood of the hilum, that the battle is most often joined ; though occasionally the cocci make a much deeper initial penetration, so that the earliest patch of inflammation is a wedge or cone nearer the peri-phery. Ordinarily, pneumococci of low virulence which reach the lungs are dealt with very much as though they were merely particles of dust, being ingested and removed by macrophages without the necessity for any polymorphonuclear leucocytic

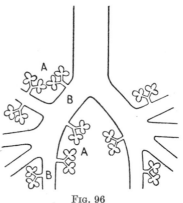

Fig. 96

Diagram to show the type of arrange-ment of terminal lung units arising directly from the large bronchi. These alveolar units (A) arise directly from the large bronchi (B), and are thus in very intimate relationship with them. (*After Gaskell.*)

activity. The patient may suffer no sense of illness at all, or at most there may be a very mild " bronchitis." If the resistance of the host is poor, however, as may happen in old people, weakly children or patients who are comatose, even these low grade organisms may not be held in check.

Organisms of a somewhat higher virulence make more headway. The inflammatory reaction then consists of con-gestion and the exudation of serous fluid into the alveoli ; the cocci are quickly destroyed by lysis in the alveolar fluid or ingested by macrophages, so they are only seen in the earliest stages, and here again, not many polymorphonuclear leucocytes make their appearance. Later, small patches of central broncho-pneumonic consolidation are seen, around which is a zone of alveoli filled as above with sterile serous exudate. The capillaries in the central patch, engorged up to the fourth or fifth day, are by the seventh day obliterated by the pressure of the mass of solidly packed cells which now fill the affected alveoli. The small bronchiole of the pneumonic zone is filled with alveolar exudate. The patches are few and localised, or many and diffuse, according to the balance struck between invasive power and resistance. Sometimes the process takes the form of a low-grade, " creeping " bronchopneumonia. Most of the cocci in the original patch are destroyed, but a few escape to other alveoli. Thus, while the first lesion heals, further successive zones of battle develop. The warfare, dying down in one place to break out elsewhere, may go on in a desultory, indecisive fashion, sometimes for months. This type of illness is occasionally seen in children or in the aged, usually because the resistance is just not good enough to hold even the poorly equipped invader.

With organisms of the next higher degree of virulence the inflammation is more severe and extensive, and the invasion harder to localise. For a time the pneumococci are able to increase themselves ; the body pours out more leucocytes and more exudate into the alveoli, and there is more fibrin in the exudate. As before, capillaries are first engorged and later obliterated. The pneumonic patches are larger, with surrounding zones of alveoli filled with sterile exudate, and soon these coalesce into consolidated areas the size of anatomical lobules (*i.e.*, about 25 primary lung units) or even larger. The bronchioles in these areas may lose their epithelium, are filled with exudate and are lost in the general solidification of the patches of what may now be called *lobular* or even *segmental* pneumonia. As the battle progresses, the lymphatic vessels become distended with serum and cell debris as they carry the exudate away from the battle area.

A still higher degree of virulence produces a *lobar pneumonia*. Here, even in the healthy young athlete, invasion cannot be kept back by the localising forces, and it advances to the periphery of the lobe until it is brought up against the comparatively avascular limiting membrane of the pleura. Even then it may after a time throw bridges across and so reach an adjoining lobe, resuming its advance. Another way in which more than one lobe may be involved is by the simultaneous invasion of them by separate columns of cocci. In the early stages there is the usual patchy reaction in the units attacked by the invading organisms, but coalescence into larger areas is very rapid. Infected, highly fibrinous exudate spills over from one alveolus to the next, via the smallest bronchioles ; the fibrin clots, large numbers of cells are entangled in the meshes, capillaries are intensely engorged and lymphatics widely distended with absorbed debris. The defence is, as it were, one " in depth," so that in a short time a diagrammatic and over-simplified picture might be given as follows (Fig. 97).

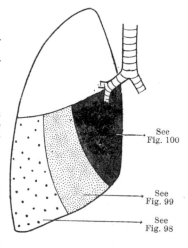

Grey hepatisation (Fig. 100)—
    Alveolar walls compressed and blood-less.
    Alveoli crowded with polymorpho-nuclear leucocytes.

Red hepatisation (Fig. 99)—
    Alveolar walls congested and swollen.
    Alveoli filled with an exudate of fibrin and red blood corpuscles, with a few polymorphs, monocytes and pneumococci.

Early congestive lesion (Fig. 98)—
    Alveolar walls markedly congested.
    Alveoli filled with serous exudate, with a few pneumococci and hardly any leucocytes.

See Fig. 100

See Fig. 99

See Fig. 98

FIG. 97

Diagrammatic representation of the three zones of the lobar pneumonic lesion.

Centrally, the polymorphonuclear leucocytes are very numerous, pneumococci there have been destroyed in large numbers, and the previously engorged capillaries are now obliterated—in other words, a central zone of grey hepatisation (Fig. 100). Peripherally to this, where the battle is at its height, there is a zone of red hepatisation, the capillaries intensely engorged and swollen, the alveoli solid with fibrinous exudate, red blood corpuscles and a few leucocytes (Fig. 99). The alveolar walls are attacked in the same way and become infiltrated with inflammatory exudate. Pneumococci are present in both walls and lumen. In these areas of hepatisation the smaller bronchi and bronchioles are involved (the changes follow those in the surrounding alveoli and are therefore secondary), shedding their epithelium, being filled with exudate which spreads from the alveoli, and merging into the general consolidation. More peripherally still, the alveoli are in process of early reaction to the vigorous advance troops of cocci, with capillaries engorged and sero-fibrinous exudate in which are numerous cocci in the alveolar spaces (Fig. 98). The whole process is rapid and dramatic. Capillaries engorged up to the fourth day are quickly obliterated by the fifth day, and cocci which are very numerous and vigorous up to the third day are mostly destroyed by the fifth day, partly by phagocytosis and partly extracellularly in the alveolar exudate. The phagocytic cells, laden with their prey, find their way either into the lymphatic channels, which by the third day are enormously distended, and so to the lymph nodes, or else into the blood stream. By the fifth day the whole lobe is in the condition of grey hepatisation. Variations in the speed and intensity of the infection may obviously modify this arbitrary picture. Within forty-eight hours of the onset of the illness, for example, a patient may die with one or more lobes wholly solid at the stage of red hepatisation.

If the battle is won by the host, **resolution** takes place, mainly by liquefaction of the solid exudate by proteolytic cellular ferments. A little of the material is coughed up, but most of it is absorbed into the lymphatics as the result of the activity of mononuclear phagocytes. There is no necrosis of bronchiolar or alveolar walls, and the lung is restored intact, so that by three weeks after the infection there is nothing there to tell of the ordeal which it has survived. It is as though a breeze had swept over a field of corn and passed on. If, however, the invaders win, blood infection occurs, and the outlook is grave indeed. Sometimes the clotted fibrinous exudate with its entangled cells is not liquefied and removed speedily enough before fibroblasts have an opportunity of invading it ; on these rare occasions the alveolar exudate becomes organised into fibrous tissue, the lobe becomes fleshy (" carnified "), and the condition is now a true *unresolved and organised pneumonia* (Fig. 101).

Pleurisy occurs to a greater or less degree with all but the mildest lesions. Over a lobular lesion which is near the surface of the lung, an area of pleural congestion and fibrinous exudate may be found, which is sterile at all stages of the pneumonic process. With more extensive lesions, the local pleuritic patch may become infected, and then a considerable pleural effusion usually develops. With lobar pneumonia there is a fibrinous

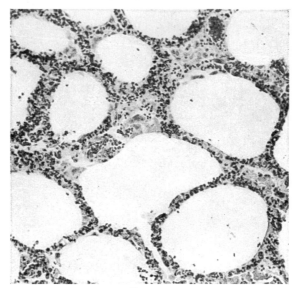

FIG. 98.
Lobar Pneumonia—early congestive lesion.

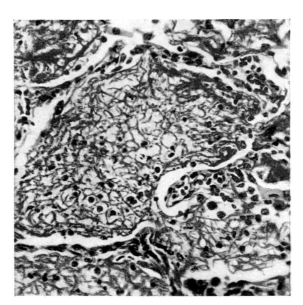

FIG. 99.
Lobar Pneumonia—red hepatisation.

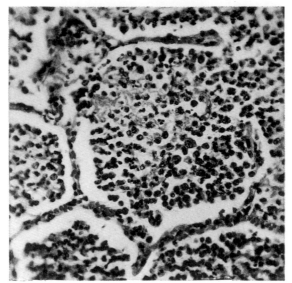

Fig. 100.
Lobar Pneumonia—grey hepatisation. (See Text, p. 207)

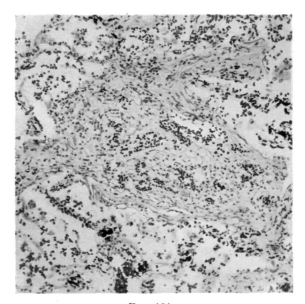

Fig. 101.
Lobar Pneumonia—organisation—in some of the alveoli, vascular
connective tissue has replaced the original inflammatory exudate.
Hæmatoxylin and Eosin. (See Text, p. 209)

pleurisy with a certain amount of effusion in the corresponding pleural cavity ; usually it occurs some time later than the initial invasion (" metapneumonic," as contrasted with the " synpneumonic " or simultaneous effusion characteristic of streptococcal pneumonia), and cocci persist in the fluid after they have been destroyed in the more central zones of the lung itself. Sometimes the pleural cocci are destroyed quickly, so that the effusion is thin and turbid, with only a moderate number of leucocytes in it. Sometimes the infection is heavier, and the call on leucocytes much greater, so that the effusion thickens to frank pus. Where the surface of the lung is not very far from the point of invasion, direct extension can be very rapid—from the root of the lung to the anterior or posterior margins, for example.

Pneumococci of the highest virulence sweep irresistibly through all defences, though it is usually possible to find an area where there is evidence of an attempt to halt their advance. The cocci spread in great numbers into intensely engorged lung capillaries, and reach the blood stream as a massive septicæmic invasion. A diffuse, patchy serous exudate teeming with pneumococci half fills the alveoli ; and numerous small hæmorrhages, scattered throughout the lungs, show where blood has been extravasated through capillary walls damaged by the intense toxic process. Within twenty-four hours of the invasion, cocci have swept through the lung into the pleural cavity, causing an acute pleurisy which may rapidly become bilateral and may spread to the pericardium. The polymorpho-nuclear leucocytic reaction is negligible. Such a *septicæmic* or *"miliary" pneumonia* occurs as a fulminating infection especially in infants, and is usually fatal within forty-eight hours ; or it may occur as part of a pneumococcal septicæmia secondary to a focus outside the lung. Similar changes occur in the other lobes when to a lobar pneumonia is added a massive septicæmia.

All these variations illustrate the varying play between " seed " and " soil," as the body tries to localise the coccal invasion. This localisation is probably more easily accom-plished in the larger lungs of adults than in the small ones of children. Broadly speaking, the younger the child the more likely is the pneumococcal invasion to spread beyond the lungs to other parts of the body, and the greater the tendency to the formation of purulent pleural effusions.

14

While the type of lesion produced depends on the virulence of the organism, it must be obvious that enough organisms have to find their way into the bronchi to start a lesion—that is, there is a " minimal effective dose." The higher the virulence of the cocci the fewer of them are needed to overcome the primary defences and initiate an invasion of the lung. The healthy adult rarely suffers a pure pneumococcal lobular or bronchopneumonia, for his defences against the less virulent cocci are so good that they have little chance of infecting his lung ; he falls only to the virulent ones, and has a typical lobar pneumonia. It is the aged, the invalid or the unconscious adult who is liable to develop pneumococcal bronchopneumonia. Though it is more often seen in children, even among them it is the weakly, marasmic, or those with upper respiratory affections who are much more likely to develop it. The aged or weakly adult who is infected by a coccus of " lobar " virulence will develop a " miliary " septicæmic pneumonia.

LOBAR PNEUMONIA

Lobar pneumonia is typically an infection by virulent pneumococci of adolescent and adult patients with a fair degree of resistance, though it can occur in children also. Most cases are sporadic, but there is no doubt that the disease has a low but real infectivity. In older and debilitated persons the infection may be endogenous, as in the Type III infections. Debilitating diseases such as diabetes, chronic nephritis, chronic alcoholism and cirrhosis of the liver may so alter the balance of forces between the " seed " and the " soil " as to determine the lobar variety of pneumonia even with cocci of low virulence. The incubation period is short—twenty-four to forty-eight hours.

SYMPTOMS

Sometimes the patient has recently had a cold, which weakens the primary defences and allows the pneumococci to break through ; but often the onset is like a bolt from the blue. He suddenly feels shivery and ill, and huddles in front of the fire, looking grey and shocked ; or he may start with a frank rigor. In young children the illness often begins with vomiting or a convulsion. The temperature rises sharply to 103° F. or more, and usually remains at about that level until recovery begins, though it may be remittent. The pulse is quickened, becoming full and bounding ; the face is now flushed and the skin burning hot. In a few hours (sometimes it is the presenting symptom) the lancinating pain of acute pleurisy makes itself felt, near the nipple or towards the axilla ; it makes him grunt and hold his side, and it stabs him with each inspiration or cough. If the pleurisy involves the central part of the diaphragm, the pain is referred to the shoulder, and if the outer surface of the diaphragm or of the lower lobe is involved it may be referred to the abdomen (see Chap. II, p. 55). At this early stage cough is sharp and painful, cut short by a grunt or even a cry of pain. With great difficulty he begins to get up a little viscid sputum ; the congestion of the lung causes it to be tinged with blood, the hæmoglobin of which may be changed to a pinkish, rusty, tawny or even bright orange colour. Because it is so scanty and loaded with fibrin, the sputum sticks to his mouth and has to be removed in a stringy mass by means of a handkerchief or dab of cotton-wool, and when it is in the sputum cup it clings tenaciously to it even when the cup is inverted. In the early days of the illness the alveoli are filled with exudate and the blood vessels still engorged ; so the breathing is rapid and shallow (the affected lung being more rigid), and there is a purplish cyanosis due to impaired aeration of the alveoli. In children the breathing may be very rapid, and may reach 60 or even 80 respirations per minute ; in both children and adults the alæ nasæ are seen to be working. This quick, shallow breathing alters the ratio of pulse rate to respiration rate (normally 4 to 1) to 3 to 1, or even 2 to 1.

In about half the cases, herpes appears, usually about the lips, from the second to the fifth day. The tongue becomes furred with a dry, dirty-brown coating, and there may be gastro-intestinal disturbances. In the seriously toxic cases severe tympanites can be very troublesome, increasing the respiratory embarrassment. In the minor forms of the illness the patient's mind may remain clear throughout ; but a combination of toxæmia and poor oxygenation of the brain may result in a delirium which varies from occasional " wandering " to a grave, maniacal condition.

These symptoms persist, with hardly any change, for some

days, and the patient remains gravely ill. The urine is scanty, concentrated, and may show a small amount of albumin, due to the cloudy swelling of the kidneys. If he is reacting well to the infection a leucocytosis of 20,000 cells per cubic milli-metre or more is found. As the strain of battle continues the pulse gradually becomes softer and smaller ; if it rises above 120 per minute the patient is beginning to lose ground. By the fifth day the capillaries in the affected part of the lung have become obliterated, so that there is little or no flow of blood through them. Poorly oxygenated blood is therefore no longer mixed with properly aerated blood from the rest of the lung, and the cyanosis is not so marked. What cyanosis there is, is now not purple but of lighter hue, because the rapid, shallow breathing has washed out of the blood a good deal of carbon dioxide (see p. 167).

Meanwhile, if the battle goes well, pneumococci are being destroyed in the lung in great numbers, until by the fifth day most of them have been killed. Their endotoxin is liberated, and antibodies begin to accumulate in the blood about the fifth day, reaching their maximum concentration on the seventh or eighth day. Then victory may come with startling abrupt-ness—by **crisis.** The patient has been struggling against the virulent infection, and the onlooker wonders if he can hold out much longer. Suddenly the whole picture changes ; tempera-ture, pulse and respiration become normal within a few hours, the skin becomes moist, the tongue begins to clean, he feels much better and drops off into natural, quiet sleep from which he wakes refreshed.* Sometimes the final victory is less dramatic, and the symptoms subside more slowly, the tem-perature taking several days to reach the normal level—termina-tion by **lysis.** In either case the lung is still solid and remains so for several days.

PHYSICAL SIGNS

The pathological changes as the invasion spreads through the lung determine the signs which may be found at the various

---

* An old lady of 76, who on the seventh day of her pneumonia looked as though she would die any minute, had her crisis, dropped off to sleep, and when she woke up said to her nurse : " Oh dear, I am so hungry ; do you know what I should like ? I want some bread and cheese and a bottle of beer. I've never tasted beer in my life, but I just fancy it now." She had her desire, and enjoyed it !

stages of the illness. The student is apt to equate "pneumonia" with the picture of full-blown consolidation, and to be puzzled if, as he often says, "the signs are not typical." But it takes anything from two to five days for the solidification to spread from the hilum to the periphery and involve the whole lobe; sometimes it is arrested before it gets that far, and is never more than a *central* pneumonia. In the early stages the pathological picture may be that shown in Figs. 102 and 103.

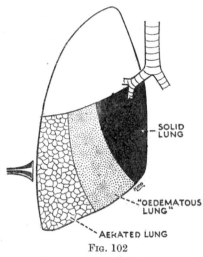

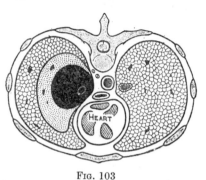

FIG. 102

Lung seen in vertical section.

FIG. 103

Lung seen in cross-section.

To show the anatomico-pathological picture in the earlier stage of lobar pneumonia. (This stage corresponds to "central pneumonia.")

Examination of the chest then reveals diminished expansion over the affected lobe, no dulness to percussion, no increase of vocal fremitus or vocal resonance, and diminished breath sounds owing to the poor movement. As the edge of the lesion advances there will come a stage when exudate begins to accumulate in the still aerated superficial alveoli; at the end of inspiration, or maybe only on deep inspiration, the moist surfaces separate and fine crepitations are heard. As the consolidation approaches the periphery there may be a stage when deep but not light percussion gives a dull note. Again, as voice sounds are louder than breath sounds and carry farther, there may be a stage when voice sounds are exaggerated (bronchophony), but breath sounds are still vesicular and faint. Then may come a period when bronchial breathing, due to the approaching consolidation, is at last heard—but distantly, for it is damped down by the peripheral layer of still partly aerated lung. Finally, the whole lobe is solid, and the "typical signs of consolidation" are un-mistakable: diminished expansion, greatly impaired percussion note (but not the absolute dulness of fluid), increased vocal fremitus, bronchophony, whispered pectoriloquy and bronchial breathing, but usually no râles, for the lobe is solid and the larger bronchi are patent and not narrowed by swelling or filled by exudate.

Very rarely a plug of viscid, fibrinous sputum may block one of the large bronchi after the consolidation is established, so that breath sounds are not heard. Solid lung does not collapse, however, to anything like the same extent as does aerated lung, so that the mediastinal traction displacement characteristic of massive collapse of the lung is not so obvious. This condition is called *massive pneumonia*. It is uncommon, and may easily be mistaken for pleural effusion, but the percussion note is less board-like, and there is no appreciable mediastinal displacement, whereas with considerable pleural effusion the displacement is away from the side of the lesion.

In the earlier stages of involvement of the pleura, friction sounds may be heard. When the inflammation involves that portion of the pleura which is in relation to the pericardium, the rub is influenced by the cardiac rhythm, producing the so-called pleuro-pericardial rub. The rub disappears as soon as there is exudation of enough fluid to separate the two pleural membranes.

With resolution, after the liquefaction and removal of the exudate, inspired air begins to reach the alveoli and smaller bronchi again, so that moist sounds in the form of fine and medium crepitations are heard. These are the *redux crepita-tions*—the heralds of the returning air. When there is more liquefied exudate, partly filling medium or larger bronchi, the crepitations are medium or coarse. If a still solidified patch happens to surround them they may be loud and consonating, giving the inexperienced the impression that dreadful compli-cations are on foot ; but in a few days they have disappeared. Expansion of the lung, percussion note and breath sounds take longer to become normal, because the usually associated pleurisy takes longer to resolve. If, however, empyema develops, the symptoms and signs of it take the place of the above clinical picture of recovery (see Chap. XXV).

The general macroscopic characteristics of the *sputum* during the illness have already been described. Microscopically, mucus, fibrin, red blood corpuscles, leucocytes, epithelial cells and pneumococci may be found. The sputum should always be examined for tubercle bacilli, so that an active tuberculous lesion is not overlooked ; it must be remembered, however, that tubercle bacilli are not likely to be found in pneumonic phthisis until the lung tissue begins to break down. If possible, the infecting pneumococcus should be typed ; this is a matter for the laboratory, not because the technique is difficult but because it is not feasible for the practitioner to keep a collection of specific testing sera.

The *blood* shows a considerable polymorphonuclear leucocytosis if the body is reacting well to the disease—a white-cell count, for example, of 20,000 to 30,000. A poor reaction (say below 12,000) or a leucopenia is usually a bad sign. The increased white-cell count should fall with the crisis ; if it persists, or if it falls and then rises again, it is probable that some complication, such as empyema, is developing. Some clinical pathologists regard an increase in the *immature* polymorphonuclears as a more certain measure of the defensive response. In the early days of the illness, pneumococci can often be found in the circulating blood ; this has sometimes been called a " spilling over " of organisms into the blood stream, but the phrase hardly defines any clear-cut pathological conception. It has already been pointed out that as the pneumococci are attacked by the body, macrophages ingest them and carry them off into lymphatic and blood channels. Some of these cocci may, however, escape death, so that by *blood culture* of considerable amounts of blood, colonies of pneumococci may be grown. By about the fifth day, in favourable cases, the invading pneumococci are destroyed, and the blood culture is wholly negative. On the other hand, if there is grave septicæmic invasion, cocci break through into the blood stream in force. If, therefore, bacteriæmia is of such a degree that it can be demonstrated in only 1 or 2 c.c. of blood even in the early stages, the invasion is serious and the outlook poor ; moreover, late invasion of the blood stream is of serious import. Accompanied by a rising leucocytosis, it may herald some complication such as empyema, pericarditis, or meningitis ; accompanied by a leucopenia, it usually indicates a fulminating septicæmic infection which is overwhelming every defence.

Radiology of the chest by a portable apparatus can be very helpful in showing the extent and site of lung involvement ; it is a matter for the expert, however, and is not usually available for the doctor practising in the homes of ordinary people.

COMPLICATIONS

The struggle may not go well for the patient. The cocci may advance and break through into the blood stream, the toxæmia may overwhelm him, or the associated anoxia may so damage vital tissues that he is placed in grave jeopardy. The inflammation may spread to other lobes of the lung, or *empyema* or *pericarditis* may develop. Cocci may be carried in the blood stream to the endocardium or the meninges, and cause *septic endocarditis* or *meningitis*. Rare complications are *diffuse septic destruction of the lung tissue, arthritis, peritonitis, venous thrombosis, severe toxic damage to the liver* and *acute toxic nephritis*.

The combination of toxæmia and prolonged anoxia may gravely damage the myocardium and paralyse the vasomotor control of the circulation. Suddenly or gradually there may be a change for the worse. The breathing becomes more and more rapid and shallow and the hitherto unaffected parts of the lungs water-logged : the face is pale and livid : the pulse " runs away," becomes thready and often irregular, and finally cannot be felt : the blood pressure falls : the skin is covered with a cold sweat : the extremities become cold : and the patient sinks helplessly down the bed in spite of the pillows which propped him up. Unconscious of his surroundings, maybe restless and muttering in a low delirium, he soon dies. In rare cases sudden death may occur as a patient makes some effort which is too much for his damaged myocardium.

DIAGNOSIS

Even in instances where the illness does not begin with chill and pain in the side, the rapid respirations and cyanosis, the diminished expansion of one side of the chest and the rusty sputum which soon follows, make the diagnosis fairly easy. With the pathological background in mind the student must try to translate the symptoms and signs which are present into a picture of what is happening—the extent, intensity and stage of the disease. He must distinguish it from *bronchopneumonias* due to other organisms (usually bilateral, with more gradual onset, an irregular and lower temperature, and diffuse and less defined physical signs ; though where the bronchopneumonic patches become confluent, the distinction may be impossible) : from *pleurisy with effusion* (see Chap. XXIV) : from *collapse of the lung* (see Chap. VII) : from *acute tuberculous pneumonia* (here, resolution does not occur, and later there are signs of breaking down of the lung with or without obvious cavitation, and tubercle bacilli are found in the sputum) : from non-infected *pulmonary infarcts* (associated with chronic heart disease, thrombophlebitis or embolus from a recent operative field, and with the spitting up of frank blood rather than rusty sputum). When lower lobe pneumonia is present and the pain of the pleurisy is referred to the abdomen, the condition must be distinguished from *acute abdominal illnesses* such as appendicitis or cholecystitis. In the differential diagnosis the appearance of the patient is often invaluable. Both in the " acute abdomen " and in pneumonia the patient has an anxious appearance, but in the " acute abdomen " he looks drawn and wan, and there is generalised pallor. In the early stages of pneumonia, if pallor is present it is circumoral. In both conditions respirations may be rapid and shallow : in the abdominal case, in order to reduce all movement of the abdomen, and in pneumonia, because of the lung changes already described. The most striking difference, however, is that the alæ nasæ are rarely seen in movement in purely abdominal states, but almost always in acute lobar pneumonia. Moreover, in unilateral pneumonia there is obvious lack of expansion of one side of the chest. It is a wise precaution to examine the chest in every case of apparent acute abdominal illness. This is more than ever necessary when the diagnosis is not straightforward, and still more particularly when the abdominal rigidity is unilateral. The lower intercostal nerves supply not only the lower part of the chest wall and parietal pleura together with the peripheral zone of the diaphragm, but also the abdomen. Pain in the lower thorax may therefore be referred to the abdomen, unilateral lack of chest expansion being accompanied by reflex, unilateral abdominal rigidity.

Other conditions which may give rise to difficulty are *acute pneumothorax* (see Chap. XXVII), *herpes zoster* (see p. 376) and *cardiac infarction*. In the latter, pain on the left side of the thorax, breathlessness and cyanosis may make the differentiation from left-sided pneumonia difficult. Moreover, if the lesion involves the anterior descending branch of the left coronary artery, blood-stained sputum caused by pulmonary emboli due to clot and necrotic debris from the right ventricle may simulate primary congestion of the lung.

PROGNOSIS

The final issue must depend largely on the interplay between " seed " and " soil," and it is not easy to disengage for purposes of analysis their relative rôles. For example, Type III pneumonia is perhaps the most fatal of all types, not because these pneumococci are in themselves the most virulent, but because they especially attack old people. Until the recent chemotherapeutic discoveries, it could have been added that for ten to fifteen patients out of every hundred, the balance could be tipped either towards recovery or towards death by the employment or not of correct treatment and careful nursing. Nowadays, however, the use of chemotherapy has appreciably diminished the death rate.

Factors which throw light on the forces of the " seed " are the virulence of the pneumococci concerned, the bacteriæmia which they may cause, the complications, and the extent of lung invaded. The " soil," the patient attacked, is conditioned by the state of the various organs, the general nutrition and the reserves which can be called upon to meet the illness. Thus chronic diseases of the lungs, damage to heart, arteries, liver and kidneys, obesity, diabetes mellitus, inferior economic conditions, wrong habits (*e.g.*, alcoholism), and especially advancing age—all go to rob the " soil " of its vitality. Poverty, economic distress and undernutrition double the death rate. Patients with cardiovascular degeneration or with renal damage fare badly ; the doctor should remember that there are two simple renal tests which can be of much help to him in prognosis—the testing of the urine for coagulable protein (albumin), especially if he finds more than the usual trace due to febrile albuminuria, and the examination of its deposit for casts of various types.

The factor of *age* deserves more detailed consideration. In childhood, pneumonia is more common and far more deadly in the first two years of life than later. In the adult over 40 (this refers to the days before more recent treatment by serum or chemotherapy), the death rate for any particular age is roughly the age figure expressed as a percentage. Osler said that to die of pneumonia is almost the natural end of old people ; a man wears out, " the soul's dark cottage, battered and decayed " develops many chinks, and age brings an added load on renal, cardiovascular, pulmonary and hepatic functions. If the age of 40 is taken as an arbitrary watershed, analysis makes it clear how serious for patients " on the wrong side of 40 " are cardiovascular disease, damaged kidneys or liver and chronic respiratory disease.

In any individual patient there are certain particular factors which need mention. Signs of peripheral vascular failure or of serious anoxia are of grave import—low and falling blood pressure, livid cyanosis, a low temperature with a rising pulse and respiration rate, marked restlessness and insomnia, and marked dehydration are all serious. So is the failure of leucocytic response ; so usually is very extensive lung involvement. A high temperature, provided that it is short of hyperpyrexia, may mean a good reaction to the disease. Certain complications are very serious ; pericarditis and meningitis nearly always end in death, empyema in infancy has a high mortality, and synpneumonic empyema (rare in pneumococcal, though common in streptococcal pneumonia) usually indicates the highly virulent, septicæmic form of invasion. Yet when all is said, the disease still has its surprises, both happy and unhappy ; here are two sentences from Hilton Fagge's remarks on prognosis, as true now as they were in 1866 : " To old people, or to those who (though not old) are worn out by overwork, dissipation or drunkenness, the disease is exceedingly fatal ; though from time to time one sees a patient recover even when the circumstances have appeared most adverse." And again : " Experience has taught me that it is never safe to speak confidently of the prospect of recovery of a patient with pneumonia, however favourable its course may be during the first few days."

TREATMENT

A hundred years ago the treatment of pneumonia was heroic.* The flushed patient with a bounding pulse and high fever needed strong measures, so it was argued, to counteract these manifestations ; he was therefore bled, purged, starved, blistered and doped with opium. Skoda (1846), realising that the disease runs but a brief course, adopted " expectant treatment," letting Nature do the work, while the doctor tried to conserve the patient's strength. He found that for every four patients who died on the older, vigorous treatment he lost only one by the new method. This principle of treatment still holds the field, and has not been displaced even by the recent successful use of chemotherapy, whereby the outlook for recovery has been enormously bettered. The doctor's attitude must be, however, not to " wait and see," but rather to " wait and foresee " ; for seven days or so he will be playing a game of chess, as it were, and he must try always to be a move ahead of his opponent. He must visualise the pathological changes as they occur in his patient, and be ever on the watch for dangers ahead.

The patient's strength must be jealously hoarded, for he is likely to have to call on all his reserves as the exhausting days go by. Fresh air and complete rest of body and mind are essential. The room should be quiet, well-ventilated but not draughty, and warmed with a fire ; and the single bed, with light bed clothing and sheets, not blankets, for the patient to lie between, should face the open window. His clothing should be loose, opening down the front † so that examination is easy ; once the diagnosis is made there is no need, for some days at least, to disturb him more than to examine the chest in the front and in the axillæ. The old-

---

* Compare, even for a less serious condition, the following extract from a letter from Dr Samuel Johnson to Dr Lawrence (20th January 1780), quoted in Boswell's *Life* : " I have been hindered by a vexatious and incessant cough, for which within these ten days I have been bled once, fasted four or five times, taken physick five times, and opiates, I think, six. This day it seems to remit."

† It should be said that many nurses prefer the loose gown which opens down the back and is tied with tapes. This is easier for washing, sponging or poulticing ; when examination of the chest is made, the gown can be pulled up from the front.

fashioned gamgee pneumonia-jacket is quite unnecessary and should not be used.

Absolute bed rest must be insisted upon. He must use a bed-pan, even if he dislikes the idea and would rather use a commode by the side of the bed ; great care must be taken in lifting him on to it, and he must not try to help himself. Nor must he reach for his sputum cup or his drinks. The mouth needs special attention ; artificial dentures should be removed, and the mouth should be rinsed every two or three hours, and also after the stringy sputum has been got up, with a pleasant mouth-wash such as glycerine of thymol. Some patients find that a drop of sweet oil inserted occasionally into each nostril is refreshing.

Skilled nursing may well turn the scales for him, so that unless he can have a day and a night nurse, he is better in hospital. It is wrong to delay the decision about this for a few days to see how he goes on, for if he is to be moved at all, the earlier the better, when the journey can do least harm. He must be shielded from worries as far as possible, and the doctor must sum up his temperament and act accordingly. It may even be wisest to tell him frankly that he has a week's battle in front of him, and to suggest that if he has any specially important business to settle he should get it off his mind and then give all his time and energy to getting better. The doctor must also make up his mind about the patient's wife ; if she is a restless, fussy person she must tactfully be kept occupied outside the sick room as much as possible. A good nurse is like the Biblical woman whose price is far above rubies. " She openeth her mouth with wisdom," and therefore usually keeps it shut in the sick room, allowing the patient to talk as little as possible, for talking makes him cough and exhausts him. Well-meaning visitors, letters and telegrams must be kept outside, but a calm, soothing member of the household who does the patient good may be allowed in occasionally. It is a good rule never to allow more than two persons in the sick room at any time, other than the patient. Shall a clergyman be allowed to visit ? That depends on whether the patient desires him and on what sort of man the clergyman is. Some patients look upon the parson as they used to look upon the oxygen cylinder—a last and desperate resort. Some clergymen take the atmosphere of the churchyard with them to the sick bed, while others bring quietness, confidence and strength. One further point about the general management : the doctor must insist on the full confidence of the patient's relatives, so that throughout the ups and downs of the illness he may be able to resist being badgered into action which is better left undone.

The patient can be nursed recumbent, semi-prone or propped up with pillows, whichever is most comfortable for him. If there is much dyspnœa he will breathe more easily propped up, as he has fuller use of his diaphragm, and also some of the blood is thereby enabled to drain from the thorax into the splanchnic area (see p. 50). On the other hand, propping him up so that he is bent at a right angle will hamper the movements of the diaphragm. At the onset of the illness, and only if it is necessary, the bowels should be moved with calomel, followed by a saline aperient ; later, a simple enema is better. Plenty of fluids must be given, and about 5 pints in the twenty-four hours are needed ; the moistness of the tongue is a good guide, for if it is dry the patient is not getting enough. He can have plain water, natural orangeade or lemonade, Imperial drink,* grapes, weak tea, and coffee (not in the evening, however), with glucose or sugar added whenever feasible. About 2, or at most 3, pints of milk in the day are usually all that are required, for the feverish patient is apt to find it unappetising ; served up as iced coffee, coffee junket or ice-cream, he may find it much more interesting. Sherry whey is a useful addition to the feeds. Sometimes he feels like eating something more solid, and can then be given thin bread and butter spread with honey, jellies, custard, stewed or tinned pears with their juice, or a lightly boiled egg. At any time during the illness abdominal distension may become very troublesome ; starchy messes such as bread and milk, arrow-root and various proprietary invalid foods are best avoided. If distension does occur, simple enemata, the rectal " flatus tube," or an injection of pituitrin may be needed. Pituitrin is dangerous, however, if the myocardium is flagging. Pyrexia is normal to the disease, and of comparatively short duration. If the fever rises above 104° F., tepid sponging is soothing and comforting and tones up the vasomotor system.

* To make Imperial drink : Lemons (or lemon substitute), 3 ; sugar, 2 oz. ; cream of tartar, 2 teaspoonfuls. Pare the rind of two lemons *thinly* into a jug, squeeze the juice of all three into it, add the sugar and cream of tartar. Then add boiling water to make 1 litre. Allow to cool, and strain.

Good sleep in the first few days of the illness is essential to the patient's chances of getting through the critical days which follow ; omnopon ($\frac{1}{3}$ gr.) or morphia ($\frac{1}{4}$ gr.) should be given the first night without hesitation, with or without a hot whisky nightcap. Later, the hot whisky may be sufficient to ensure it, though if the patient is restless the opiate may be repeated the following night. The early distressing cough can be made easier by warm alkaline drinks and a codein linctus ; the cough is exhausting, especially so if he has pain from pleurisy. The treatment of accompanying pleurisy is dealt with on p. 384.*

The introduction in 1938 of sulphapyridine, and later of other **sulphonamides,** has greatly lowered the death rate from pneumococcal pneumonia. The drop has been very marked in patients under 40, while even in those over 40 the previously high mortality has been at least halved. The drug acts bio-chemically and directly, preventing the multiplication of the cocci by blocking a special enzymic action concerned with the utilisation of a substance, p-aminobenzoic acid, necessary to their support. The invading cocci become like a bogged army whose supplies and reinforcements cannot reach them—easy prey for a strong opponent. It is essential to obtain as quickly as possible an effective concentration of the drug in the blood and body fluids, and to maintain it until the battle is won. The action of the sulphonamides is quantitative, and it is therefore vital to intervene before the organisms can multiply into a great and overwhelming host. Sulphathiazole, sulpha-diazine and sulphamezathine are the drugs in common use. They are excreted through the kidneys as acetyl derivatives of comparatively low solubility, and if the patient is dehydrated or is passing little urine because his fluid intake is low, they may be deposited as crystals in the renal tubules and pelvis of the kidney, causing renal irritation and haematuria. Sulpha-mezathine is the least insoluble, and therefore the most suitable for routine administration. In any event, a large fluid intake must be insisted upon during the course of treatment—ideally, one pint of bland fluid for every gram of sulphonamide in the daily dose. The best measure for the patient's safety is to ensure a daily urinary output of *at least* 1$\frac{1}{2}$ litres. When

---

* For the details of poulticing, see p. 183.

sulphathiazole or sulphadiazine are being given, a further safe-guard is to give enough sodium citrate to keep the urine just alkaline, a medium in which their excretion-derivatives are less insoluble.

It is worse than useless to fiddle nervously with small and ineffective doses, for not only do they fail to influence the disease but they may also result in making the cocci " drug fast," so that even much larger doses thereafter have no effect on them. For an adult, the initial dose should be 2 to 4 gm., followed by 1 gm. four-hourly. The tablets should be crushed, taken into the mouth and washed down with two or three ounces of water or milk. The administration of the drug should be continued until the temperature has been normal for two or three days. By the above intensive method the temperature in most patients falls to normal within forty-eight hours of the initial dose, and there is an obvious and often remarkable clinical improvement. An apparently desperately ill man may be well enough to want to see the morning paper twenty-four hours after his first dose of sulphonamide. Exhibition of the drug is short and sharp, so reducing the danger of toxic mani-festations which may occur if it is given over a longer time. If no clinical effect is seen within four or five days the diagnosis probably needs revision, and it is useless and may be dangerous to go on with the drug.

Sulphonamides have certain effects which in some patients may be troublesome. They may be depressing, and they some-times cause nausea or vomiting. If vomiting persists, it may be necessary to give the drug as the sodium salt by intravenous injection for a time, preferably in a continuous drip of glucose saline. Intravenous administration may also be necessary in fulminant infections, for which especially rapid concentration of the drug in the blood is desirable. Toxic manifestations due to the drug are not common, and seldom serious, especially if the principles of administration set out above are properly observed. They consist of cyanosis due to the formation of methæmoglobin (if it is severe, 0·5 to 1 gm. of methylene blue given in the twenty-four hours may counteract it), granulocytopenia (usually from prolonged administration), morbilliform rashes and " drug fever." This latter comes on some three or four days after the start of treatment, and it may mislead the doctor into persisting with sulphonamide because the temperature has not subsided. If he is aware of this uncommon possibility he will see that a pyrexia of 102° to 104° F. persists even though the patient is obviously much better from his pneumonia, and he will stop the drug. If the temperature does not then fall he must look for some complication such as empyema.

Most pneumococcal infections are satisfactorily combated by sulphonamides. Taken over a wide field of patients suffering from pneumococcal pneumonia, **penicillin** is about equally effective. Owing to the ease of administration, sulphonamide remains the drug of choice in the great majority of instances ; but once more it must be emphasised that dosage must be adequate and not half-hearted, and the principles of adminise tration must be fully observed. Sulphonamide therapy may fail, either because the infection is so severe that a concentration of drug sufficient to combat the infection cannot be achieved in time, or because the organism is for some reason resistant to sulphonamides. Patients in whom the prognosis is grave from the start (by reason, for example, of extreme toxæmia or old age, or infancy, especially prematurity, or heavy pneumococcal bacteræmia) should be given penicillin, with or without sulphonamide, according to the indications. Thus, patients known to be sulphonamide-resistant should be treated by penicillin only. So, too, should those with an initial leucopenia or severe anæmia, or in whom there is reason to believe that the urinary excretion of sulphonamide is likely to be impaired (*e.g.* patients suffering from congestive heart failure, acute or chronic nephritis, or cirrhosis of the liver). The severe diabetic who has pneumonia will probably be better served by penicillin treatment. Moreover, in any pneumococcal pneumonia where pyrexia has not been appreciably lowered, and where the clinical condition has not improved after about 30 hours of sulphonamide therapy, treatment by penicillin should then be substituted.

Whenever possible, penicillin-sensitivity tests should be made on the organism responsible for the infection, though these bacteriological investigations should not delay the institution of treatment if clinical judgment supports its desirability. Intermittent intramuscular administration at three-hourly intervals is the method of choice, the initial dose being 30,000 to 60,000 units or more, according to the severity of the illness.

15

This should be followed by 25,000 units, three-hourly, day and night. In favourable cases, treatment needs to be continued for about five or six days, although subsidence of the pyrexia and of toxic symptoms may be obvious within 24 to 48 hours.

For infants, the dosage is 2000 to 4000 units per lb. of body weight in the 24 hours, according to the severity of the infection.

As yet the practical details of penicillin therapy are by no means finally established. Probably for the convenience of both patient and attendants, there is now a tendency to give much higher doses (in order to prolong the period of effective blood concentration) at less frequent intervals. This may prove of advantage in ensuring that the patient's necessary sleep is not unduly disturbed.

Once solidification of any part of the lung is established, the natural processes of resolution have to be brought into play before the lung recovers its anatomical integrity. Therefore, while the illness may be cut short by the treatment and the invasion slowed down, the signs of consolidation still take their usual time to disappear. There is no evidence that resolution is delayed by sulphonamides. It is probable that clear or turbid pleural effusions are discovered somewhat more frequently than in the old days, the reason being that in the days before chemotherapy these patients would have suffered a far more intense infection and probably died early of the septicæmic form of the disease, with synpneumonic empyema.

If in spite of treatment the illness progresses unfavourably, cyanosis and peripheral vascular failure are likely to be the outstanding indications of the combined toxæmia and anoxia. Cyanosis calls for the *early* administration of oxygen (see Chap. XIII). Adequate oxygenation of the brain is the best treatment for restlessness and lack of sleep, and the best safeguard against respiratory and vasomotor failure, while proper oxygenation of the heart muscle helps to prevent myocardial damage and cardiac failure. Congestive cardiac failure with engorged jugular veins and other typical signs is very uncommon in pneumonia ; if—and only if—it occurs, venesection may give temporary relief. Save for the complication of auricular fibrillation, digitalis is of no proved value in pneumonia and should not be given merely as a routine. Peripheral vascular failure has sometimes been called " medical shock." It would seem reasonable to treat it by measures similar to those adopted for other forms of shock, such as blood transfusion or plasma transfusion. The patient is already worn out by days of struggle with the disease, and the myocardium is enfeebled and toxic, so that there is great danger of overloading it. In America, considerable success has been claimed after treatment by blood transfusion. Anæmia, however, is not a feature of lobar pneumonia, except in patients already suffering from nutritional or other anæmias ; transfusion of blood plasma would therefore appear to be preferable. It is obvious, however, that this form of treatment cannot as yet be recommended, even for what is always a desperate situation. If previously adequate treatment by oxygen and other measures has not prevented circulatory failure, it is hardly likely that a late transfusion will save the patient. There is no indication for vasoconstrictors such as adrenalin or pituitrin, for the peripheral vessels are constricted already. Warm drinks sweetened with glucose should be given in abundance and the patient kept warm. Strychnine and digitalis are useless, but nikethamide (coramine) may help.

If at any time in the later stages of the illness it appears vital to get the patient some sleep, and if oxygen and alcohol are not sufficient to secure it, either 20 gr. of chloral hydrate * or 2 drachms of paraldehyde by mouth, flavoured with syrup of orange (and also with whisky if the patient likes it), or double the dose per rectum, may be successful. Expectorants are wasted, for they will not enable him to cough up the solid fibrinous exudate ; in any case recent work suggests that, short of emetic doses, they are ineffective. With resolution, if there is a productive cough, a mixture containing sodium iodide and tincture of lobelia, together with warm alkaline drinks, will help to get up any sputum there may be.

Empyema is so common a complication that the medical attendant must be especially watchful for evidence of its development. If pyrexia recurs after the crisis, or if it persists after the twelfth day : if there is an increase in the leuco-cytosis : and if an area of board-like dulness develops, empyema should be suspected. The only convincing method of diagnosis is to explore the chest with a needle (see Chap. XXV).

In a straightforward case convalescence is usually rapid.

* Chloral hydrate is often given with bromide. Single doses of bromide are useless, however, for the drug is ineffective as a soporific until it has been given in such amount and for such a period as to displace chlorine ions from the blood.

Unless there are signs of myocardial weakness the patient may be allowed to sit up in bed a week after the illness is over, as a preliminary measure before being allowed up.   Fresh air, good food and a simple tonic will probably see him fit enough in about three weeks' time for a holiday either in the country or at the seaside.

CHAPTER XVIII

THE PNEUMONIAS (2)

PNEUMOCOCCUS LOBULAR PNEUMONIA

IT has already been shown that a pure pneumococcus infection can cause patchy bronchopneumonia, and the pathology of it has been described (p. 203). It would be better to speak of it as a *lobular pneumonia*, for here it is only secondarily that the bronchioles are filled with alveolar exudate. The clinical picture, too, is altogether different from the bronchopneumonias due to other organisms or to mixed infections ; there is usually no antecedent bronchitis, the attack is of sudden onset and short duration, the temperature usually remains persistently high, there is no marked tendency to relapse, and the termination is often by crisis. The clinical picture is thus akin to that of lobar pneumonia, though the lesion simulates a bronchopneumonia by being lobular in distribution. Moreover, as in lobar pneumonia, while the respirations are rapid and shallow, there are no signs of obstructed breathing.

At this point it is worth recalling another type of lesion which in its lobular distribution resembles bronchopneumonia—*septic embolic consolidation*. Each anatomical lobule is, as it were, a lung in miniature, with its own bronchus, artery, vein and lymphatic vessels. A septic embolus, say from an area of acute osteomyelitis, may be carried by the blood stream to various lobular arterioles and cause patchy areas of inflammation which finally become suppurative.

Pure pneumococcus lobular pneumonia is typically seen in children in the first two years of life, though it is not confined to any age period. Usually the child has been in good health when he is struck down with the illness. Indeed, if an apparently healthy child *suddenly* falls ill with " bronchopneumonia " it is likely either that the infection is purely pneumococcal, or (rarely) that the precipitating factor is an as yet unrecognised attack of measles or influenza—in which case the rash of measles may perhaps surprise the doctor by appearing a few hours later. The physical signs vary according to the amount of lung involved. There may be small areas of dullness, or none at all ; the sudden onset and the relatively short duration of the illness, and the usual absence of a preceding bronchitis or specific fever are characteristic, so that the symptoms and course are much more informative than the physical signs.

THE BRONCHOPNEUMONIAS

Here, again, the balance of "seed and soil" largely decides the issue. Bronchopneumonias have been classified as "primary" and "secondary," but this is merely to say that in the first instance the soil has been prepared for invasion by constitutional debility, in the second by an actual preceding disease. Leaving aside the pure pneumococcus infections which have a pathology and clinical picture of their own, the essential feature of the disease is that pathogenic micro-organisms gain access to the smaller bronchi and initiate an inflammation there which spreads to the neighbouring lung parenchyma. The periods of greatest incidence are in early childhood and in old age ; the contagious diseases of childhood (especially if the child is weakly), and the weakness of old people subject to bronchitis are here the predisposing factors (see Chap. XIV). The infection is usually a mixed one ; organisms normally present in the upper respiratory tract are concerned—especially streptococcus, Hæmophilus influenzæ and staphylococcus, together with certain non-epidemic strains of pneumococcus ; one particular organism probably being predominant in numbers or virulence.

The importance of constitutional debility is underlined not only by the factor of old age but also by social and economic factors. There is a close correlation between the mortality from pneumonia and poor social conditions ; in Glasgow, for instance, it was found that in children under 5 years of age the mortality in the industrial districts was four to seven times greater than in the residential. Diseases of poverty and ignorance, such as rickets and nutritional iron deficiency, conduce to minor (and therefore major) respiratory infections.

Almost any specific infectious disease of childhood may be complicated by bronchopneumonia, though the commonest antecedents are measles and whooping-cough. Epidemic influenza attacks persons of any age, and prepares the way for secondary invaders (Chap. XII) ; so also may the common cold, bronchitis and bronchial damage due to irritant gases. Bronchopneumonia may also follow the inhalation of infected material by accident, or during anæsthesia or coma. As for the " seed," the degree of virulence of the infecting organisms will clearly help to determine the intensity and extent of the lesion ; a good illustration of this will be seen later in the section on streptococcal pneumonia.

PATHOLOGY

The clinical picture in any particular patient depends so intimately upon the pathological manifestations that the student must try to visualise the various possible lesions. For one reason or another the primary defences of the lung are penetrated, and pathogenic bacteria reach various lobular bronchi and terminal bronchioles, causing an inflammation (bronchiolitis) which spreads to the adjoining lung tissue, both directly into the related alveoli and indirectly through the bronchiolar wall into contiguous alveoli. Usually both lungs are affected, especially the lower lobes. Being related to scattered small bronchi, the alveolar consolidation is patchy. It is irregular in both distribution and severity, the lesions being at different stages in different areas. The whole of a lobule, or only part of it, may be involved. The consolidated patches may coalesce into larger areas, and sometimes this *confluent bronchopneumonia* is so extensive as to involve the whole, or almost the whole, of a lobe. Blocking of the smaller bronchi by exudate causes collapse of the corresponding air cells ; there may be compensatory emphysema elsewhere, and even emphysematous bullæ due to " one-way obstruction " may occasionally be seen on the pleural surface. Thus on the pleural surface may be seen areas of consolidation, with a thin layer of fibrin over them : areas of collapse : areas of emphysema : and more or less normal areas of aerated lung. Similarly, when the lung is cut across, its mottled appearance is due to the same four possibilities—isolated or confluent reddish grey areas of consolidation standing out against the dark red background of the congested lung, bluish depressed patches of collapse, distended alveoli and aerated areas. Tiny beads of pus can be squeezed from the bronchioles, which form the centre of the consolidated areas.

Microscopically there is an intense inflammation of the bronchiolar walls ; they are swollen, thickened and infiltrated with leucocytes. Purulent exudate fills the lumen, with shed epithelium, leucocytes and bacteria, but there is little fibrin. Around the bronchiole is a zone of peribronchial inflammation, then a ring of alveoli filled with inflammatory exudate, beyond this again, a zone of inflammatory œdema, and beyond this again there may be compensatory emphysema of the alveoli.* The inflammation spreads to alveolar walls and along the interlobular septa, and there is an *interstitial inflammation* ; in severe infections, this inflammation may produce purulent infiltration of greater or less degree, and microscopic examination may reveal lymphatic vessels distended with pus. Blood and lymph vessels are greatly engorged, and if the inflammation is intense, hæmorrhages may be dotted about the area (Fig. 106). Fulminant infections may cause sufficient necrosis of tissue to lead to abscess formation (see Chap. XIX).

The pathological aspects which particularly colour the clinical picture are these : the infection sweeps rapidly or creeps slowly down the bronchial tubes, and on to the finer tubes. To the bronchitis of the larger tubes is thus added a bronchiolitis which forms the centre of the lesion, and a secondary localised, surrounding pneumonia. Here there may be an area of associated alveolar collapse, there a zone of emphysema. If the inflammation is widespread, so many bronchioles are occluded by exudate that a slow asphyxia develops ; hence the term " suffocative bronchiolitis." Moreover, damage to the bronchial walls and the interstitial tissue of the lung is likely to leave permanent damage, even if the patient recovers. Suppurative interstitial changes, even though they may be microscopic rather than macroscopic in size and extent, prolong the illness, and may explain why many of these lesions respond but poorly to chemotherapy.

Obviously the pathological and clinical picture may vary enormously, because of the various and complex factors which are concerned in the onset and in the development of the disease. The infection, for example, may be fulminating or mild, the lesion hæmorrhagic or œdematous, fibrinous or purulent (septic), according to the type and virulence of the

_____

* This states the matter " diagrammatically "—the areas are not necessarily so clear cut.

predominant organism in what is usually a mixed infection. In the septic pneumonias, abscesses may develop, miliary in size or quite large, according to the amount of lung destruction. When putrefactive organisms are present, the abscess is putrid. Recovery may be fairly rapid, or very slow, so that the pneumonia might be described as acute, subacute or chronic. There is therefore no single picture of bronchopneumonia ; a score or so might be drawn, and labelled according to the predominant organism, the distribution of the lesions, the course of the illness and the results of the inflammation. The student —and the physician—who bears this in mind will try to discern the exact character of the underlying lesion rather than be content with the label " atypical pneumonia."

In sporadic bronchopneumonia, with its mixed infection by invaders of low virulence, it is not easy to define the exact part played by each, particularly as one which is predominant at first may later be displaced from that rôle by another. In epidemics, however, one particular organism may run riot, its virulence enormously increased by passage from patient to patient, and the resulting pneumonia has fairly well-defined characteristics. This point has already been touched upon in the chapter on Influenza (Chap. XII).

STREPTOCOCCUS PNEUMONIA

Streptococci of low virulence in a feeble patient may produce a bronchopneumonia of the type already described. The β-hæmolytic strains, on the other hand, when they have once gained a foothold in a tissue, tend to spread diffusely, causing damage and destruction as they go. A striking illustration during the 1914–18 war was the epidemic of streptococcus pneumonia which followed the outbreak of measles in U.S.A. army camps in 1917-18. At first the predominant secondary invader, the coccus grew in virulence and soon appeared in epidemic form independently of measles. Later still it appeared again, this time as a virulent secondary invader in the pandemic of influenza. According to the resistance of the host, it took one of two main forms of attack, both very serious, but one fulminatingly so. In both instances the infection spread rapidly down the upper respiratory tract, giving rise to an intense inflammation of the throat, larynx, trachea and bronchi. In the terminal bronchioles the cocci were found in great numbers, causing destruction of the epithelium and plugging of the lumen with hæmorrhagic and purulent exudate, infiltrating the walls and producing a marked mural and peribronchial inflammation. The inflammatory reaction spread into the lymphatics of the bronchial walls and into the interlobular septa, and the cocci passed rapidly along the lymphatic channels to the pleural lymphatic plexus, with a resulting streptococcal effusion into the pleural cavity. The patchy bronchopneumonia, sometimes confluent, was in this way quickly accompanied by a thin, turbid *synpneumonic* empyema which might be blood-stained (see Chap. XXV). If, however, the cocci were exceedingly virulent, or the resistance negligible, they swept through the lung and into the blood stream almost without sign of opposition. There was then little effective inflammatory response ; the lungs showed zones of œdematous exudation, large hæmorrhagic patches and areas of necrotic tissue—all of them teeming with myriads of cocci. The œdema, hæmorrhages and widespread necrosis, together with the early purulent pleural effusion, were very characteristic of the desperate bronchopneumonias of the last influenzal pandemic.

When the invasion was not so overwhelming, the patient might survive long enough for some of the septic pneumonic patches to disintegrate into abscesses, which might rupture into the bronchi or the pleural cavity or both. Moreover, a striking infiltration of alveolar walls and interstitial tissue by macrophages occurred early, and was soon accompanied by the formation of new connective tissue. Patients with influenzal bronchopneumonia who died on the ninth day already showed a widespread fibroblastic reaction in the bronchiolar and alveolar exudate, the bronchial and alveolar walls and the interstitial tissue. Obviously, therefore, a patient who suffers a virulent streptococcal pneumonia will have a hard struggle to survive, and if he does so, is unlikely to emerge without badly scarred lungs.

HÆMOPHILUS INFLUENZÆ PNEUMONIA

The most virulent form of attack produces an intensely hæmorrhagic consolidation and œdematous reaction in patches which quickly become confluent. The leucocytic exudation is marked around the bronchioles. If the infection is somewhat less virulent, or the host's resistance is greater, the nasal sinuses and larger bronchi are filled with purulent secretion, the bronchioles are heavily damaged, their epithelium desquamated, their walls thickened and infiltrated with inflammatory exudate, their muscular layers degenerated and they are filled with pus. The adjacent alveoli are consolidated, with the usual surrounding areas of œdema, collapse, emphysema and, maybe, hæmorrhages. The lymphatics and interstitial tissue are not seriously invaded, so that the intensity of the inflammation is concentrated round the bronchioles. The lesions are therefore nodular and peribronchial, giving a " focal bronchopneumonia " ; the small nodules look somewhat like miliary tubercles, and may be mistaken for them by the inexperienced eye (see also p. 166).

STAPHYLOCOCCUS AUREUS PNEUMONIA

Pure staphylococcus infections tend to be localised at the point of entrance, creating an intense concentric inflammation, which ends in abscess formation. As a predominating secondary invader of the lungs, staphylococcus aureus is uncommon. When it occurs it is usually in association with an epidemic of influenza, though, very rarely, sporadic cases of what appear to be primary pneumonia are seen. The fulminating type produces a necrosing tracheo-bronchitis, with hæmorrhages, œdema and multiple foci (" clusters ") of suppuration in the lungs. The illness is fatal within a day or two of the onset. If the organism is not quite so virulent, and the patient survives, the multiple abscesses may discharge into bronchi, leaving cavities in the lungs, or they may open into the pleural cavity with resulting pyopneumothorax, or they may slowly heal with scarring. Clearly, even if the patient recovers, such an illness must be a prolonged one.

Friedländer's bacillus pneumonia—This is very rare, forming not more than 1 per cent. of all pneumonias. The organism may give a confluent, pseudolobar pneumonia, or a patchy bronchopneumonia, usually in the elderly or weakly.

The mortality is very high. If the patient survives the acute attack, he is almost certain to emerge with serious residual lung damage. In the acute stage there is widespread destruction of lung tissue, with necrosis which goes on to multiple abscess and cavity formation. The alveolar exudate is slimy and tenacious. As the upper lobe is very often affected, the condition simulates tuberculosis of the lung, but tubercle bacilli are never found. Once the acute stage is passed and death does not occur, the disease settles down into a long and indolent course, which may continue for many tedious months. As the abscesses are in the upper lobe, bronchial drainage may be reasonably effective. In the acute stage the bacillus may be found easily in the sputum ; later on, other secondary invaders are apt to overgrow them.

It is clear that in the serious pneumonias due to mixed infections, as in epidemics, the possible combinations and permutations of lesions must be considerable. In the sporadic bronchopneumonias where the organisms are of low virulence, and the resistance of the host more or less feeble, the lesions may be equally diverse. In this latter group particularly, the course of the disease may be acute, subacute or chronic, depending on the balance between the " seed " and the " soil." The word " bronchopneumonia " is apt to be associated only with an acute or fairly acute illness, and any prolongations of it put down either to complications or to " atypicality." But sometimes the battle moves slowly one way or the other with neither side making much headway for a long time, until finally either the disease wears down the patient or his processes of healing wear down the infection. A possible analogy, though it must not be pressed too far, is chronic pulmonary tuberculosis. These **chronic bronchopneumonias** may show themselves in many different guises, according to the various lesions in the lung—suppurative, non-suppurative, œdematous, hæmorrhagic, cavitated and fibrotic ; while the results of any obstructive bronchiolitis (collapse and emphysema) have to be added to the general picture.

Tuberculous bronchopneumonia is so common in children that it must always be borne in mind by the doctor or student confronted with a young patient suffering from bronchopneumonia. It will be considered in more detail in the section on tuberculosis of the lung (Chap. XX).

SYMPTOMS AND COURSE

Apart from epidemics (see Chap. XII) the *onset* of bronchopneumonia is usually gradual. The symptoms of the antecedent disease, if it exists, alter slowly or rapidly, for the worse.

An infant who has had bronchitis for some days begins to look drawn and distressed, has a sudden rise of temperature, and the *alæ nasæ* are seen to be working ; within a few hours it is clear that he is acutely ill. An old man with a recent exacerbation of his chronic bronchitis may gradually and almost imperceptibly fail over a period of a few days ; there is perhaps a slight increase in fever, his cough becomes more troublesome, he breathes more quickly and he goes a little blue. If the pyrexia of a patient with bronchitis persists longer than four or five days, the possibility of bronchopneumonia should always be borne in mind.

The extension of the inflammation usually sends up the *temperature*, which is then remittent in type. If the resistance is poor, as in marasmic infants or greatly enfeebled old people, there may be no pyrexia at all, even when the disease is to prove fatal. Where the progress is favourable, the fever may last for about a week, and then fall by lysis ; but if the bronchopneumonia has a subacute or chronic course, or the infection passes to suppuration, or if a succession of bronchi become obstructed or infected by " spill over " of secretions, pyrexia may persist for many weeks, or even months.

As the inflammatory exudate fills the bronchioles and adjacent alveoli, it causes obstruction to the free entrance of air into the alveoli. The extent of the involvement determines the degree of this suffocative process. The more extensive it is, the more serious the anoxia, resulting in purplish *cyanosis*, which later may become the livid cyanosis already described on p. 167. In all but the mild cases the breathing is rapid, and in children especially the obstructed respiration is made clear by the indrawing of the soft parts of the chest wall and the use of the accessory muscles of respiration. " The patient sits up, with chest heaving and with nostrils quivering, unable to utter more than two or three words at a time, using his shoulders and arms in violent efforts to breathe. On carefully inspecting the thoracic movements one finds that obviously there is a great obstacle to the entrance of air into the lungs. The epigastric and the hypochondriac regions of the abdomen recede at every inspiration ; in children, all the lower ribs and the lower part of the sternum may be forcibly sucked in. The supraclavicular and the suprasternal spaces also recede, but on the other hand the upper ribs often remain almost motionless in a position which is that of a forced inspiration, giving to the corresponding part of the chest a vaulted shape " (Hilton Fagge).

There is thus a severe strain on the muscles of respiration. Seeing that in the sporadic types of the disease at least, the patients are usually feeble, whether they are infants or old people, the cough reflex has little power. The bronchial tubes are therefore not easily cleared, and more or less extensive areas of collapse are liable to occur. The infant is often too fully occupied with the effort of breathing, or too weak, to cry loudly ; crying is apt, therefore, to be replaced by a low, distressed moaning.

Cough is usually present—dry during the congestive stages of the pneumonia, loose when there is much secretion, its power depending on the patient's strength. The *expectoration* is variable ; at first it may correspond to the antecedent bronchitis, or it may consist of frothy mucus, sometimes blood-stained. Later, if the patient survives, it becomes muco-purulent, and may contain an obviously predominant micro-organism. Often, however, all that is found is a mixed flora of no particular significance, comprising the common inhabitants of the upper respiratory tract. In moribund patients, cough ceases, and the secretions accumulate and flood the lungs. *Gastro-intestinal symptoms* are common, especially in children. Appetite is lost and digestion impaired by the toxæmia and the anoxia—a point which should warn the doctor against over-medication or any attempt to overfeed. Flatulence and tympanites may be troublesome, especially if they are sufficient to impede the action of the diaphragm. The *blood* usually shows a leucocytosis, but if the organism is very virulent or the resistance low, there may be leucopenia. In contrast to lobar pneumonia, a fair degree of anæmia is common, probably because in bronchopneumonia the " soil " is so often poor. If the toxæmia is prolonged, the anæmia may become very marked. As the disease progresses, *dehydration* may become serious ; * the tongue is dry, the mouth sore, the skin wrinkled and inelastic and the abdomen scaphoid. Nervous symptoms which are due to the combined toxæmia and anoxia are sleeplessness, restlessness, mental excitement and delirium. Convulsions

---

* It should not be forgotten that rapid, shallow breathing may markedly increase the loss of water from the body as water vapour in the breath.

may occur in children, but they are not so common as in the
more acute, pure pneumococcus pneumonias.

In the milder cases pleurisy is not common ; it is more
likely to occur in the small lungs of infants and in streptococcus
pneumonias.   In fatal cases death is usually due to peripheral
vascular failure, the features of which have already been
described (p. 216).   If the infection is very prolonged, however,
the patient may die of sheer exhaustion.

PHYSICAL SIGNS

In the earlier stages the infection is spreading down to
the smaller tubes, and therefore medium and fine crepitations
are heard.   The fine crepitations reveal the inflammatory
exudate in the bronchioles and their adjacent alveoli, and
they are discovered most frequently at the bases of the lungs,
below the angles of the scapulæ.   Usually both lungs are
involved, and therefore there may not be any noticeable
difference in the expansion of the two sides.   Dulness to
percussion is only present if the areas of consolidation are
large.   By the same token, bronchial breathing is not heard
very easily, except where there is confluent or pseudolobar
pneumonia.   As collapse of the lung is also a frequent complication, it is clear that the breath sounds in various parts of
the lungs may be apparently normal, or bronchial, or absent.
It is therefore the fine crepitations, localised and persistent,
which are the most important, and may be the only physical
signs of bronchopneumonia.

DIAGNOSIS

At first there may be difficulty in deciding whether a patient
with bronchitis or some acute specific disease has developed
bronchopneumonia.   The increase in the seriousness of the
symptoms and the development of fine crepitations indicate
the spread to the bronchioles and so inevitably to their alveoli.
The insidious onset, the remittent fever, the physical signs
and the mixed flora of " potentially pathogenic " organisms
natural to the upper respiratory tract help to distinguish it
from *lobar pneumonia*.   The diagnosis from *tuberculous bronchopneumonia* may be extremely difficult until tubercle bacilli

are found in the sputum, and this may not occur for some time (see Chap. XX). *Acute miliary tuberculosis* may present the same difficulties, but here the spleen is often enlarged, and there is no marked leucocytosis. *Passive congestion of the lungs* may show medium and fine crepitations at the bases, but is not usually accompanied by remittent fever. So-called *hypostatic pneumonia* is a form of passive congestion of the lungs, to which is added a low-grade bronchopneumonia.

PROGNOSIS

The disease is always serious, and is particularly dangerous in infants and in the aged. As has already been seen, it can also be extremely fatal in epidemics such as those of measles or influenza, where the secondary invaders may develop a high virulence. Unfavourable features are, firstly, those of a poor " soil "—infancy, old age, marasmus, rickets, underlying tuberculosis of the lungs or chronic lung disease such as bronchiectasis, weakness from a recent operation, defences enfeebled by coma or a prolonged anæsthetic. If the predominant organism is the pneumococcus, the outlook is probably better than if it is the streptococcus, other things being equal. The effects of " seed " on " soil " are indicated by the toxæmia and anoxia, and by the extent of the lung involvement, all of which have an important prognostic bearing. It may also be measured by the type of the disease. Prolonged chronic bronchopneumonia, such as has already been described, may wear out the patient until he finally dies of exhaustion ; nevertheless the doctor can here take comfort from the old cliché, " While there's life there's hope," for even when, after months of unsuccessful treatment, he is in despair, his patient may begin to recover.

Recovery may often exact the price of permanent damage to the lung. The dangers of absorption collapse, with resulting bronchiectasis as the most likely result, have already been described (Chap. VII). Fibrosis may be another important sequel, with its troublesome mechanical effects ; often, too, it conduces to later inflammatory exacerbations. Such fibrosis may be localised to the peribronchial tissue, or it may involve more or less extensively the parenchyma of the lung.

TREATMENT

So serious is bronchopneumonia that every effort should be made towards **prevention.** Proper treatment of the common cold or of simple bronchitis would go far towards reducing the incidence of bronchopneumonia. This in turn calls for prophylaxis against these simpler diseases, by the avoidance of contact infection, by isolation of those infected, and by the treatment of chronic affections in the nose and pharynx. The student and the young doctor will learn by experience of practice how often specific fevers such as measles and whooping-cough are still regarded as visitations which of necessity will run through the children of a household. Certainly a child suffering from one of these diseases should be isolated in a warm room and kept in bed during the acute stage and the early days of convalescence. But quite apart from ignorance, the poor have no rooms to spare for isolation and convalescence. All too often the child " runs about the house," infecting his brothers and sisters, and is liable himself to get chilled. The relation of bronchopneumonia to poverty and poor social conditions has already been stressed.

The *general management* is very much that laid down in the chapters on Bronchitis and Lobar Pneumonia (Chaps. XIV and XVII). This disease, however, is drawn out longer, and the doctor's " game of chess with the infection " may well tax to the utmost his patience, watchfulness and ingenuity. *Feeding* is more important than in the short, sharp attack of pure pneumococcus pneumonia, especially as many patients with bronchopneumonia start the race with a nutritional handicap. At the same time, the dangers of upsetting digestion in this longer illness are very real in weakly children and old people, so the diet must be easily digested, with large amounts of fluid to prevent dehydration. For adults, about 5 pints of fluid in the day are required, for the infant about 2 pints, the measure of need being dryness of the tongue and the condition of the skin.* The fluids may comprise weak tea, coffee with milk, diluted fruit juices, all sweetened with glucose or sugar, and plain water. Milk can be citrated, given with Ovaltine or Bourn-vita, put into milk puddings, custards, junket, icecream, vegetable soup or gruel. Jellies, honey, syrup, vegetable purees, eggs, thin bread and butter, and tinned pears or peaches

* In the infant the degree of depression of the fontanelle is also a helpful guide.

16

with their juices all help to make up an adequate diet. Sick children often need tempting with their food, and much resource may be needed by the nurse or the mother. Small amounts every two hours do not exhaust the child or his interest as may larger, less frequent feeds.

The indications for *early oxygen treatment* are the same as for lobar pneumonia, and the need, as a rule, is even greater. It reduces restlessness and delirium, so conserving energy, and combats the development of grave anoxic symptoms. Actually, in the days before the discovery of the new sulphonamide drugs, F. C. McDonald of Boston reduced the mortality of pneumonia in infants under 2 years of age from 30 to 4 per cent. by giving oxygen and sedatives liberally, ensuring an adequate intake of fluids and nourishment by good nursing, and combating anæmia and serum protein deficiency by early blood transfusion. He used morphia as a sedative, a drug which I would not recommend in bronchopneumonia unless there was a strong and clear indication for it. His results, however, do emphasise the prime importance of combating anoxia and dehydration, and preventing the patient from exhausting himself.

The state of the digestion must be closely watched and the feeding adapted to it ; if there is much flatulence, spaced doses of calomel for adults, $\frac{1}{8}$ gr. every hour for eight doses (or hydrarg. cum creta $\frac{1}{2}$ to 1 gr. at night, for children), can be very helpful. An unproductive cough which racks and exhausts the patient should be eased by hot drinks and a codein linctus (for children, a paregoric linctus) ; but cough associated with tenacious sputum calls for something to help expectoration and reduce bronchial spasm—hot alkaline drinks and a mixture containing iodide and lobelia, with the addition of ephedrine if necessary. For children, moistening of the air by means of a steam tent helps to loosen the secretions and to prevent absorption collapse of the lungs, but care must be taken to avoid overheating inside the tent. Changes of position may ease the breathing and help to bring up the sputum. If there is pleural pain, linseed or kaolin poultices may be sufficient to abolish it ; if it is too severe, opium may be necessary. But here its use is dangerous, especially if there is much secretion in the lungs, or if the patient is cyanotic. It should be given, therefore, in doses of $\frac{1}{8}$ gr. of morphia with $\frac{1}{100}$ gr. of atropine, while he is fully under the effect of oxygen therapy. If in spite of the basic treatment by oxygen and plenty of fluids the patient is restless, sleepless or has delirium, tepid sponging followed by 10 gr. of aspirin and a hot drink of whisky and water may be sufficient to quieten him and give him sleep : otherwise an appropriate dose of chloral hydrate may be necessary. Paraldehyde (2 drachms by mouth, or 3 to 4 drachms emulsified with normal saline and given by rectum) is safe but nauseating. The treatment of circulatory failure has been discussed elsewhere (see p. 226).

CHEMOTHERAPY

W. F. Gaisford gives the following scheme for the suggested maximum dose for infants and young children : **the figures refer to tablets, not grammes, each tablet containing $\frac{1}{2}$ gm.**

	Initial Dose.	Total in First Twelve Hours.	Subsequent Four-hourly Dose.
Weight—			
5 lb.	$\frac{1}{4}$	1	$\frac{1}{4}$
10 ,,	$\frac{1}{4}$	$1\frac{1}{2}$	$\frac{1}{4}$
15 ,,	$\frac{1}{2}$	2	$\frac{1}{4}$
20 ,,	$\frac{3}{4}$	3	$\frac{1}{2}$
Age—			
2 years	1	5	$\frac{1}{2}$
3 ,,	2	6	$\frac{3}{4}$
4 ,,	2	7	1
5 to 10 years	3	8	1
10 to 15 ,,	4	10	2

Quicker saturation is obtained by two-hourly doses in the early stages of treatment. The initial dose is usually double the subsequent ones—*e.g.*, a 15-lb. baby may be given $\frac{1}{2}$ tablet when first seen, then $\frac{1}{4}$ tablet two-hourly for six doses, and then $\frac{1}{4}$ tablet four-hourly till the temperature falls. Similarly a 3-year-old child may be started with 2 tablets, and given four doses of 1 tablet three-hourly. In all cases the dosage should be reduced when the total given in column 2 is reached.

Seeing that bronchopneumonia is usually due to a mixed infection, and that the poverty of the " soil " rather than the virulence of the " seed " is so often the determining factor, it cannot be expected that sulphonamides will have the same dramatic effect as in pure pneumococcus pneumonia. Nevertheless they should be given sulphanilamide if the infection is predominantly streptococcal, sulphathiazole if staphylococcal, sulphamezathine or sulphathiazole if the infection appears a mixed one without an obviously predominating organism. No specific effect is obtained against H. influenzae, and very little against Friedländer's bacillus, though against the latter large doses of sulphadiazine may occasionally succeed. Children are more tolerant than adults to sulphonamides, and they can be given half as much again as the dose calculated for age on the usual formula.

Penicillin is much more reliably effective against staphylo-coccal infections than is any sulphonamide. It is also effective against pneumococci and streptococci, but not against Friedländer's bacillus or most strains of H. influenzae. The great majority of bronchopneumonias, however, are caused by organisms sensitive both to sulphonamides and to penicillin. In severe infections, however, in which some degree of interstitial and alveolar pulmonary suppuration is present, penicillin has the great advantage of effective action even in the presence of pus. To patients with bronchopneumonia, therefore, both drugs should be given, if possible—certainly for the severe case, or for the case in which sulphonamide has brought no response within 30 hours.

If during the course of the illness relapses occur, the treatment of the relapse is the same as that of the initial acute stage. The prophylaxis and treatment of complicating pulmonary collapse is dealt with in Chapter VII.

Convalescence may be tedious, and while there is any physical or radiological evidence that the lungs are not fully recovered, the patient should be kept under the doctor's watchful eye. The lungs after bronchopneumonia should be as carefully watched as the heart after acute rheumatism. A month's convalescent holiday in the country or at the sea-side is advisable.

Little has been said in this chapter about radiology. Interest in *subacute and chronic bronchopneumonias*, septic or otherwise, has been reawakened, however, by the discovery that they may give X-ray pictures which are very similar to those of pulmonary tuberculosis. Indeed, they are often diagnosed as tuberculous, though tubercle bacilli are never found in the sputum. The modern use of chest radiology has not in this instance been sufficiently accompanied as yet by an eagerness to turn to pathology for the solution of clinical puzzles, and there is still much to be learned about these different patterns of prolonged and troublesome broncho-pneumonia.

Another problem still to be solved is whether certain viruses can directly cause pneumonia or whether they merely prepare the ground for secondary invaders. The question is discussed in Chapter XXI.

" **Post-operative pneumonia** " is a term somewhat loosely applied to a number of conditions following operation—mild bronchitis, mild or severe bronchopneumonia due to inhalation of micro-organisms or to aspiration of infected foreign material, and massive collapse of the lung. It is not always easy to differentiate post-operative inhalation bronchopneumonia from infarction due to septic emboli from the field of operation.

Oil aspiration pneumonia—Accidental aspiration of oil into the lung may set up a chronic proliferative inflammation which varies with the kind of oil inhaled and the secondary invaders which may be carried with it. Milk fat, liquid paraffin, cod-liver oil and the medicated nasal oils may all produce it. Macrophages which ingest the oily globules appear in the alveoli and the alveolar walls. The condition is mentioned here particularly as a warning against the indiscriminate use of oily nasal drops in weakly children or in feeble recumbent old people ; and against clumsy or forced feeding with milk or cod-liver oil of premature or semi-comatose children, or comatose adults.

In war-time, instances of this form of pneumonia are seen following the torpedoing of a ship and the aspiration of Diesel oil constituents into the lungs of survivors who have to swim in the contaminated water.

Traumatic pneumonia (see Chap. XXXII).

CHAPTER XIX

ABSCESS OF THE LUNG

ABSCESS of the lung is but the later stage of invasion by certain organisms whose access is usually by the air passages but may on occasion be by the blood stream. Infection associated with any form of septic bronchopneumonia, or following inhalation of a foreign body (Chap. VIII), or associated with bronchial obstruction due to new growth (Chap. X) or to aortic aneurysm, or due to straightforward streptococcal or other organismal invasion, may result in abscess formation. Septic emboli carried to the lung may produce metastatic abscesses which have a lobular distribution (see p. 229).

It is comparatively seldom that frank suppuration follows an ordinary bronchopneumonia due to infection by organisms unassociated with the inhalation of foreign matter ; examples have, however, been described in the preceding chapter. It is the *inhalation of infected material* such as may occur in septic conditions in the nose and pharynx, or during operations on the teeth, nose or throat, which is the determining factor. After tonsillectomy, for example, blood can be found in the bronchial tree in more than half the cases, and is especially likely to reach the more distal bronchi if the operation is done with the head at a higher level than the trunk. Nevertheless the defences of the lung can usually cope with this danger, for the incidence of lung abscess after tonsillectomy (with the head lowered) is much less than 1 per cent. Both in ordinary and in " inhalation " bronchopneumonia the development of lung abscess depends partly on the virulence of the infecting organisms, partly on poor bodily resistance, and partly on the seriousness of the interference with the normal defences. Such interference is seen, for example, when there is obstruction of one of the larger branches of the bronchial tree by a plug of blood clot, mucus, mucopus, infected debris or neoplastic tissue.

The essential pathological picture is that of an intensely destructive bronchopneumonia which goes on to purulent softening in and around the smaller bronchi or the terminal bronchioles of the affected areas. If the bronchopneumonia is patchy in distribution the necrotic areas are patchy also, and the resulting abscesses are small and multiple. If the necrotic areas run together into larger patches, the result may be one or two larger abscesses, or even a single large abscess. The latter may follow either confluent necrosing bronchopneumonia or, more commonly, extensive bronchopneumonia following obstruction of a segmental bronchus by a plug of septic material. Around the area of suppuration, large or small, there is a zone of consolidation. If the invasive advance is stemmed, the surrounding consolidation becomes occupied by fibroblasts, so that eventually the abscess cavity may be ringed round with fibrous tissue. When the necrotic material is liquefied it may be evacuated partially or completely via the bronchus which supplies the area. The fact that it is often coughed up with dramatic suddenness, leaving behind an aerated cavity (which can be clearly seen in an X-ray picture), strongly suggests that an occluding slough or plug in the bronchus has disintegrated and given way. Very rarely the bronchus remains permanently closed, and the abscess, if it does not rupture into the pleural cavity, becomes a distended purulent cyst.

Seeing that the essential lesion is a septic bronchopneumonia, it is clear on anatomical grounds that the larger abscesses must involve a considerable number of terminal bronchioles, with their related alveoli. Such abscesses soon approach the surface of the lung, therefore, and determine an adhesive pleurisy. Less commonly, the pleurisy is accompanied by effusion, which at first may be sterile, but which rapidly becomes infected. The clear, sterile exudate is given the name of " **reactionary effusion.**" It is, therefore, possible to withdraw pleural fluid which to-day is clear and sterile ; yet another sample obtained twenty-four hours later may be turbid and purulent. As a rule, by the time effusion is suspected and diagnostic paracentesis is performed, empyema is already present. Moreover, the effusion may, on occasion, be loculated, one loculus containing clear sterile fluid and an adjacent one pus. If the abscess communicates freely with a bronchus as well as with the pleural cavity, not only is air present as well as pus (pyopneumothorax), but the patient may expectorate copious amounts of sputum, continuing to do so as long as the empyema is undrained.

When the abscess is discharged through a bronchus its evacuation is often incomplete, the small bronchioles being too narrow for adequate drainage ; both they and the larger segmental bronchi become, moreover, considerably obstructed by swelling of the mucous membrane and by the formation of granulation tissue. Since the non-cartilaginous smaller bronchi are dilated by inspiration and contracted by expiration, it follows that when there is swelling of the mucous membrane the lumen may become completely closed during expiration and also, therefore, during the expiratory phase of coughing (see Fig. 104).

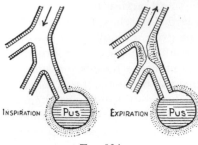

FIG. 104

To show the occlusion during expiration of narrowed bronchus supplying the abscess, with consequent failure of drainage.

When the abscess is completely evacuated via a bronchus, especially if the resulting cavity is small, healing may take place with fibrosis. More frequently, however, the evacuation is only partial. The relief of tension in the abscess may at first produce an appreciable degree of improvement in the condition of the patient ; nevertheless the persistently inadequate drainage results in the disease settling down to a prolonged subacute or chronic course. This is dangerous, not only because of the local chronic pulmonary suppuration, but also because at any time the pus may " spill over " into healthy zones of lung and cause suppurative bronchopneumonia there.

PUTRID ABSCESS OF THE LUNG

The old distinction between abscess and gangrene of the lung is perhaps more conveniently expressed by the terms " non-putrid abscess " and " putrid abscess," for the contrast is between simple necrosis and necrosis with putrefaction. Putrid abscess forms a considerable proportion of the lung abscesses of adults. The pathogenic organisms concerned are those associated with oral sepsis and pyorrhœa—anærobes, of which the most important are fusiform bacilli and spirilla. It has long been noticed that the odour of dental caries is identical with that of putrid lung abscess. The modern view is that these organisms are themselves the cause of the original bronchopneumonia and abscess, and not merely secondary invaders of a pneumonia or abscess already present.

Obvious occasions for the aspiration of unclean material from the mouth—ulcerating cancers, general anæsthesia, operations on the mouth, nose and throat, dental extractions, coma and immersion—account for less than half the cases. In the rest, the illness begins as an apparently severe influenza or bronchopneumonia, and the diagnosis is only revised or amplified when the patient begins to cough up large amounts of fœtid sputum. Sometimes the onset is rather insidious, with tiredness and malaise as the main features ; in these patients the infected material is most probably inhaled during

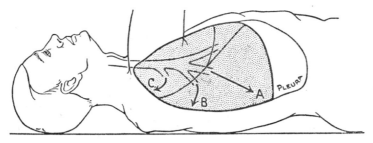

Fig. 105

To show the most usual sites of lung abscess following inhalations in the recumbent posture. B is the most likely site, then C, and then A (compare Fig. 26, p. 26).

sleep. It is known that a small amount of lipiodol left in the mouth at bedtime can be seen by radiograms to have entered the lung by the next morning. These abscesses are usually single and of fair size, involving a segmental zone of the lung ; the organisms are carried into the bronchial tree in a small occluding piece of particulate debris, the usual site of arrest being one of the smaller bronchi of the fourth or fifth order. It lodges in the right lung more often than the left, and the position of the thorax at the time of inhalation largely determines the segment of lung affected. If a patient lies on his back, foreign material is likely to flow into posterolateral segment of the right upper lobe and into the dorsal segments of the lower lobes. If he lies on his side, it gravitates into some part of the " axillary " region of the dependent upper lobe. As might be expected in the recumbent person, arrest may occur in branches of the posterior basic bronchus, of the dorsal bronchus of the lower lobe or of the posterior branch of the posterolateral division of the upper lobe (Fig. 105, A, B and C). The middle lobe or even the anterior part of the upper lobe may on occasion be involved.

The essential lesion is the same as that of a non-putrid abscess, namely, an intense, necrosing bronchopneumonia, in which the putrefactive organisms make their own foul-smelling addition to the clinical picture. Beyond the point where the lumen of the bronchus is occluded by necrotic debris, the septic bronchopneumonia passes on to necrosis and then to putrid liquefaction. The resulting abscess consists, therefore, of blood-stained, foul-smelling necrotic and purulent debris, maybe with a certain amount of gas produced by the anaerobes. Around it is a zone of bronchopneumonia, its extent depending on the intensity of the infection and on the resistance to it. As the infection is situated towards the periphery of the lung, pleurisy is likely to be an early feature, often resulting in thick pleural adhesions which obliterate the pleural space over the region of the abscess.

Meanwhile not only does the tension rise inside the abscess, but the occluding mass in the bronchus also gradually disintegrates and liquefies, so that by the tenth to the fourteenth day the plug is free of the wall, and is coughed up, followed by a large amount of foul sputum from the abscess itself. For a day or two before the bronchial lumen is thus reopened, gases may diffuse from the cavity through the occluding plug of debris, so that when the patient coughs, a whiff of fœtid air may be noticed even though as yet there is no sputum.

Following drainage through the bronchus, the stage is reached of a localised putrid abscess cavity, which is usually of comparatively large size and reaches close to the surface of the lung ; it is now partially filled with pus and partially with air. Around the cavity there is a more or less extensive zone of consolidation. As with non-putrid abscess, there may be accompanying adhesive pleurisy, "reactionary effusion" or putrid empyema.

When the invasion is overwhelming and the resistance poor, the necrosis and bronchopneumonia spread diffusely, with little or no attempt at localisation ; the affected lung tissue is soft and mushy, with small, ragged cavities in the middle of it.

If, in the less fulminating cases, there is a wide bronchial channel for the escape of the pus, the cavity may be completely evacuated, with eventual healing at the cost of scarring. In children, the greater elasticity of the lungs helps the obliteration of any type of abscess, provided that it is well drained. When drainage is incomplete, however, the lesion may spread either directly or by " spill over " to other bronchi, or it may remain apparently stabilised for weeks or even months, to break down again later. Other abscesses may then develop near by, and may come to communicate with the original one, so that in these more chronic cases a multilocular abscess may be finally seen in the midst of dense fibrous tissue. The " spill over " may even be into the bronchi of the opposite lung, causing secondary abscesses there.

Embolic abscesses—The pyæmic deposits are usually staphylococcal or streptococcal, multiple and small, and arise from such lesions as osteomyelitis, lateral sinus infection which complicates otitis, and infective thrombophlebitis in the pelvis or elsewhere. As most of the deposits are subpleural in site, the danger of rupture into the pleural cavity is considerable, with consequent empyema or pyopneumothorax. Rarely they may discharge into a neighbouring bronchus, and then cough and expectoration develop. Most commonly, however, the condition in the lung is overshadowed by the fulminating systemic infection, so that the abscesses in the lung are found only at autopsy.

Abscesses by extension may occur from suppuration in adjacent organs such as the vertebræ or the mediastinum. Those which follow *subdiaphragmatic infection* or liver abscess are discussed in Chapter XXVI. *Bronchiectatic abscess cavities* are described in Chapter IX. *Post-traumatic abscess* may follow bruising, crushing or penetrating injuries to the chest (Chap. XXXII). The ragged necrotic *abscess following the breakdown of neoplastic masses* has been referred to in Chapter X.

SYMPTOMS AND SIGNS

A typical history of the onset of lung abscess is as follows : two or three days after tonsillectomy or other operation in which there is a risk of inhalation of infected material, the patient feels a sense of malaise which gradually increases. The temperature rises, irregular pyrexia continues and he may have a rigor. A short, irritable and unproductive cough develops, which may be accompanied sooner or later by a sharp pain in the side of the chest. At first the condition is liable to be regarded as a simple bronchitis or bronchopneumonia following the anæsthetic. Soon, however, frank pleurisy is established, with breathlessness, drenching sweats, and maybe cyanosis. The patient is now very ill and a diagnosis of acute broncho-pneumonia may be made. After ten days or a fortnight of grave illness the medical attendant may notice, if the under-lying abscess is putrid, a foul smell when the patient coughs, even though there is as yet hardly any expectoration ; or the patient himself may complain of a filthy taste in the mouth. Meanwhile, owing to the intense bronchial inflammation and ulceration, hæmoptysis is common, either in the form of blood-streaked sputum or as a more profuse hæmorrhage. Rarely, ulceration of a large artery or vein causes bleeding which is fatal.

A day or two after the foul odour has been detected in the breath, the patient has a bout of coughing which is accom-panied initially by a blood-stained plug of sputum, and then by the evacuation of a large amount of pus—yellowish-green if the abscess is simple, dirty and stinking if the abscess is putrid. Evacuation of a non-putrid abscess is not preceded by diffusion of foul gases through the occluding plug. The filthy taste of the pus from a putrid abscess may lead the patient to describe it as " like a midden," or in other such expressive terms. If empyema is also present, together with a bronchial fistula communicating both with the pleural cavity and the lung abscess, the patient may expectorate not only the contents of the abscess but also a considerable portion of the empyema ; as much as a pint or more of pus may thus be evacuated over a short period of time. Occasionally the bursting of an abscess and empyema into the bronchial tree floods the lungs and suffocates the patient.

Sometimes the illness presents itself apparently as a pneumonia obviously complicated by pleural effusion or em-pyema. The fluid may be clear, straw-coloured and sterile ; such cells as are found in it, after centrifugalisation, are poly-morphonuclear leucocytes. Within a few hours, the period varying according to the severity of the pulmonary infection, a further diagnostic paracentesis reveals that the effusion has become purulent. Often, however, the diagnosis of fluid in the pleural cavity is not made until after the stage of " reactionary effusion " ; paracentesis then reveals a turbid or frankly purulent fluid.

In cases with a more insidious onset, the clinical picture is liable at first to be regarded as one of influenza. As the illness takes its course, influenzal bronchopneumonia is suspected. Finally, the diagnosis becomes clear when the patient suddenly coughs up a large quantity of pus, with resulting cavitation seen on the X-ray film.

The **physical signs** in the chest depend on the situation and size of the abscess, and on the surrounding infiltration. In any case they are usually slight and unconvincing in the early stages of the disease. There may be a pleural rub, a local area of dulness to percussion and weak breath sounds. Owing to the congestion and œdema around the abscess, crepitations may be heard, or more rarely the signs of consolidation may be discovered. After evacuation of the pus and the formation of a sizeable, aerated cavity, the signs of cavitation become evident, provided that the bronchus is open and allows the entry and exit of air during respiration. Small abscesses do not necessarily show the signs of cavitation, being lost in the surrounding consolidation ; nor do larger abscesses, when the bronchus of supply is occluded by granulation tissue. The tiny disseminated abscesses of pyæmia show either no local signs at all or else the signs only of the surrounding patches of bronchopneumonia. When pleural effusion develops, the signs of fluid in the pleural space overshadow those of the underlying pulmonary lesion (see Chap. XXIV).

Clubbing of the fingers occurs early in patients in whom the drainage of the abscess is inefficient ; as a rule it is established within the first six or eight weeks. Except in fulminating infections where there is no resistance, the *blood count* shows a polymorphonuclear leucocytosis of 20,000 to 30,000. The *sputum* contains many pus cells, with a mixed growth of organisms, though sometimes the predominant infectors are obvious ; elastic tissue and pieces of necrotic lung are found in the acute destructive phase.

THE COURSE OF THE DISEASE

To sum up, the course of the disease may take one of three main directions. The suppurative necrosing bronchopneumonia may advance relentlessly, and death comes before there is any effective localisation. In the less fulminating cases there is free drainage, the abscess being coughed up through a wide bronchial communication ; the surrounding infiltration subsides, the cavity is gradually obliterated by scar tissue, and a cure follows. In many cases, however, there is a limited degree of recovery only : drainage is inadequate and the resistance of the patient is poor : the acute phase passes gradually into the **subacute** or **chronic** stage. With large abscesses, and especially with putrid abscesses, the last of these three courses is the usual one. Irregular fever then continues. There may be periods when the pus is locked up in the cavity, and then fever is high and persistent, toxæmia is severe, while the cough and expectoration diminish. Later, the retained pus may be discharged, suddenly or gradually, with consequent increase of cough and expectoration, and diminution of pyrexia and toxæmia. The cough may be paroxysmal and brought on by a change of position by which some of the pus may flow from the abscess into the bronchial tree. From time to time hæmoptysis may occur. Once localisation has taken place and the abscess become chronic, dyspnœa may be comparatively slight, save on exertion. Sooner or later intense fatigue from toxæmia, loss of weight and strength, and profound secondary anæmia become prominent.

Although the patient in the subacute or chronic phase may hold his own for a time, eventually he dies from a fresh attack of bronchopneumonia, from cerebral or other metastatic abscesses (the septic embolus originating in thrombosed vessels in the wall of the cavity) or from amyloid disease. Not many patients with chronic lung abscess, especially of the putrid type, survive longer than three years from the onset.

Radiology is of the utmost help and may be the only way of clinching the diagnosis. In the acute phase the dark shadow of bronchopneumonia and necrosis, with the surrounding infiltration, establishes the site of the lesion but does not throw much light on its nature. Not until pus is discharged and air enters can cavitation be recognised. A " fluid level " in the cavity shows that pus is still present and that drainage is therefore incomplete ; this fluid level varies according to the amount of pus contained in the cavity. As the condition improves, the surrounding shadow of pulmonary infiltration diminishes. It must be borne in mind that an abscess in the dorsal lobe shows as an apparently hilar lesion in the anterior or posterior X-ray film, but a lateral film reveals the true situation (compare Figs. 22 and 23, p. 24). This is but one illustration of the importance of taking both anterior and lateral films for the localisation of an abscess. Furthermore, it must be remembered that a collection of small cavities seen on the film may in fact represent the several loculi of a single multilocular abscess.

Lipiodol does not, as a rule, enter the opaque area or the abscess cavity, for the communicating bronchus is usually obstructed by œdematous swelling, granulations or pus.

Bronchoscopy is necessary in almost every case, even when the abscess is still acute, for it is vital to make sure that there is not an underlying foreign body, and wise to exclude a primary bronchial neoplasm. It may also help in accurate localisation of the abscess by demonstrating the particular bronchus from which pus is oozing ; the bronchus which communicates directly with the cavity cannot usually be seen, being a smaller one (or more) which drains at one or two removes into the visible bronchus.

Exploration of a lung for suspected abscess by needling through the chest wall and possibly a still uninfected pleural cavity, is thoroughly bad practice ; it may produce empyema, pleurobronchial fistula and serious infection of the chest wall.

DIAGNOSIS

The actual dividing line between the original bronchopneumonia and the formation of an abscess is not easily recognised at the bedside. The clinical picture is at first that of a severe bronchopneumonia. The fever persists and becomes " septic " in type. One or two weeks after the onset of the disease there is usually a sudden, considerable increase in the amount of sputum. This sudden coughing up of a considerable amount of pus containing elastic tissue and maybe pieces of necrosed lung is the most suggestive diagnostic feature. The course of *acute tuberculous bronchopneumonia* with subsequent cavitation may be mistaken for that of septic bronchopneumonia followed by lung abscess ; but with caseation and breakdown of lung tissue, tubercle bacilli are found in the sputum. *Foreign body in the bronchus* and *bronchial neoplasm* must always be excluded even when an abscess is obviously present.

Bronchiectasis following absorption collapse of the lung may become secondarily infected, so that finally actual abscess cavities are formed (Chap. IX) ; here, however, the pus is usually discharged easily by postural drainage, after which lipiodol flows readily into the cavities so that they are well delineated in the X-ray film.

Sterile pleural effusion ("reactionary effusion") has to be differentiated from acute *tuberculous pleurisy with effusion*. The reactionary effusion rapidly becomes purulent, often in a few hours. *Pyothorax* or *pyopneumothorax* are so often the result of an abscess which is near the pleural surface that this possibility must always be kept in mind. The typical symptoms and course of pulmonary abscess are of great help in diagnosis ; as also is radiology, especially after the abscess has been coughed up or the empyema drained. Sometimes it is possible to demonstrate the existence of a pleural fistula by means of lipiodol.

Interlobar empyema has to be regarded, for purposes of treatment, as a form of lung abscess. If it ruptures into a bronchus, the expectorated pus does not contain elastic fibres unless there has been accompanying destruction of adjacent lung tissue. Radiologically it appears towards the hilum in the anterior film, and along the line of the interlobar fissure, usually about the mid-zone, in the lateral view (see Fig. 109, p. 391).

Other forms of pulmonary cavitation are not, as a rule, difficult to distinguish from lung abscess. In practice, the most difficult problem is to decide, not whether an abscess is present, but whether or not it is part of the picture of bronchial carcinoma (see p. 137). Hence the importance of bronchoscopic examination before treatment is undertaken.

PROGNOSIS

The chances of spontaneous healing depend largely on the extent of the necrosis and the existence of a wide bronchial channel of drainage. If an inhaled foreign body is the cause, its early removal is often followed by complete cure. Abscesses in the upper lobes obviously can drain continuously and well, by reason of gravity, provided that there is no obstruction to the outflow, and so they are more likely to heal spontaneously than those in the middle or lower lobes. Whenever the drainage is poor, by reason of swelling of the mucous membrane or of obstructing granulation tissue, healing is unlikely, and the abscess becomes subacute or chronic. It has already been said that the outlook is best in children, always provided that the bronchial drainage is good ; their younger, more elastic lungs can compensate adequately for the subsequent scar of healing. At most, however, only one in five putrid abscesses heals spontaneously ; unless healing occurs within a month or two of the initial expectoration of the pus, it is unlikely to do so later. The rest, if untreated or wrongly treated, become chronic and usually kill the patient within three years. Rupture of a small abscess into the pleural cavity sometimes results in healing of the lung, provided that the resulting pyothorax is properly drained, though the patient passes through a stormy illness and is fortunate to survive.

TREATMENT

The pathology of the disease gives the best guide to treatment. Initially the illness is a bronchopneumonia, the only stage at which sulphonamides can be effective. Once necrosis has occurred, or pus formed, it is idle to expect these drugs to cure an abscess, though they may help to prevent the spread of pneumonic infiltration around it. Early in the illness, it is impossible to know whether the initial bronchopneumonia will become a necrotising one, leading to lung abscess (putrid or non-putrid). This makes it all the more important to treat any patient suffering from bronchopneumonia with early and adequate doses of sulphonamide, or if this fails, with penicillin. Most non-putrid lung abscesses are caused by the hæmolytic streptococcus ; adequate chemotherapy given during the initial bronchopneumonic phase might well prevent many of them.

Non-putrid abscesses do not contain sloughs of lung tissue, which so often interfere with proper drainage of a putrid abscess. The likelihood of spontaneous cure following discharge of the abscess contents via a bronchus, with subsequent obliteration of the cavity, is therefore much greater than in the putrid abscess. For this reason, the physician can afford to give a much longer time to the hope of recovery without surgical interference.

Once a pulmonary abscess is formed, treatment is conditioned by the efficiency or otherwise of the bronchial drainage. If there is a sufficiently wide channel communicating with the abscess cavity, postural drainage will probably empty it, and keep it empty ; the patient must adopt the position most suitable for the outflow of the pus, and therefore an accurate localisation of the abscess is essential. If this fails, broncho-scopic drainage will almost certainly fail also, for the barrier to adequate drainage is likely to be beyond the range of bronchoscopic manipulation. The first diagnostic broncho-scopic examination may sometimes disturb the occluding plug, and good results are then immediate. A jolting journey on a stretcher or in an ambulance, or heavy percussion of the chest, may have the same effect.

A young man was sent into hospital with the diagnosis of tuberculous pleural effusion. Some weeks before, he had been operated upon for perforated gastric ulcer, and later he developed pulmonary symptoms and a sterile pleural effusion at the base of the right lung. During a ward clinic the patient was demonstrated to a group of clinical clerks, several of whom were allowed to percuss his chest. The group retired from the bedside to the middle of the ward to discuss the diagnosis. The alternatives of tuberculous pleural effusion, and lung abscess with " reactionary effusion " following abdominal infection, were being thrashed out, when the man obligingly started to cough, bringing up a gobbet of blood-stained sputum. Paroxysmal coughing over a period of about half an hour then brought up a large cupful of frank pus.* He had had a subphrenic infection which had passed through the diaphragmatic lymphatics to the lung (see Chap. XXVI), developed a septic bronchopneumonia at the right base and finally two or three abscesses in the parenchyma of the lung, one of which was of considerable size. The pleural effusion was a sterile " reactionary effusion."

Inadequate drainage is indicated by the persistence of pus in the cavity (shown on the X-ray film by a fluid level) after two weeks, and by the continuance of an obviously

* This happy issue—for it finally cured the patient—hardly justifies the student in percussing with a mutton fist. Wilfred Trotter wrote the following : " When you ask a patient if you are hurting him, nine times out of ten he will reply with touching cheerfulness, ' Not yet, Doctor.' What a succession of iron thumbs is disclosed by that answer ! Some extremists have thought that the man who has the handling of sick human bodies should make himself ambidextrous. I do not subscribe to that, but I sometimes think the student would do well to limit himself to the possession of only one left hand."

considerable zone of infiltration around it. This may happen
even though, owing to partial drainage and the relief of tension
in the abscess, the clinical condition of the patient appreciably
improves. It is not enough, however, to convert an acute
abscess into a subacute or chronic one ; the gravity of the
prognosis remains, even though the disease is not immediately
fatal, and though there may be periods of long remission of the
most serious symptoms. Once the condition is diagnosed the
doctor must be content only if its course is set to complete
healing. If the disease spreads, or even if it merely " hangs
fire," the sooner the abscess is drained externally the better
for the patient, especially if it is of the putrid variety. Here,
the sloughs of lung tissue behave much as does a dead bony
sequestrum in osteomyelitis. They keep up the chronic suppuration, with all its risks of spread of infection elsewhere in
the lungs, and until they are removed, recovery is impossible.
Such chronic suppuration often results eventually in a lobe
which consists almost wholly of dense fibrous tissue riddled
with cavities filled with pus—a rubbery, sponge-like purulent
mass, impossible to drain effectively, and necessitating a difficult
and hazardous surgical excision of the whole diseased area.
Penicillin, therefore, must not become a substitute for sound
surgical principles.

Within a few weeks it will become clear whether the abscess
is likely to heal with medical treatment and postural drainage.
If the infection is obviously spreading, external drainage done
early may save the patient. Surgical access is through the
adhesions between the pleural layers which lie over the infected
area, or through adhesions artificially induced. The acute
lesion with diffuse septic bronchopneumonia and necrosis, at
the centre of which many small abscess cavities are found, is
often dealt with by coagulation and excision by means of the
diathermy loop. The less acute abscesses with a defined wall
are drained by a free opening. Chronic abscesses with thick
fibrous walls of long standing may need excision of the whole
lobe. If well-formed pleural adhesions are not present the
operation must be done in two stages, the first stage being
devoted to ensuring that adhesions are formed ; for the dangers
of allowing infected material to reach a free pleural cavity are
so serious that they must be avoided at all costs. At the same
time the skin, subcutaneous and muscle layers are sewn together

at the edges of the wound, so as to reduce the danger, during drainage, of grave cellulitis in the chest wall.

More and more it is becoming clear that for putrid abscess early operation is in the best interests of the patient ; the time for it is when medical treatment ceases to show clear progress towards complete recovery. Later, when healing has taken place, there may be so much fibrosis that relaxation of the affected lung becomes advisable ; this can often be obtained by phrenic paralysis. Artificial pneumothorax has no place in the treatment of lung abscess. It may increase the pressure in it, thereby increasing the toxæmia ; or it may tear apart pleural adhesions and cause a fatal pyopneumothorax.

CHAPTER XX

PULMONARY TUBERCULOSIS

IT has been said that if a teacher were allowed one subject only wherewith to teach the principles of medicine, tuberculosis would be the disease of choice. It is a meeting ground of pathologist, radiologist, medical officer of health, physician and surgeon ; nor can its medical problems be disentangled from the economic and social life of the human community.

THE MICRO-ORGANISM

A full description of the types and characteristics of tubercle bacilli may be read in bacteriological textbooks. Here it is sufficient to emphasise certain points. In the tuberculosis of human beings the human and bovine types of bacilli are the only ones which matter. They are aerobic and non-motile. Whatever the variety, they stain with difficulty. They contain a waxy substance which is resistant to acids and alcohol after coloration with certain aniline dyes ; thus they are " acid-fast." They can be cultured only on special media and grow very slowly. In culturing material such as milk, where numerous other organisms may be present, these latter may crowd out the more slowly growing tubercle bacillus and prevent its development on the medium ; use is therefore made of the high susceptibility of the guinea-pig to tuberculosis for diagnostic guinea-pig inoculation. The bacillus contains a protein which determines allergic reactions, and a polysaccharide which is a factor in certain humoral reactions ; these latter are as yet of no particular clinical interest. Except to direct sunlight, the bacillus is (apart from spore-bearing organisms) one of the most resistant pathogenic micro-organisms known, the more so when it is protected by a mucoid envelope of sputum. Being so tenacious of life, it is a widespread infector. The bovine bacillus grows differently and less readily on culture than the human. It is more virulent for cattle and most other lower animals than for man ; inoculation into rabbits is used as a convenient way of distinguishing the two types.

MODES AND PORTALS OF ENTRY

Sputum is the primary source of the human type of tuberculosis ; the bacilli are spread through droplet infection, by infected dust, or by ingestion from the fingers and mouth. The latter is especially important in children who play on dusty floors and convey infection from fingers and toys to their mouths, whence the bacilli are swallowed into the alimentary tract or inhaled into the lungs. Milk and its products (butter and cheese) are the great source of infection by the bovine bacillus ; the lesions occur particularly in young children, and involve sites infected from the alimentary tract—cervical glands which drain the pharynx, the intestine, the peritoneum and the abdominal glands. It has been estimated that some 40 per cent. of cattle in this country have tuberculous lesions somewhere in the body, and that about 10 per cent. of all samples of milk contain living tubercle bacilli. The domesticated cow may in its career produce some 2000 gals. of milk, as against the 150 gals. of the wild cow ; the high incidence of bovine tuberculosis is no doubt Nature's nemesis for human exploitation. The prevention of this menace at the source by building up tubercle-free herds is a matter of long-term national agricultural policy. Here and there individual attempts are made to produce clean, tubercle-free milk from tuberculin-tested cows, encouraged partly by the demand from intelligent parents and partly by Governmental recognition of different grades of milk ; but they hardly touch the surface of the problem. Meanwhile the dangers of dirty milk containing living tubercle bacilli can be lessened only by pasteurisation (at 143° F. for thirty minutes) or by boiling.

Obviously the incidence of human infection with the bovine bacillus will vary from country to country, according to the amount of tuberculosis in cattle and of the consumption of raw milk. If the figures available are examined it will be seen that lesions due to the bovine bacillus are, on the whole, less severe, and tend to be localised to the glands of the neck, to the tracheo-bronchial glands, or to the glands of the abdomen. Nevertheless there is a serious amount of bone and joint, meningeal and generalised tuberculosis of the bovine type in infancy and early childhood.

Inhaled into the lung alveoli or ingested into the pharynx or intestine, the tubercle bacillus may produce a lesion where it lodges ; this is usual in the lung, but not so common in the alimentary tract. In any case the bacilli are treated by the body as foreign particles, engulfed by wandering macrophages and carried through the tissue spaces into the lymphatics, eventually to reach the corresponding lymph nodes. The initial lesion depends partly on the virulence of the organism (and for practical purposes this is entirely a matter of its type) and on the dose, and partly on the resistance of the host. The results of this interplay will be discussed later.

THE INTERACTION OF " SEED " AND " SOIL "

Tuberculosis is no longer " the captain of the men of death." Over the last hundred years its mortality has been steadily falling, and there is no longer the same universality of infection. At the end of the nineteenth century almost every-one, certainly in the cities, became infected by tuberculosis sooner or later, though the great majority never developed clinical signs of active disease. Looked for by the tuberculin test or at autopsy, tuberculous infection was found to be almost universal among adults. It was estimated, for example, that in densely populated areas some 15 per cent. were infected in the first decade of life, 30 to 60 per cent. in the second, and 99 per cent. by the sixth or seventh decade. Most tuberculous infections, however, become quiescent and heal, unrecognised by the patient or his family. Obviously the power of the body to withstand the infection is very great. Why is it that less than one in sixty of the persons nowadays infected by tubercle bacilli fall ill with clinically recognisable, progressive tuberculous disease ?

The answer lies in the interplay of " seed " and " soil." It may be that the " seed " is now less common than it was, possibly because (as some think) we are coming towards the end-phase of an epidemic of tuberculosis which has extended over a period of a century or more. There is no doubt, how-ever, that given sufficiently intimate contact with tubercle bacilli, infection is almost inevitable, and this is underlined by the fact that it is particularly a " family disease." Where preventive measures and health education have been widely adopted, they are now bearing fruit in the reduction of opportunities for contact with infecting tubercle bacilli. It has already been noted that while the human type of bacillus is more virulent for man than the bovine, there is little if any difference in virulence among bacilli of the same type.

Of the factors which influence the " soil," environment is the most important. It is not established whether inherited differences of resistance (racial, familial or individual) exist or not. The periods of greatest stress are undoubtedly the most dangerous for the development of active tuberculous disease. Puberty, pregnancy, lactation and the menopause may all lower natural resistance ; so also may excess of work or play, prolonged exhaustion and any grave physical, mental or emotional strain. The decline in the death rate from tuberculosis has one outstanding exception which emphasises the seriousness of environmental stress : it does not hold for females between 15 and 25 years of age, a time when girls emerge into womanhood and enter the rough and tumble of industry, or the period of full reproductive power, with its consequent domestic cares. Modern war with its resulting fatigues of body and mind, and poverty with its malnutrition, bad housing, overcrowding, and poor hygienic and medical facilities, contribute gravely to impoverishment of the " soil." Industrial diseases such as silicosis, and debilitating illnesses, of which diabetes mellitus and influenza are outstanding examples, also play their part.

The " soil " may be further modified by the reaction of the body itself to tuberculous infection, particularly by the development of acquired immunity and of allergic sensitivity to tuberculo-protein.

TUBERCLE BACILLI AND THE TISSUES

Wherever the point of entry of the bacilli the same fundamental types of reaction may occur. The bacilli may be overcome before they can do any damage, or they may multiply and produce a lesion, slowly progressive or fulminant according to the strength of the defensive reaction. If they gain a foothold they damage the surrounding tissue cells and also destroy some of the leucocytes which have ingested them. The resulting microscopic collection of dead tissue and leucocytes then attracts phagocytic cells ; these large mononuclear macrophages, the so-called "epithelioid cells," ingest the dead material and many of the tubercle bacilli, and form a *cordon sanitaire* round the focus. Some of these cells become multinucleated to form giant cells which are typical of inflammation around a foreign body. Outside this *tuberculous follicle* there may develop an irregular zone of infiltration with lymphocytes. A single follicle, or a coalescing group of smaller ones, may at length become large enough to be visible to the naked eye as a compact greyish nodule which later may become cream-coloured—the *miliary tubercle*. The change in appearance from grey to cream is due to coagulation necrosis (*caseation*). The necrosis is caused partly by the avascularity of the tubercle, but mainly by toxic substances derived from tubercle bacilli in the nodule.

This is the fundamental pattern of the clash between the invading tubercle bacilli and the body, but obviously it must vary according to the balance between the attack and the defence. If the invasion is feeble (few bacilli, especially if they are of the less virulent bovine type) and the bodily resistance good, the bacilli may be killed outright, or a tubercle which has developed may be completely absorbed, or it may be walled off by fibrosis. Even a small area of caseation may be removed by macrophages and leave no trace ; usually, however, it is either replaced by scar tissue or more commonly it undergoes calcification. Even so, the lesion cannot be regarded as absolutely healed. Some bacilli may still remain alive inside the imprisoning fibrosis or the calcium deposit in the lesion or in the neighbouring lymph nodes, and are able to resume their evil activities, perhaps years later, if bodily resistance breaks down or if some injury bruises or tears the tissue.

If, on the other hand, the invasion is heavy and the resistance poor, a limiting barrier of macrophages and fibrous tissue is never established ; the bacilli multiply rapidly, are carried through the feeble defences and fan out into the surrounding tissue. The only evidence of an attempt at defence is an acute inflammatory exudate containing some mononuclear macrophages, many bacilli, much fibrin and maybe red blood corpuscles. Caseation (coagulation necrosis), without the formation of tubercles, spreads rapidly through the affected tissue.

Tuberculo-protein liberated from dead bacilli produces **allergic sensitivity,** which takes about six weeks to develop and which henceforward profoundly modifies the reactions of the body to further doses of tuberculo-protein, in this way altering the quality of the " soil." It is probably due to an antibody accumulated on the surfaces of cells, which in contact with the antigenic tuberculo-protein forms a poison which damages or kills the cell. Thus there is produced an œdematous or exudative allergic inflammation, and, if the reaction is severe, marked necrosis of tissue wherever the bacilli lodge. This allergy determines the positive reaction to tuberculin tests. In children especially it may manifest itself at a distance in the form of pleural effusion, erythema nodosum, *lichen scrofulosorum* or phlyctenular conjunctivitis.

Another factor which modifies the " soil " and influences the response of the body to tuberculous infection is the development of a certain degree of **immunity.** Immunity is quite distinct from allergy, and is not due to the allergic inflammatory reaction. It depends essentially on a combination of cellular (mononuclear, " epithelioid " phagocytes) and humoral (agglutinating antibody) reaction, whereby the invading bacilli are fixed at the point of entry, and then killed and digested by macrophages.

It is clear, therefore, that the reaction of the body to a first invasion of tubercle bacilli will differ from that to a reinfection. Depending on the strength of the invading force, first infections usually result either in trivial lesions which heal almost without symptoms, or in rapidly progressive and diffuse lesions with a grave prognosis. On the other hand, provided that an overwhelming dose of bacilli does not produce an intense, necrotising allergic reaction, reinfections are more likely to produce tuberculous formations which, because of the enhanced resistance of the body, are limited and chronic. For this reason reinfections are apt to develop insidiously, a factor which helps to explain why some 85 per cent. of cases of pulmonary tuberculosis of the " adult " type are not diagnosed until the disease has become extensive.

Immunity is, unfortunately, far from absolute. It modifies rather than prevents reinfection, and can be readily nullified by anything which impoverishes the " soil," or by excessive doses of infecting bacilli.

INFECTION OF THE LUNGS WITH TUBERCLE BACILLI

A first infection on " virgin soil " may occur at any age, though most first contacts with the organism are likely to occur in children. The First World War provided a striking example of widespread infection at a later age. Senegalese troops hitherto uninfected with tubercle bacilli (only about 2 per cent. of them reacted positively to the tuberculin test) came to France. Subjected to exposure to already infected Europeans, and later to each other, in crowded barracks and elsewhere, large numbers of them developed rapidly progressive pulmonary tuberculosis, many of them dying from generalised miliary dissemination.

Tubercle bacilli aspirated into the lungs usually reach the periphery, so that one or more subpleural lesions form at the site of implantation—the **primary focus.** Involvement of the bronchial lymphatic nodes and of the hilar glands draining the area follows. The primary focus (*Ghon's focus*) is usually a rounded, discrete subpleural lesion up to 1 cm. in diameter, and may be situated in any of the lobes. This lesion, together with the tuberculous lymphangitis and the infected hilar glands, form the **primary complex.** A similar primary focus may occur in the abdomen, the pharynx or, rarely, the skin, with enlargement of the corresponding lymphatic glands.

The results produced by primary infection of the lungs depend to some extent on the age of the subject and on his natural resistance, but mainly on the size and frequency of the infecting dose. An infant withstands it far less than an older child, and adults of " non-tuberculinised " communities (native races, for example) are liable to suffer severely. The death rate of children below the age of 1 year infected with tubercle bacilli is at least 36 per cent., as contrasted with 4 per cent. in the age group 3 to 7 years and 0·8 per cent. in the group 7 to 16 years. With minimal doses of bacilli, complete recovery may take place without any obvious infection of the bronchial or hilar glands. In mild or only moderate degrees of infection a primary focus is formed, the corresponding glands are infected, and later, as allergy develops, a perifocal inflammation may occur. Usually this eventually subsides and the primary focus heals by means of encapsulating fibrosis and the later deposition of calcium salts in the caseous centre (*calcification*). Healing takes considerable time—several months at least, and maybe two to four years. Caseous glands heal even more slowly.

In most children, therefore, particularly after the age of 2 years, the infection is arrested and healed at the stage of the primary complex, and there is little disturbance of health. Sometimes the child does not thrive for a time, and sometimes he develops a recognisable mild fever about six weeks after the primary infection. The first warnings may be illnesses which manifest a localised sensitivity to tuberculo-protein. In infants and young children under 3 years it may be *phlyctenular conjunctivitis*, which occurs some two to three months after the primary infection. Another manifestation which is rare in children under 3 but common in later childhood and adolescence is *erythema nodosum*, appearing about six weeks after the infection. *Lichen scrofulosorum*, appearing especially on the trunk, may also occur as a response to high sensitivity. *Allergic pleural effusion* is most commonly seen some six to twelve months after the initial infection.

Within two to three months after the primary infection, therefore, the primary complex has been formed and allergy established. When the lesion is not arrested at this stage the disease becomes progressive, and spreads in one or more ways which are determined by the anatomy of the lungs. It may infiltrate through the defences locally. It may advance along the lymphatic channels. Caseous material may be discharged into one of the smaller bronchi, from the lung (leaving behind a **cavity**) or from a peribronchial gland, and be coughed or sucked into other parts of the lungs. A caseating gland at the hilum may ulcerate into a large bronchus, so that the portion of lung supplied by it is flooded with tubercle bacilli which then cause a massive tuberculous bronchopneumonia. Erosion of a blood vessel may result in the dissemination of bacilli through the circulation—into the lung capillaries if a branch of the pulmonary artery or a vein such as the azygos is involved, and elsewhere over the body if the discharge is into a pulmonary vein. The former mechanism explains the occasional development of miliary tuberculosis confined to the lungs : usually fatal, but which rarely may become chronic and even heal. The latter mechanism may result in generalised miliary tuberculosis, and in more isolated systemic lesions such as tuberculous disease of bones and joints, kidneys or brain and meninges.

It must be remembered that, though bone and joint tuberculosis may follow infection with the bovine type of bacillus, it is more frequently caused by the human type. In England three out of every four cases in children under the age of 5 years are due to the human bacillus, and four out of every five in children over 5 years. In Scotland, where there is more bovine tuberculosis, the proportion is less. Healing of a tuberculous lesion of bone is very slow, and until this is achieved the danger of wider dissemination and especially of tuberculous meningitis remains. In the brain small tuberculomata result from dissemination through the systemic circulation ; if the local resistance is ineffective, submeningeal deposits rupture into the subarachnoid space and cause meningitis. Most attacks of tuberculous meningitis occur about one to two months after the first manifestation of the primary infection, and both it and generalised miliary tuberculosis seldom develop later than three months after it. It has been seen, however, that this rule is not absolute. They may occur at any time during the prolonged course of bone and joint tuberculosis, and also during the rare but again protracted activity of tuberculosis of the kidneys. Wallgren, the Scandinavian physician, who has done so much to establish the true picture of tuberculosis in childhood, has a dictum that there are " two essentially different danger periods "—a statement which is generally true, but with exceptions. The first period is the first three months after the onset of primary tuberculosis, children under the age of 3 years being especially threatened. When the child has safely passed this danger he enters into a rather harmless stage which lasts until the beginning of puberty, when the second danger period begins. It follows, then, that if a child does not develop a progressive lung lesion or complication (in bone, meninges or kidney particularly) within six months of its primary infection, the primary complex is well on the way to healing and is clinically quiescent, and the danger of meningitis or other tuberculous lesions of childhood can reasonably be regarded as past.

Very rarely infection passes into the lungs from a primary abdominal lesion. Sometimes it is carried by the systemic circulation to the heart and thence to the lungs; rarely it is borne along the lymphatic channels into the thoracic glands, one of which later erodes a bronchus and so discharges tubercle bacilli into the bronchial tree.

"**Epituberculosis**" is the name given to an afebrile and benign form of pulmonary lesion characterised by a radiological shadow suggestive of consolidation. It is accompanied by few or no symptoms, and the shadow slowly clears, maybe after many months, leaving a calcified nodule behind at its centre. In effect, "epituberculosis" is a radiological diagnosis which is supported by the subsequent benign course of the condition. In practice the term is liable to be used to cover various pathological conditions—a low-grade tuberculous broncho-pneumonic infiltration, a perifocal allergic inflammation or exudate, or collapse of a portion of lung following tuberculous bronchitis or pressure of an enlarged gland on a bronchus.

" CONTACT INFECTION "

While tuberculosis in childhood is usually benign, the same cannot be said for the period of infancy and the first two years. Infancy clearly affords the greatest opportunity for massive and repeated doses of bacilli, coughed up often unsuspectingly by a mother, father or old " bronchitic " grandparent. " There is more than one way of telling whether or not an adult has an open tuberculous lesion : one can find the bacilli in his sputum, or one can find the infection in his baby " (Park). There are still many households like that of the Brontë family. Mrs Brontë died of consumption when Charlotte was 4 years old, and all but one of her children eventually died of the disease.

Whatever the age, however, it is important to recognise tuberculous infection as early as possible. The significance of the tuberculous allergic illnesses has already been noted ; they are rare in infancy and are therefore not often available as diagnostic signals. There are two guiding principles which will help : to take heed of any known exposure to infection, and to watch for the development of sensitivity to tuberculo-protein.

The key to the former lies in the family ; infecting " chance contacts " are relatively uncommon. Whenever a member of the family is found to be suffering from pulmonary tuberculosis the other members should be examined for infection, especially the children. A tuberculin test should be made and an X-ray film of the chest should be taken. As an example of the importance of such investigations, Opie found that 75 per cent. of children under 5 years who had had contact with a " sputum-positive " case were sensitive to the tuberculin test, and 37 per cent. of them had lesions revealed by a radiogram ; whereas only about 30 per cent. who had had no known contact with a patient with open tuberculosis (that is, with tubercle bacilli discovered in the sputum) had a positive tuberculin test, and only 1·2 per cent. had a lesion shown on the X-ray film. Moreover, since some of these children had been in contact with patients with a " negative sputum," it is possible that they had encountered occasional tubercle bacilli coughed up but not discovered in the sputum. Of those exposed to known infection, one in three developed calcified nodules in the lungs, and one in five suffered from progressive pulmonary lesions. Other figures suggest that at least 40 per cent. of children who show a positive tuberculin test before the age of 2 years die from acute tuberculosis before the age of 5. It is obvious, therefore, how foolish is the idea that it is better not to try to shield a child from infective persons or infected milk in the hope that he will develop immunity ; in any case, there can be no control of the dose of tubercle bacilli administered, and immunity is an insecure reed on which to lean.

The detection of contact infection, and the subsequent steps necessary, concern at least three interested parties—the individual and his family, the family doctor, and the community (represented by the doctor of the tuberculosis services). It is a difficult team to harness together. Whatever the present " spirit of the age," the family remains the fundamental social unit, whereas State and municipality are but convenient instruments for promoting and supplying certain social needs. For various reasons the family doctor has now but little part in dealing with the disease ; nor can his colleagues of municipal and State services be content with the frustrations inherent in the present arrangements for combating it. It is wrong that all too often the family doctor and the " tuberculosis doctor " are so apart in the field. The result is an unsureness of approach and a lack of co-ordination in thought. The clinician devotes himself by training and tradition to caring for the one sheep that is lost, leaving the ninety and nine in the wilderness in order to do so. The medical administrator, responsible finally to hard-headed politicians who represent the community, is almost forced to deal in mass methods, which appear to pay a good dividend, rather than to study the needs of each individual sufferer.

There are various methods which have their partisans : " isolation " of adult sufferers ; " immunisation " by Calmette and Guérin's B.C.G. vaccine, not yet generally accepted as sound ; " environment," in the sense of placing the family under the ideal conditions of such village settlements as Papworth, but which in future ought to be widened to include economic and social adjustments ; and " separation," the removal of the child from the home, as by the *Œuvre Grancher* * in France. Family, economic and social needs vary so much that probably all four methods have their place at various times and in varying proportions. At all events, if the student and doctor understand the various aspects of what is a complex problem of human lives, they can resolve to work for that " body of knowledge " which has yet to be achieved, and which will inspire and direct right action.

Meanwhile the family doctor has still, by the very nature of his calling, a key position in prevention, for he more than anyone can educate his people in the fundamental facts of the disease. He can combat the old yet still widespread heresy that tuberculosis is hereditary, an error which monopolises attention which should be given to the real dangers of contact and milk-borne infection. He can establish close co-operation with the Tuberculosis Officer, seeing that the latter can bring into play the resources of the State. To the many patients who are ignorant of the dire risk of infecting their children and of the scrupulous and detailed care necessary to avoid it, he should be the best and most trusted person to give instruction and guidance.

THE TUBERCULIN TEST

The investigation of allergy to tuberculo-protein by means of the tuberculin test is called for not only when there has

* The L.C.C. and certain other authorities have similar schemes.

been exposure to infection or an allergic tuberculous illness but also when there is any reason to suspect tuberculous infection ; for example, the onset of any unexplained illness, especially if the infant or young child ceases to thrive or if there is persistent pyrexia.

The most convenient method of testing is by the *Vollmer percutaneous patch test*. Three squares of filter paper are set on a strip of adhesive plaster ; the two outer squares are saturated with undiluted old tuberculin (O.T.), the centre one with glycerin broth to act as a control. Recently a tuberculin jelly prepared from purified tuberculin has been used for patch testing, and it is claimed that more satisfactory results are obtained from it than from the old tuberculin preparation. The skin over the sternum is cleaned with acetone and dried, and the patch is then applied. It is removed in forty-eight hours, and twenty-four hours later the result is read. A positive reaction is shown as a raised red area, or alternatively as a series of discrete pinhead papules. The result naturally varies with the sensitivity and also to some extent on the type of skin, but not on the severity or extent of the disease.

In children below the age of 5, a negative patch test can be accepted without re-testing.* In older children it should be followed by the Mantoux intradermal test, because there is a small group of " sensitives " who react only to 1/100 O.T. intradermally. Moreover, in this latter group there will always be a small group of " pseudo-positives " who, on repeating the 1/100 Mantoux test, will prove to be negative. In children the patch test and the intradermal test agree closely ; routine adoption of the patch test spares many children the prick of a needle. In adults the patch test is less satisfactory and the Mantoux reaction should be used.

The Mantoux test (which has largely taken the place of the original von Pirquet test) is made by intradermal injection of old tuberculin, beginning with 0·1 c.c. of 1/10,000 solution and re-testing with 1/1000 and, if necessary, 1/100 when the weaker dose fails to give a positive result. If there is good reason to expect active tuberculosis (especially in children) it is wise to begin with an even weaker dilution, 1/50,000, lest too severe a reaction occur. A positive reaction is indicated by an area of œdema surrounded by a zone of erythema appearing at the site of injection in about twenty-four to forty-eight hours.

* This holds good only if the testing material is perfect and the technique of the test is scrupulously carried out. In view of the conflicting results obtained owing to faulty material or to an insufficient time being allowed for the reading of the test, it is perhaps safer in practice always to follow a negative patch test with a Mantoux test.

18

A positive reaction to the tuberculin tests signifies that the subject has at some time or other been exposed to infecting tubercle bacilli, and that he has a tuberculous focus in his body ; it does not indicate, however, when the focus developed, where it is, what is its extent or whether it is healed or active. Its greatest value is that it sieves out those who need further investigation. Moreover, periodically repeated tests may define the limits of time between which the initial infection must have occurred when an earlier negative reaction changes later to a positive one.

It should be noted that even after tuberculous infection the skin test may be negative not only for the short period between infection and the development of sensitivity, but also in acute miliary infection, after certain fevers (particularly measles), and in the last stages of the disease.

DIAGNOSIS OF THE DISEASE IN CHILDREN

The diagnosis of active pulmonary tuberculosis in children is never easy. Sometimes the disease presents itself in the form of an illness with persistent pyrexia for which no obvious explanation can be found. Under such circumstances a tuberculin test should be done, together with an X-ray film of the chest. Sometimes a typical clinical picture is seen, to which has been given the name of " the wheezing, wasting syndrome of infantile tuberculosis." The wheeze, which is due to the pressure of an enlarged tuberculous gland on one of the larger bronchi, is heard especially during crying or feeding.

In older children the first indication of tuberculous infection may be one of the allergic illnesses which have already been described. On the other hand, the disease may assume one of the forms commonly described in adults. Acute lesions such as tuberculous bronchopneumonia or caseous pneumonia (" pneumonic phthisis "), with or without cavitation, may be difficult to distinguish from simple acute bronchitis or the non-tuberculous pneumonias. Confronted with an infant or a young child suffering from bronchopneumonia, the doctor should always bear in mind the comparative frequency of tuberculous bronchopneumonia in children. Moreover, it should be noted that tuberculous bronchopneumonia sometimes directly follows measles or whooping-cough, and the differentiation from simple bronchopneumonia is then even more difficult than usual. It is caused by the aspiration of caseous material, usually from the breaking down of a gland which ulcerates into a bronchus. This is determined by the diminished bodily resistance caused by the initial infectious disease. When, therefore, an apparently simple pneumonia does not respond to chemotherapy, a chest radiogram is called for and the sputum (obtained if need be by laryngeal swab or by gastric lavage) should be examined for tubercle bacilli. Tuberculous, in contrast to other types of pneumonia in children, is apt to be insidious and less dramatic in its course, but it nearly always progresses relentlessly to a fatal ending.

The picture of fibrocaseous phthisis with cavity formation may occasionally be seen even in infancy. Tuberculous pleural effusion is uncommon in the early years of childhood ; at that period a collection of fluid in the pleural cavity is likely to be an empyema. The grave complications of miliary tuberculosis, tuberculous meningitis and tuberculous disease of bones and joints have already been mentioned. Generalised miliary tuberculosis presents the picture of an acute general infection of the " typhoid " type, with enlargement of the spleen ; both it and acute miliary tuberculosis of the lungs involve so much of the lung parenchyma in tuberculous formations and accompanying œdema that dyspnœa and cyanosis are intense.

To sum up : the primary infection (often called " the childhood type ") prepares the ground for the reinfection or " adult type " of tuberculosis. This it does partly by establishing the necessary primary focus and partly by determining allergic and immunity changes which henceforward modify the reaction of the lung tissue. Everyone, therefore, who has recovered from a first infection is a candidate for the adult type of tuberculosis, though happily the percentage of failures is high ; obviously, however, it is wise to keep a watchful eye on all such susceptibles. The sooner, therefore, the discovery of primary tuberculous infection in a child can be made, the sooner can measures be taken to prevent further exposure to infecting bacilli and to guard and build up his general resistance. Once a child has been infected by the tubercle bacillus special care is needed to protect him from infectious diseases such as measles and whooping-cough, which may wreck any healing or immunity he may be in process of developing. This is particularly important during the critical six months when, as has been pointed out earlier, most of the crippling or fatal complications of tuberculous infection are likely to occur.

POST-PRIMARY LESIONS

Primary infections in adults do not differ in any material way from those in children ; it is the primary nature of the lesion and not the age of the patient which determines their character. Unless this is clearly understood the use of the terms " childhood type " and " adult type " of pulmonary tuberculosis are misleading, even though they have a certain rough-and-ready clinical convenience. Strictly speaking, once allergy is established any further production of tuberculo-protein may cause a " post-primary " lesion. Unless the invading tubercle bacilli are destroyed by the initial proliferative reaction before the advent of allergy, the tuberculo-protein poured out by the surviving bacilli will contribute to a new type of tissue response conditioned by allergy on the one hand and by immunity on the other. It is clear, therefore, that a primary lesion may be arrested at an early stage and either become absorbed or be replaced by fibrous tissue. On the other hand, there may be caseating necrosis of the primary focus and the associated lymph nodes. This caseous focus may still heal, with eventual calcification, or the destructive damage may extend. The final result obviously depends on the dose of bacilli and on the resistance of the patient. Primary and post-primary lesions may form part of a continuous illness, as, for example, in the progressive lesions of young children ; or there may be a distinct and often long interval between the primary and the later infections, as in the majority of types of the disease seen in adults.

There is no common agreement on whether *exogenous re-infection* (that is, a fresh infection by bacilli from without) or *endogenous exacerbation* (that is, a local recurrence or " flare-up," usually of an old quiescent process) is the more usual mechanism in the development of later post-primary lesions. Obviously both can occur. The reawakening of a " healed " pulmonary lesion may be caused in various ways. Bacilli still alive in the old scar or in the calcified nodule of the primary focus or lymph node may be carried out into healthy tissues by leucocytes, following the lowering of local resistance or the occasional reabsorption of calcium. Here intercurrent inflammation of the lung may sometimes be a factor, or the fibrous capsule of the lesion (often only partly calcified) may be ruptured by trauma, and so allow the escape of living bacilli into the lymphatic or the blood stream.

The resultant disease depends largely on the balance between the allergic response (itself dependent largely on the newly infecting dose of bacilli) and the bodily resistance (which is partly conditioned by the acquired immunity). The former determines the degree of exudative or necrotic reaction, the latter the power to limit the disease by fibrosis. The lesions may vary, therefore, from the acute and highly destructive to the chronic and markedly fibrotic. The different pathological processes of spread or healing, which have been described earlier, make it clear that the clinical picture of pulmonary tuberculosis can be of almost infinite complexity and variety. The main clinical forms classified for convenience of description are thus only samples of a host of possible pathological combinations.

ACUTE FORMS OF POST-PRIMARY PULMONARY TUBERCULOSIS

Miliary tuberculosis, whether generalised or localised to the lungs, is a post-primary form of the disease. It follows the sudden discharge, from a tuberculous gland or other focus into the blood stream, of material with a high content of tubercle bacilli. The particles are arrested in the same areas as experimentally injected particles are arrested in animals—in the lungs, spleen, liver and bone marrow especially, and hardly at all in muscle, skin or brain (the small tuberculomata of brain, which when they rupture, produce meningitis, are not the direct and immediate result of hæmatogenous infection of the meninges, but are much older caseous foci). Occasionally tubercles " seeded " in the choroid can be recognised by means of the ophthalmoscope. The disease, when generalised, may arise as a complication of an already obvious tuberculous lesion in the body. Often, however, the original tuberculous lesion is not recognised, and the onset of miliary tuberculosis is somewhat insidious. The illness is characterised by a gradually increasing pulse rate and pyrexia. Headache, malaise, drowsiness and weakness may suggest an enteric infection. The pyrexia may be continuous or remittent. Frequently it is " inverted," the temperature rising high in the morning and remitting in the evening. In infants an illness of this type should always arouse suspicion of tuberculosis. In differential diagnosis the possibility of acute pyelonephritis should especially be borne in mind, for unless an examination of the urine is made this condition may easily be overlooked. In adults the differential diagnosis becomes that of a " pyrexia of uncertain origin," though the most usual difficulty is to distinguish it from either enteric fever or infective endocarditis, especially as in all three conditions the spleen may be enlarged.

With miliary dissemination throughout the lungs (see also p. 268) local reactionary œdema is considerable, and dyspnœa and cyanosis may be intense. Sputum is scanty, for death usually occurs before the lesions break down and liquefy, and there may be little or no cough. There is no treatment likely to alter the grave course of the disease, and symptomatic measures are all that can be adopted.

Acute tuberculous pneumonia results from the discharge of caseous material, usually from a gland or a pre-existing cavity, into one or more of the larger bronchi. According to the distribution and to the severity of the reaction the condition may be one of discrete patches of tuberculous bronchopneumonia ; or of confluent bronchopneumonia involving a whole lobe (pneumonic phthisis).

Pneumonic phthisis begins as an apparent lobar pneumonia. There is no effective response, however, to chemotherapy, and the temperature remains high, without any promise of a crisis. After about a week of illness, empyema may be suspected, especially as the temperature tends to become remittent. If paracentesis is done, however, no pus is found. The pyrexia does not subside, there is marked sweating and rapid emaciation, and if a leucocyte count is made a leucopenia and not a leucocytosis will usually be found. Finally, when caseous matter from the confluent tuberculous pneumonia is at length discharged via a bronchus into the sputum, tubercle bacilli are discovered. Occasionally hæmoptysis may indicate the ulceration of a fair-sized blood vessel.

The outlook is grave. Most patients die within three months of the onset of the illness, many of them before there has been sufficient breaking down of the lesion to produce tubercle bacilli in the sputum.

Tuberculous bronchopneumonia is more common than pneumonic phthisis, and is often bilateral. At first the symptoms are those of acute bronchitis, with cough and scanty expectoration. Later, patches of bronchopneumonia may be discovered.

A patient recovers from a simple bronchopneumonia usually within three to six weeks ; in tuberculous bronchopneumonia the illness persists, with a high remittent temperature, marked dyspnœa and cyanosis, and the development within about six weeks of some degree of " beaking " of the finger nails. Sweating, rapid emaciation, and maybe hæmoptysis accompany the progress of the lesions. As in pneumonic phthisis, the patient may at length expectorate caseous material containing tubercle bacilli, the quantity of sputum increases, and the development of pulmonary cavitation may be recognised in the X-ray film. He may not, however, survive long enough for this to happen.

The condition is always serious, though obviously the smaller the area of lung involved the better the chance of recovery. The treatment of these tuberculous pneumonias is that of any grave pyrexial illness, with *absolute* rest in bed. There are no specific drugs which can modify the illness. If the acute condition subsides an artificial pneumothorax, instituted very slowly and carefully because of the danger of discharging caseous material into the opposite lung, is sometimes worth trying, though it is usually a counsel of desperation if the lung is extensively involved. If the patient does survive the immediate illness he is likely to be left with a considerable amount of destruction of the lung. A similar acute bronchopneumonia may develop also as a sequel of severe hæmoptysis. It is due to aspiration of blood and pus in a patient already suffering from chronic pulmonary tuberculosis.

Tuberculous pleurisy with effusion will be dealt with in a later chapter (see Chap. XXIV).

CHRONIC FORMS OF POST-PRIMARY PULMONARY TUBERCULOSIS

These can occur at any time after the primary infection, and, therefore, at any age. They are not common, however, under the age of puberty. Afterwards they increase in frequency, determine the high mortality from tuberculosis in young adult life, and remain prevalent, especially in the most chronic forms, right up to senility.

The varying degrees of resistance and allergic sensitivity, the spread of bacilli by various routes and at various times, and the production of areas of collapse by plugs of thick sputum may all combine to determine lesions of great complexity and variety. For the purposes of clinical description they are usually classified into three groups : the " early " subapical lesion, chronic ulcerative phthisis and fibroid phthisis.

THE " EARLY " LESION

As a rule the " **early** " **lesion** begins in the upper lobe, in the subclavicular region, as a focus some 1 to 2 in. in diameter (*Assmann's focus*). No convincing reason is available to explain why the subapical part of the lung is so frequently the site.* This " early " or " incipient phthisis " of the older physicians is not always a lesion of short duration. The corresponding hilar glands are not appreciably enlarged, partly owing to the tendency to local fixation of the bacilli because of immunity, and partly perhaps to the less active lymphatic drainage with increasing years. If the infection is heavy or the bodily resistance poor the lesions tend to caseate and break down. If the infection is slight and the bodily resistance is good the tendency is towards localisation of the disease by fibrosis. All too often, however, the fibrous barrier is incomplete, and fresh tuberculous deposits may then be found outside it. If the inflammatory process spreads near to a bronchiole it causes a local bronchial catarrh, with irritating and almost non-productive cough. Later the bronchial wall may be eroded, with the result that tubercle-infected material is discharged into the sputum, which may then be found to contain tubercle bacilli, pus, red blood corpuscles, caseous debris and maybe fragments of pulmonary elastic tissue.

CAVITATION

When resistance to the infecting tubercle bacilli is poor the local lesion progresses, individual tubercles coalesce, caseation

---

* Recent work by R. C. Brock suggests that it is due to inhalation of bacilli into the zone of a posterior bronchial division at the apex.

takes place, caseous material is eventually discharged into the bronchial tree and cavitation is thus established. The boundary wall of the cavity is formed in part by fibrous tissue (provided that there is a certain degree of resistance), and in part by consolidated lung with a poor vascular supply due to inflammatory endarteritis. The centrifugal pull of elastic fibres in the surrounding intact lung tissue tends to keep the walls apart and the contour of the cavity roughly spherical. The inside lining of the cavity is ragged and has a greyish sloughing appearance due to the caseating tubercles. Sometimes strands of tissue containing small bronchi and blood vessels traverse the lumen. These vessels are usually obliterated by thrombosis; occasionally, however, they remain patent and constitute a source of danger, for owing to direct ulceration or to aneurysmal dilatation they may bleed and give rise to serious and maybe fatal hæmorrhage.

There may be one or more small bronchi opening into the cavity. If the opening is dependent and free, the cavity is adequately drained and remains dry. If the opening is not dependent or is blocked, secretions accumulate within the cavity, demonstrable on an X-ray film as a " fluid level." Imperfect drainage increases infectivity, both tuberculous and by secondary organisms within the cavity. This not only leads to an increase in the absorption of toxins, but it may also provoke a pneumonic reaction (consolidation) around the cavity. Another factor which may contribute to the thickness of the wall of a cavity is collapse of the surrounding lung tissue, due to occlusion of the finest bronchioles and of the alveoli. This collapsed lung tissue is capable of re-expansion, thereby compensating in part for the diminution in size of a cavity, if and when the latter becomes reduced in size or obliterated by absorption of the contained air.

The bronchi draining the cavity are as a rule implicated, at any rate in its vicinity. There may be allergic or inflammatory œdema, caseous change or fibrosis. It sometimes happens that occlusion of the bronchus leading to the cavity supervenes, either because of the intrinsic bronchial changes, or by extrabronchial fibrosis, or by plugs of secretion or debris from the interior of the cavity itself. If the occlusion is complete and permanent the air inside the cavity is absorbed, the walls fall together, and eventually the processes of healing may bring about its final obliteration. More often, however, the occlusion is incomplete and acts like a valve, allowing air to get in but not out. A distended spherical " tension cavity " then develops, with a positive pressure inside it. Its size may vary from time to time, according to the balance of absorption of air from it and the inspiration of air into it.

Small recent cavities with thin walls (provided that they are not of the " tension " variety) may heal completely, following a period of strict and prolonged rest. It must be borne in mind that even recent cavities may have thick walls, by reason of surrounding consolidation or of collapse of lung tissue. Older cavities, as a rule, have thicker, more fibrotic walls, and are obliterated with difficulty, if at all. The mechanism of the production of giant cavities associated with lobar or segmental collapse has been described in Chapter VII, p. 100.

The formation of a cavity, even though it may be very small in size, immeasurably increases the menace of the disease. It has been calculated, from a study of the after-history of these patients, that of those with a cavity 4 cm. or less in diameter, 50 per cent. will be dead in four years ; of those with a cavity 5 to 10 cm. in diameter, the percentage rises to 75. The discharge of large numbers of tubercle bacilli into the sputum may result in *laryngeal tuberculosis*, due to the persistent falling back of infected sputum into the inter-arytenoid area. Sputum may be swallowed and cause *tuberculous enteritis* or *fistula in ano*. Infected material may be aspirated during coughing into other parts of the bronchial tree and so spread the infection widely throughout the lungs. It may block a bronchus, produce collapse of the lung and lead later to bronchiectasis.

CHRONIC ULCERATIVE PHTHISIS

The chronic progressive lesion with cavitation spreads by direct extension to adjacent lung tissue, by the lymphatics, and by aspiration along the air passages. With each new extension of infection to some other part of the lung there is an immediate inflammatory reaction. If the number of bacilli involved in bronchial spread is considerable the reaction is severe and acute, expressing itself clinically as an attack of tuberculous bronchopneumonia. The course of chronic ulcerative phthisis is, therefore, apt to be dotted with acute exacerbations, and as the lungs become ever more extensively involved the opportunities for further spread are proportionately increased. Eventually the lungs show a most complex picture of lesions at all stages of development, together with attempts at limitation.

The surprising feature is not that these extensions occur, but that the incidence of them is not more frequent and more extensive. An essential fact to be remembered is that acute exacerbations can occur even when the patient is under the strictest sanatorium treatment : at any time, that is, until the disease in the lung is under complete control. This applies not only to patients with chronic ulcerative phthisis but also to those with fibroid phthisis.

FIBROID PHTHISIS

In a fairly large number of patients the attempts at healing are the predominating feature, and the lung or lungs become the seat of extensive fibroid change. Fibroid phthisis usually affects the upper third or so of the lung, though sometimes the whole lung is involved. Often there is a densely walled cavity or cavities, and the pleura is almost invariably thickened and usually adherent. The shrinkage of the lung in the course of time becomes even more striking when a large bronchus becomes stenosed, with resulting collapse of the lobe or segment of lung supplied by it, and later secondary bronchiectatic changes, which may be very extensive. The tuberculous disease may become arrested, or it may advance so slowly that tubercle bacilli are not found in the sputum at this stage. Because of the bronchiectasis, however, expectoration is abundant and purulent, and frequent hæmoptyses may occur. Gradually and progressively the fibrosis causes strain on the right side of the heart, and eventual right heart failure.

SYMPTOMS AND SIGNS

Pulmonary tuberculosis is an infective disease causing a local lesion, which in its turn produces secondary constitutional disturbance. The lesion in the lungs may give **focal** symptoms and signs, such as cough, expectoration, hæmoptysis, pleurisy, or occasionally spontaneous pneumothorax, all of which direct attention to the lungs. The **general constitutional symptoms**

are toxæmic and are due to the absorption into the circulation
of tuberculo-protein, and also tissue disintegration products
derived from the local lesion.

Although the local lesion precedes and is responsible for the
constitutional symptoms, the focal symptoms and signs may
be so insignificant or ill-defined that the constitutional symptoms
are evident and paramount for months, or even years, prior
to the recognition of the primary focal lesion. When, as so
often happens, the toxæmic symptoms precede the local manifestations, they may not arouse suspicion of pulmonary disease,
and may even be largely disregarded by the patient or by his
doctor. The patient usually has his own simple explanation
for such common symptoms as tiredness or irritability, or for
a liability to frequent colds. He thinks that he is " run down,"
that he is working too hard, that he needs a holiday, or (if
these symptoms are accompanied by a persistent cough) that
he is smoking too much. He is apt to feel that these complaints
are too trivial for a visit to his doctor, and unfortunately the
doctor, when consulted, frequently confirms him in this belief.
On the other hand, the spitting of blood usually frightens him
into immediate action, but here again the doctor too often
calms his fears by making light of it, or attributing it to the
rupture of a capillary vessel in the pharynx. If blood is coughed
or spat up, it must *always* be regarded as coming from the lung,
and therefore having a serious import, *unless and until some
other cause is demonstrable.*

A young woman in apparently good health had a bout of coughing after a spell
of vigorous exercise and brought up an eggcupful of blood. Very frightened, she
went to see her doctor, who examined her carefully, told her that he could find no
evidence of tuberculosis, and relieved her fears by assuring her that she must have
burst a small blood vessel in the throat. She carried on with her usual mode of life
and work, until eighteen months later she had another sharp hæmoptysis. By this
time there was extensive tuberculous disease, with cavitation, of the right upper
lobe, together with patchy lesions in the left upper lobe. Sputum and radiological
examinations undertaken after the first hæmoptysis, and repeated at intervals if
necessary, would certainly have revealed the disease at a much earlier stage.

A minimal tuberculous lesion may give no symptoms until
sensitivity to tuberculo-protein is established. If the allergy
is not severe the symptoms may be indefinite and equivocal.
For example, *recurrent slight febrile attacks*, labelled " colds "
or " influenzal attacks," may be due to tuberculous intoxica-
tion ; and, as might be expected at this stage, a few days'
rest in bed will cause the pyrexia to subside. *Tachycardia*

may be erroneously regarded as nervous or thyrotoxic. In war time it may be labelled " D.A.H." (disordered action of the heart, " effort syndrome ") ; the after-history of patients with this diagnosis reveals that about 5 per cent. of them eventually develop obvious pulmonary tuberculosis. *Fatigue, irritability, sleeplessness, neurasthenia* and even *nervous breakdown* may similarly be due to toxæmia, but they are apt to be put down to the pace or worries or overwork of modern life ; in any case the usual rest cure may well give temporary but misleading relief. The young servant girl or typist with *dyspepsia* may be suffering from a toxæmic upset of the digestion. Her indigestion may easily be regarded, however, as " functional " or as due to irregular scamped meals and too much strong tea, or even to true peptic ulcer. *Loss of appetite, loss of weight, anæmia, amenorrhœa* and *excessive sweating* (for example, the " dripping axillæ " seen during the medical examination of the patient) may likewise be expressions of tuberculous toxæmia.

Of the localising symptoms, *cough* is the most common and persistent. It depends on the nearness of the lesion to or actual involvement of a bronchus rather than to the severity of the disease. Many patients accept it as due to a " cold" which they cannot throw off, or to smoking, but it should be a rule to suspect any cough which persists for longer than a month, and to investigate thoroughly its cause. *Expectoration* is at first due to irritative bronchial catarrh ; later, when the lesion erodes a bronchus, the sputum will contain tubercle bacilli and other material evacuated from the caseous focus. *Hæmoptysis* (see also p. 53) is rarely dangerous. The smaller blood vessels in the neighbourhood of the lesion undergo endarteritis obliterans, but this is not always complete. The sputum may be stained pink owing to the seeping of a few red blood corpuscles into the lumen of a bronchus, or there may be obvious streaks or clots of blood, which continue for a few days. Sometimes, even at a very early stage, a fair-sized vessel is eroded, with the result that in an apparently healthy person a copious hæmoptysis of a cupful or so of bright red blood may occur—" out of the blue," as the patient often expresses it. This may happen even before there is any X-ray evidence of a lesion, or long before tubercle bacilli are discovered in the sputum. In a young person it should always be taken as due to an active tuberculous lesion, unless full investigation reveals some other cause. Very rarely a small but exceedingly acute lesion may erode a large vein or fair-sized artery and kill the patient by loss of blood or suffocation ; usually, however, these massive hæmorrhages occur later, when cavitation is established and a large vein in the wall of a cavity is ulcerated, or when an aneurysm which has developed in the weakened wall of an artery crossing the cavity finally ruptures. It must always be remembered that when the disease is advanced and the patient becomes greatly enfeebled, even a small loss of blood may be the last fatal straw. *Pleurisy with effusion* may be an early manifestation of tuberculosis, and is discussed in detail in Chapter XXIV. *Thoracic pain* is not always due to pleurisy (see p. 376) ; it may follow the muscular strain of persistent coughing, for example, or result from spontaneous pneumothorax. In the later stages of the disease bilateral pain may be the result of traction on the mediastinum, as a result of fibrotic shrinkage of a lung. Pain may also be caused by fibrotic traction on the diaphragm ; it is referred more frequently to the shoulder, less often to the abdomen.

As the lesion progresses, the character and intensity of the general and local manifestations follow suit. The symptoms and signs of acute tuberculosis have already been described. In chronic ulcerative phthisis *pyrexia* of every type may occur. If the disease advances slowly the temperature may remain normal ; or it may rise from normal or slightly below normal to about 100° F. by the late afternoon,* and then gradually fall again ; or it may be inverted. Sometimes the only rise of temperature demonstrable is during the period immediately preceding menstruation. Extension of the disease at any time may be marked by a rise of temperature to 101° or 103° F., a change which persists as a continued or remittent pyrexia until the exacerbation subsides. The discharge of the contents of a cavity into a bronchus often causes a fall of temperature. Small variations may be due to periods of exertion or excitement. In the more advanced cases the temperature may be remittent or intermittent, types of pyrexia which have been

---

* The absence of any rise of temperature when taken by the doctor during a morning visit may, therefore, be wholly fallacious as a test of pyrexia. By the late afternoon the temperature may have risen to 101° or 102°.

described as the result of secondary infection ; but secondary infection of moment has been found to be much less common than used to be thought. The oral temperature is sufficiently reliable provided that the mouth is closed for at least five minutes before the insertion of the thermometer. *Fatigue* (lack of endurance) is usually very striking in all but the earliest stages of the disease, and may be out of all proportion to the extent of the lesion. *Anorexia* may be an early symptom, and is caused by the effect of toxæmia, both generally and locally, upon the stomach. *Tachycardia* at rest is always an important sign, though it is not specific for tuberculous infection ; it may precede a rise of temperature and provide the first evidence of an extension of the disease. *Dyspnœa*, marked on exertion, may at first be caused by toxic damage to the myocardium ; later the destruction of lung tissue becomes a predominant factor. *Persistent gastro-intestinal symptoms*, especially the diarrhœa of the moderate or advanced chronic ulcerative case, are usually due to intestinal tuberculosis, and autopsy reports show that some 60 to 80 per cent. of patients who have died of phthisis have by that time a tuberculous enteritis or colitis. Reflex vomiting may occur, especially with left basal lesions.

In the more chronic fibroid types of the disease the secondary changes in the lungs often dominate the picture. The two outstanding types are, on the one hand, those in which bronchiectatic dilatations are present, accompanied by typical copious mucopurulent sputum, and often by frequent small hæmoptyses. In spite of the copious sputum it may be difficult or impossible to find tubercle bacilli. The other type is one of apparent chronic bronchitis and emphysema, most misleading in older patients unless the sputum is tested and an X-ray film of the chest is taken. As the fibrosis and emphysema involve more and more of the lung parenchyma, dyspnœa becomes very marked, the right side of the heart begins to dilate, and finally congestive cardiac failure supervenes.

During the earliest stage of the development of the lesion **physical signs** of it are almost invariably absent, and this may be so until the lesion has a size considerable enough to surprise the student when he sees its shadow on the X-ray film. Most commonly the first, and maybe for long the only sign is *a diminution of expansion of the affected side*. It is not a finding specific for tuberculosis, but it should always challenge the doctor to investigate its cause. It should be remembered that this sign is obtained by comparing one side of the chest with the other, so that when the disease becomes bilateral it is possible for expansion to be equally impaired on the two sides. There must be few general physicians or practitioners who at some time in their experience have not been humiliated by making a provisional diagnosis of carcinoma of the stomach when faced by a cachectic, emaciated patient suffering from advanced bilateral phthisis. The chest expands equally on both sides, there are no other convincing physical signs, the man " looks malignant," the history may have been unreliable or accepted with a shade of bias ; but the radiologist, who has learned always to take a film of the chest when doing a gastro-intestinal investigation, reports advanced bilateral phthisis.

With the establishment of allergy, varying degrees of œdematous inflammatory reaction may occur. *Râles* (usually medium crepitations, but varying according to the physical condition of the underlying lung) which persist in one of the upper lobes or are increased by coughing are therefore significant ; these and the diminished expansion may be the only signs of an extensive lesion which is never sufficiently confluent to produce the signs of consolidation. Occasionally, however, a patch of bronchopneumonic consolidation can be recognised. Many cavities are quite " silent " ; they may be small, with sufficient lung tissue lying between them and the stethoscope to mask their presence, or for various reasons they do not act as a resonating chamber (see p. 85). The " silent " cavities can sometimes be detected, however, by the trained ear, by recognising the soft inrush of air occurring during an inspiration following on a cough. The dramatic signs of cavitation (" typical signs of cavity ") described in the old textbooks —cavernous breathing, post-tussive suction, layers of fluid and air, and the rest—are very late manifestations of cavities of considerable size ; the patient possessing one is already beyond effective medical aid. Even with extensive chronic phthisis, the student may be puzzled and disappointed by the few changes he can elicit by percussion ; he must remember, however, the considerable compensatory emphysema which masks the lesion. In chronic fibroid phthisis, with marked unilateral fibrosis, the chest wall may be drawn in and the trachea and apex beat of the heart displaced towards the more affected side. Very occasionally the traction on the trachea is so severe that it causes stridor. The pleura over the fibrotic lung may be greatly thickened, with the result that the percussion note is dull.

After reading the previous paragraphs the student may feel that physical signs are of little value in the diagnosis of pulmonary tuberculosis. This, however, is not true. While the modern practitioner's problem is to diagnose the disease at a much earlier stage than that represented by the " typical " physical signs of the Victorian physicians, eyes, hands and ears still need training. They may discover the clue which, in practice, may put the examiner on the right scent. The discovery, for example, of nothing more than diminished expansion of a lung, with or without medium or fine crepitations, should lead to an examination of the sputum and a radiogram. Moreover, during the course of the disease alterations in physical signs are of the utmost importance, both for diagnosis and treatment. In order to understand the clinical features of the disease the doctor has to learn to correlate the history, the symptoms, the physical signs (even when they may seem to him disappointingly few) and the radiological appearances. He is likely to encounter patients at all stages of the disease, and from all these factors he can learn much about its natural history.

THE BACTERIOLOGICAL DIAGNOSIS OF TUBERCULOSIS

The routine Ziehl-Neelsen method of staining a film of sputum is of great value, but unfortunately it fails to detect tubercle bacilli in a certain proportion of specimens because it is not sufficiently sensitive. Before bacilli can be detected in the smears something like 100,000 of them must be present in a cubic centimetre of material examined. By various *concentration* methods from three to seven times as many bacilli can be obtained than by direct centrifugation of the same specimen of sputum. *Direct cultivation* of the bacillus on Loewenstein's medium or some modification of it (the basic ingredients are egg, asparagine and Congo red or malachite green) results in colonies of human bacilli appearing within about fourteen days, whereas bovine colonies do not appear until after thirty days.

19

The Ziehl-Neelsen technique should first be employed on suspected sputum, and if tubercle bacilli are not found after a diligent search lasting for not less than fifteen minutes, at least three different specimens of sputum should be tested. If the bacilli are still not found, the result should be regarded not as negative but as inconclusive. The next step is to try to cultivate the bacilli on the suitable medium. Taking a series of different samples of sputum, cultivation is successful in finding tubercle bacilli in an additional 25 per cent., when compared with routine staining of a smear. This is important not only for diagnosis but also for the assessment of " quiescence " after treatment. It is obvious that statistics based on the old cruder routine tests may prove to be unreliable. The method of cultivation is time-consuming and demands expert technique, and unsuitable specimens (mere saliva, for example) will waste the time of the bacteriologist far more seriously than the routine film-staining method. In expert hands cultivation gives nearly as many positive results in similar samples as does *inoculation of suspected material into a guinea-pig,* results of which are not available for about six weeks. Only in a few instances, therefore, may animal inoculation be necessary for final confirmation.

Radiological examination is essential. It may, in some patients, reveal a minimal lesion long before the advent of symptoms or signs : it indicates the extent and often the character of the disease : and it is a guide to the progress or healing of the lesion, though in this respect it is of considerably less value than the clinical symptoms and signs. Interpretation of X-ray films is a matter for the expert, but the student should seize every opportunity to learn the value of radiology in all chest conditions by comparing X-ray films with his clinical findings. He will see, for example, that tuberculous disease of the lungs is nearly always far more extensive than the physical signs would lead him to believe. Above all, he has to learn that while clinical acumen enables him to recognise certain danger signals, pulmonary tuberculosis is unfortunately not detectable by physical examination unless the lesion has certain characters and is near the surface of the lung. In the past clinical teachers have hoodwinked themselves and their students into believing that " incipient " phthisis can be diagnosed by the man who is skilled enough to recognise minute differences in percussion note

or in breath sounds. The doctor must learn, however, to suspect tuberculosis when there has been contact with an infective
patient, or when he is confronted by the toxæmic symptoms
described (see p. 284). He must then waste no time before
instituting fuller investigations. If the patient comes to him
with slight physical signs already detectable, he must not wait
until they are so obvious that they proclaim extensive disease.
Radiological and sputum examination, undertaken at the first
awakening of suspicion, may avert many a tragedy of crippling
or death.

THE IMPORTANCE OF EARLY DETECTION

The decline in the mortality of pulmonary tuberculosis is
due more to a decline in the incidence of new cases rather
than to improvement in their prognosis. The best type of
sanatorium treatment ensures that 20 per cent. more patients
are alive at the end of five years, compared with those who have
not had it. There, however, the improvement has stopped,
for as Hartley and others have shown by a study of the Frimley
figures, the prognosis of the average case has not materially
changed in the last thirty years, except that in a small selected
group of patients suitable for and treated by artificial pneumothorax the outlook has considerably improved. The earlier,
therefore, the diagnosis the sooner can treatment be instituted
with good effect on both the immediate and ultimate prognosis ;
for, speaking broadly, the prognosis of chronic pulmonary
tuberculosis depends directly on the extent of lung involved
at the time of diagnosis, although there are individual exceptions.

At present something like 85 per cent. of cases are moderately
or well advanced by the time diagnosis is made. It is true
that for a time, during what has been called the " prodromal "
stage, the disease is symptomless and silent. Then comes
a period of " early symptoms," and several studies have shown
that these symptoms remain unattended far too long. The
patient naturally takes little notice of what to him are trivial
ailments ; or if he is really frightened he shrinks from the
economic consequences of illness. If he goes sick he will lose
his job, and what will happen then to his family ?

The doctor, on his part, often not adequately educated in
the natural history of tuberculosis, waits for clear-cut percussion

or stethoscopic signs, and waits too long ; or he may sympathise with the patient, hoping to defer a tragic decision, or hesitating to alarm him. He therefore orders a holiday in the country, or a sea voyage, or a change of occupation. Sometimes he appears ignorant of the strenuousness of open-air occupations as compared with sedentary ones. In some parts of the country, apart from free examinations of sputum, specialised means of investigation (especially radiology) are still not available for his help ; this constitutes a reason or excuse for post-ponement of fuller investigation and of the necessity for facing unpleasant possibilities. In about half the cases of a series which I myself studied even examination of the sputum had been neglected.

Once again it must be emphasised that every young person who complains of repeated colds, of fatigue, listlessness, undue nervousness, shortness of breath, palpitation, anæmia, loss of weight or of appetite, excessive sweating or indigestion, which have come on during the previous six to eighteen months, *may* be suffering from pulmonary tuberculosis. Every case of hæmoptysis is probably due to this disease, save when it is a symptom of some equally serious pulmonary lesion. Failure to detect physical signs may be due to inexperience or to lack of practice, but it may equally be due to the disease being still in the " silent " stage. For all these reasons, therefore, it is essential, in justice to his patient, that the practitioner explains the necessity of an X-ray examination, and of the testing of the sputum, if there is any available. If, after this, no con-clusive diagnosis can be made, the patient should be kept under periodic investigation.

There is no doubt that earlier diagnosis is possible. It will be made much more easily when it ceases to represent an economic tragedy for the sufferer and his family. The fear which leads him to procrastinate would then be considerably lightened. It will be easier, too, when student and doctor are adequately trained in the broad aspects of tuberculosis. It is a fundamental truth that to be a hearer of the word is educationally not enough ; one has also to be a doer. With earlier diagnosis better treatment will follow. For there is this prognostic paradox to be said about pulmonary tuberculosis : while at present it must be considered as largely an incurable disease, yet if it can be treated in its earlier stages it usually yields readily to rest. Amberson has shown that as many as 90 per cent of *minimal* lesions heal with adequate bed rest, without the necessity for further therapy such as artificial pneumothorax. Here is a challenge to early diagnosis, and a promise of hope in an otherwise tragic disease.

The ideal is for the disease to be discovered before the sufferer has symptoms of ill-health, during the " prodromal " or " preclinical " stage, when radiology is the only method which will reveal it. If tuberculosis were as dramatic and startling a disease as epidemic typhus, no effort or expense would be spared in stamping it out, for every member of the community would realise that he himself might be the next victim.* Its more prolonged course, however, smooths out the starkness of its outlines and enables its ravages to be to some degree hidden from the community. It is therefore not taken as seriously as it should be. This was well illustrated in the early days of the recent war when sanatoria were emptied to provide beds for huge numbers of expected air-raid casualties However grave an emergency, it is not easy to envisage any authority daring to turn loose upon their fellows large numbers of patients with typhus or diphtheria.

If X-ray photographs of the chests of apparently healthy young people are taken in factories or workshops, from one to four in every thousand are found to have " preclinical," active tuberculous lesions. Now that convenient methods of " mass radiography " are available, it is possible to make periodic examinations of every young person between the ages of 15 and 25, and so take a big step towards eradicating the disease. Meanwhile the least which might be done is to investigate all those who are exposed to exceptional risks— home contacts, nurses and students in hospitals, students in universities, young adults in State-controlled employment, in the Fighting Services and in factories. The difficulties to be surmounted are obvious. They are difficulties of organisation, of finance, of psychology ; but to overcome them will, in the long run, give a rich dividend in human life and communal safety. The tuberculin test may be used for preliminary sieving. A negative Mantoux test in a young adult indicates that

* In peace time there are about a quarter of a million patients in the British Isles suffering from tuberculosis. It is already clear that in war time the number has increased.

he has not yet been infected, and need not be subjected to serial radiography until periodic testing shows that it has become positive.

Early and effective diagnosis, then, is primarily a matter for action by a community determined to rid itself of a constant menace and willing to pay the price for it. Meanwhile the family doctor, faced with his own patients, can resolve that he at least will not be responsible for wasting vital time.

PRINCIPLES OF TREATMENT

The individual sufferer from pulmonary tuberculosis should be told frankly what is the matter with him, in order that he may know how he stands and undertake the difficult task of "making his peace with events." He should be given hope, based rightly on what can nowadays be done for the disease ; but there should be no glossing over the seriousness of his position, or the importance of his full co-operation in, and acceptance of, whatever length of treatment may be necessary. Prognosis in this disease is notoriously uncertain, and the wise doctor will not attempt to forecast, beyond telling his patient that even at best he must reckon in terms of months. It is a mistaken kindness to buoy him up with false hopes, such as by telling him that a month or two at a sanatorium will put him right. He may take the doctor at his word, only to find out later that all his arrangements, financial or otherwise, were based on utterly wrong premises. Nor is it fair to medical colleagues whose future responsibility is to advise and care for him. It must always be remembered that so many of these patients are young people, plunged suddenly into tragedy—the tragedy of shattered hopes, ambitions and human relationships. They need all the faith and courage which they can muster if they are to face without despair the necessary reorientation of their lives and the long weary journey back to health ; but faith and courage cannot be built on falsities.

The aim of treatment is not only to stop the progress of the lesion and restore the patient's capacity to live and work but also to prevent him from infecting his associates. The basis of treatment has long been fresh air, good food and rest ; in the minds of the laity fresh air and climate are still given priority and regarded as especially applicable to tuberculosis. The proper attitude, however, is to understand them as natural bounties essential for a healthy body, and therefore essential ingredients of Nature's *vis medicatrix* when the body is sick. *Fresh air* can be got both in the open country and in a well-ventilated room. Its health-giving properties depend on its free circulation, on its cleanliness and on its freedom from dust, germs and excessive moisture. Its tonic action is rather on the skin than on the lungs, and therefore the patient must be sensibly clothed. Excessive clothing is detrimental. There is no need for flannel chest protectors or layers of woollen sweaters, which induce excessive perspiration and lead to chilling of the body when they are removed. The lighter and freer the clothes, therefore, the better, so long as the patient is comfortable. If he has to lie out of doors, extra rugs or wraps will guard against excessive cold. Women patients should be forbidden to wear unsuitable corsets, which by reason of their size and material encourage excessive sweating, or which may interfere with the free movements of respiration.

For the tonic effect of fresh air the rich man does not need to go into a far country nor the poor man to tramp the town's public parks and open spaces until he is exhausted with the effort. The city clerk, used to a sedentary life, does not need to seek it in the country at the cost of the gruelling work of forking hay or of running a chicken farm. A man can get almost if not all that is necessary in his own bedroom by making it strictly " functional " (in the sense given to the word by modern architects). He should clear it of hangings and bric-à-brac, open the windows wide both top and bottom, sleep near the window and have just enough bedclothes to keep him warm. In this way the body will soon become adapted to cool, fresh air and enjoy it. Similarly, *good food* means an adequate, well-balanced diet, adapted to the patient's needs, digestible, and with proper first-class (animal) protein and vitamin content.

The importance of **rest** cannot be exaggerated. It is the foundation of all treatment. Other medical and surgical methods are only additional to it ; they can never be substitutes for it. It is true that " rest " has come to mean, for some patients, not only rest of body and mind but also local rest of the diseased lung, achieved by pneumothorax or by surgical methods of pulmonary collapse. The value of this additional local rest may be judged when it is remembered that even with strict rest in a bed a man breathes about 25,000 times a day. If one thinks what would happen to a tuberculous joint which suffered such movement, it is astonishing that any pulmonary lesion heals at all under ordinary circumstances. Rest in bed ensures quiet, shallow respiratory movements, encourages healing and reduces tuberculous toxæmia. It must be prolonged, a necessity which should be explained to the patient in order to obtain his willing co-operation. He should realise that for some time after the disappearance of the more obvious symptoms of toxæmia his lesion is not yet sufficiently healed to allow him to undertake any exercise.

As soon as the diagnosis of pulmonary tuberculosis is made the patient should be put to bed, whether or not there is pyrexia, and complete rest rigidly enforced for a period which will be determined by the seriousness of the disease. This enables the body to be built up again and to recover from the fatigue and strain caused by work or other activities persisted in during a period of toxæmia. Moreover, it enables the doctor to assess to some extent the reaction and the response of the patient to treatment. As long as toxæmia continues, with its harmful effects on the heart and other organs, rest is essential.

It is often said that if proper nursing facilities are available the initial treatment by complete rest may justifiably be carried out at home, provided that periodic (preferably monthly) X-ray films of the chest can meanwhile be taken. Practical experience shows, however, that this is rarely satisfactory and that the more rigid discipline of a good sanatorium prevents many elasticities of regime which can hardly be avoided at home. At home, for example, it is difficult to shut out daily domestic, family or business worries, telephone messages, or visitors who have come from a distance and who cannot conveniently wait or come again at a more convenient time. Such disturbances, each one little enough in itself, may add up to produce serious interference with the daily routine of treatment, and especially with what should be the sacrosanct and strictly observed periods of absolute rest. For the poorer patient with inadequate home conditions, there is no doubt whatever that hospital or sanatorium is the best place, though in many districts, unfortunately, there is a serious shortage of beds available for the prompt treatment of this stage of the disease.

If the lesion is acute, with rapid invasion of lung tissue, *absolute* bed rest is called for until the disease is under control. Ideally, the patient should not talk, or read, or write, but this counsel is unjustifiably drastic for most human beings, and in practice is likely to do more harm than good. Visitors are forbidden. Every form of muscular exertion is avoided. He must not even wash or feed himself. Clearly, this means strict supervision, with adequate nursing help. Pyrexia, tachycardia, or other evidences of toxæmia will call for at least six to eight weeks of absolute rest. Not until pyrexia and toxæmia have subsided should this strict regime be relaxed, and then only very gradually, and with a careful watch upon the patient to see the effects of any increase in his activities.

He can now be allowed a visitor for a short time. As he improves he can feed and wash himself and move about in bed. When the temperature and pulse rate have become normal, the X-ray film has shown a satisfactory degree of healing, symptoms of toxæmia (especially fatigue and lassitude) have subsided, the sputum has become negative for tubercle bacilli and the sedimentation rate (see p. 306) has become normal he may be allowed on to a couch. If this evokes no rise of temperature or increase in the pulse rate the period can be extended until he is out of bed for two, four, or eight hours in the day. Any pyrexia or other evidence of increased activity of the lesion (for example, hæmoptysis) calls for a return to more rest and less exertion. The greater the exudative factor in the lesion the longer as a rule must be the period of rest in bed.

When the patient is well enough to be up for the whole day he must avoid the temptation of over-exertion or of over-taxing such reserves as he may possess. This stage of **sanatorium regime** is of particular value, for treatment in a good sanatorium teaches the patient how to conserve and build up his strength under proper medical supervision. The good sanatorium not only provides open air and good food ; its success depends mainly on its medical and nursing care. This determines the standard of the detailed supervision of the patient's daily regime and his education in the principles by which henceforward he must live.

This education is not assimilated in a day, and as a rule a stay of not less than three months in a sanatorium is advisable. In the sanatorium the times devoted to meals, to rest, to

exercise, and to recreation are all carefully regularised. At
least two periods of absolute rest in the day must be observed
by every patient, whatever his condition. Exercise is supervised, the daily amount being controlled by the condition of
the patient, especially as revealed by the pulse and temperature chart. The details of the various programmes of work
and exercise generally accepted as suitable for patients at this
stage can be found in books especially devoted to pulmonary
tuberculosis. The student will be wise, however, to seek the
opportunity of seeing for himself how a good sanatorium deals
with this aspect of treatment.

In spite of rest and strict regime the lesion may fail to
heal or it may progress. The infection may be heavy or the
patient's resistance may be poor. The very process of healing,
with its cicatrisation, may eventually produce mechanical
tensions and distortions which result in troublesome symptoms
such as persistent, irritable cough or pain ; or it may prevent
the collapse and healing of cavities. For such patients it may
be possible to supplement the essential methods of increasing
bodily resistance already described by some method of collapse
therapy.

THE PRINCIPLES OF COLLAPSE THERAPY

The student and general practitioner should be aware of
the indications for and against the various types of collapse
therapy, even though they are best left to the experienced.
The aim is to relax and reduce the volume of the diseased
lung and to fix it against the mediastinum. This reduces the
movement of that lung, obliterates cavities and spaces, and
thereby prevents the accumulation of secretions and lessens
toxæmia. It also results in passive hyperæmia and in lymph
stasis, factors which favour healing. The choice of method
depends on the type of lesion present, though every case must
be assessed on its own merits. Speaking generally, exudative
and caseous lesions, with or without cavitation, are suitable
for artificial pneumothorax ; older lesions with considerable
fibrosis and cavitation can only be adequately collapsed by
surgical procedures which allow of falling-in of the chest wall.
Any serious impairment of vital capacity, whether by reason
of extensive bilateral involvement of the lungs, or of chronic
bronchitis and emphysema, or of cardiac or other disease,

contraindicates treatment by collapse, which itself aims at reducing the respiration of one lung. For these procedures to be applicable, therefore, the lesion must be mainly unilateral, though a limited amount of healed or healing disease in the contralateral lung does not necessarily forbid them.

Intercurrent disease (apart from that which affects the vital capacity) may influence the indications for or against collapse therapy. Serious complications such as tuberculous disease of the bowel, of bones and joints, or of kidney, as a rule contra-indicate it. Ulceration of the larynx may be benefited by it because of the reduction of the amount of sputum passing over the laryngeal mucosa. In patients with diabetes and tuberculosis the reduction of toxæmia following collapse treatment may favourably influence the sugar tolerance.

Artificial pneumothorax—The introduction of air into the pleural space allows the lung to relax. The intrapleural pressure is usually allowed to remain negative, and the collapse of the lung is therefore obtained by a reduction of intrapleural tension and not by direct compression, which has certain dangers, notably the tearing of a pleuro-pulmonary adhesion. This form of treatment is applicable to the more acute and subacute types of lesion (caseous and exudative) rather than to the fibrotic. In such cases cavitation is an urgent indication for collapse therapy ; indeed, it can be assumed as a general rule that progressive disease is almost inevitably associated with cavity formation. Artificial pneumothorax may also be used to control severe hæmoptysis, provided that it is possible to decide which lung is the source of the hæmorrhage. The technique of artificial pneumothorax is comparatively easy, but it needs judgment in the initial selection of patients suitable for it, in the after-care once it is induced, and in the balancing of certain risks of treatment against the risks of the disease.

If, therefore, a patient is suffering from acute or subacute exudative disease in one lung ; if, in spite of rest, the disease progresses or the general condition does not improve ; if cavitation is present ; or if, after healing, the unilateral disease becomes reactivated, an attempt should be made to induce an effective pneumothorax. Even if the disease is more chronic, provided that it is mainly unilateral, the attempt should still be made, though adhesions between the lung and pleura are much more likely to prevent adequate collapse. Control by X-ray films of the chest is essential during the whole course of the treatment. For this reason, and also because the patient must be kept under skilled observation from day to day, the early stages of treatment (until the pneumothorax is well-established) should be carried out in a hospital or sanatorium.

Various complications may arise which call for changes in, or maybe abandonment of, the treatment. At the stage of induction pleural shock or air embolism may occur, but they are exceedingly rare if the proper technique of the operation is scrupulously carried out. During the first few weeks of the treatment a slight loss of weight is common. Sometimes, however, the loss is steady and progressive, and the pneumothorax may have to be abandoned. Other indications for abandoning it are the failure to produce collapse adequate to control the symptoms (due to adhesions between the two pleural layers, whether complete or partial, or to fibrotic, resistant cavities) ; excessive strain on the contralateral lung or on the heart (often due to shifting of the mediastinum) ; excessive reactions, with rise of temperature after each refill ; or severe dyspnœa (due to serious impairment of the vital capacity).

To a considerable extent the reactions after introduction of air into the pleural cavity depend on the temperament of the patient. While some patients feel no effects at all, others suffer discomfort, pain, mental distress, rise of temperature or nausea. Occasionally a patient has to be regarded as unsuitable for pneumothorax largely because of temperamental disability.

The commonest complications are pleural. *Pleural effusion* is frequent and is caused by tuberculous pleurisy resulting either from tearing of an infected adhesion or from extension of the disease to the pleura. Though annoying, it does not necessarily frustrate the immediate treatment ; the ultimate result, however, may be serious thickening of the pleura and mediastinal displacement, so that it may be necessary to persist with refills and never allow the intrapleural air to be absorbed, lest still more severe traction on the mediastinum ensues. Occasionally the effusion develops into a *tuberculous empyema*. In a certain number of patients pleural effusion is followed by *obliterative pleurisy* which gradually and pro-gressively reduces the pleural space, so that eventually it is impossible to introduce air into it. *Spontaneous pneumothorax* is due usually to the tearing of an adhesion, with associated rupture of lung tissue ; it is a particularly grave complication when it arises in the course of bilateral pneumothorax (see p. 420). Moreover, it may determine the onset of a pyopneumothorax. *Spread of the disease to the contralateral lung* may so reduce the respiratory reserve that unilateral pneumothorax can no longer be carried out with safety. Sometimes the collapse obtained by pneumothorax causes *occlusion of the outlet of a cavity*, as the result either of kinking the bronchus or of blocking it by evacuated caseous or viscid material. If the occlusion persists with a valve-like action, the cavity remains distended and the pneumothorax ineffective. Finally, there are some patients in whom the mediastinum has not been fixed by adhesions. In them, it may be possible to obtain an effective collapse only at the cost of such displacement of the *mobile mediastinum* that the opposite lung and the great vessels are compressed. The resulting symptoms are so serious that it is impossible to continue the pneumothorax treatment.

In a small number of carefully selected patients **partial bilateral artificial pneumothorax** is feasible and justifiable. The normal lung reserve is so great that it is possible to collapse each lung to about half its volume without putting the patient in jeopardy. Any supervening accident which seriously impairs respiratory reserve (spontaneous pneumothorax, acute pulmonary infections) may obviously have grave consequences.

THE TECHNIQUE OF ARTIFICIAL PNEUMOTHORAX

While it is true that artificial pneumothorax should be undertaken only by or under the supervision of someone experienced in the treatment of tuberculosis, nevertheless the student should be familiar with the apparatus used, especially as he may later be called upon to take intrapleural pressure readings in a patient suffering from spontaneous pneumothorax. The simplest and most commonly used apparatus consists of two bottles connected by a siphoning tube. As fluid is siphoned from one bottle into the other, air is displaced from the second bottle, through a rubber tube and a hollow pneumothorax needle, into the pleural cavity. The second bottle is graduated in cubic centimetres, and the amount of air displaced is measured by the rise in the level of the fluid in this bottle. Along the course of the rubber tube is an air-filter. A T-piece junction allows another connection to be led off to a water manometer. The intrapleural pressures can be read off on the manometer after clipping off the delivery tube leading from the bottle.

By using the apparatus in the reverse direction (that is, by siphoning fluid from the second bottle into the first and thus creating a vacuum in the second bottle which sucks air from the pleural cavity) air can be withdrawn from a positive-pressure (tension) pneumothorax (see p. 433).

With these principles in mind the student should find an opportunity to watch an induction or a refill of a pneumothorax. This will not only help him to understand the technique but will also illustrate graphically the intrapleural negative pressure and its variations during the inspiratory and expiratory phases of respiration.

In order to avoid the accident of air embolism, induction is made by allowing air to be sucked into the pleural space, after it is seen (by the negative pressure and proper respiratory excursions revealed by the manometer needle) that there is a free pleural space. Once satisfactory collapse of the lung has been established, periodic refills of air are essential in order to replace the air which is absorbed from the pleural cavity. Treatment must usually be maintained for at least two years, or maybe considerably longer if the disease is extensive and cavities are present. The suitable interval between refills is that which maintains " optimum collapse " (that is, collapse of the lung sufficient to control the disease without producing adverse reactions), and prevents undue expansion of the lung. As a rule, the amount of air introduced at each refill should not be more than 500 c.c. It is clear that if it is found that fortnightly refills of 500 c.c. maintain an optimum collapse, monthly refills of 1000 c.c. would allow far too much variation in the volume of the lung, which would behave like a concertina. This would nullify the whole object of collapse therapy.

There are many patients in whom it is possible to establish a pneumothorax, yet it is impossible to achieve satisfactory collapse of the lung because of adhesions between the lung and the chest wall. At times a single band of adhesions holds out a pulmonary cavity, preventing its collapse. Radiograms are of great help in showing that adhesions are present, but it is quite impossible to gauge accurately from X-ray films either their size or number, or whether it is practicable to divide them. The thoracoscope, introduced into the pleural space through a cannula no wider than a lead pencil (local anæsthesia of the chest wall being sufficient to render the operation painless), allows the surgeon to see for himself the site and size and nature of the adhesions, whether they contain lung tissue which has been drawn out towards the chest wall, and whether they are in intimate relation with important structures such as the subclavian artery. He is then able to decide which adhesions are divisible, and whether he can free the lung sufficiently to ensure adequate collapse.

Intrapleural division of adhesions (**internal pneumolysis**) is done by the electric cautery, under direct thoracoscopic vision. They are divided as close to the chest wall as possible.

It is not a very great exaggeration to say that the treatment of phthisis is the treatment of cavitation, if prevention as well as obliteration of them is included in the phrase. It is true that some acute cavities will heal spontaneously after months of strict rest in bed, but this does not apply to many types, especially to the more chronic ones with a fibrotic wall. These latter rarely heal without some form of operative treatment ; adhesions to the chest wall are frequently present over them, and artificial pneumothorax may fail completely to collapse them. Even after division of the adhesions it is likely to fail because of the fibrosis surrounding the cavity, and some other form of surgical treatment is then necessary.

Whatever the lesion, even expectant treatment must be accompanied by careful supervision and frequent radiograms for comparison, for there is always the danger of extension of the disease to healthy parts of the lungs, or of the breaking down again of a cavity which has apparently healed. Every decision about the best form of treatment must be considered on the merits of the individual case, taking into account the nature, extent and activity of the disease, the family history, and the social, economic and psychological background of the patient. It may be said in general that the more acute exudative phthisis of young adolescents is so dangerous that collapse therapy is abundantly justified if X-ray examination and sputum tests show any breaking down of the lesion. Here any theoretical disadvantages of artificial pneumothorax cannot compare with the risks of rapid extension of the disease. In somewhat older persons (of " early middle age ") a period of preliminary observation with monthly X-ray and other studies is often justified. If a lesion shows no signs of healing, more active treatment must be undertaken, for the exudative forms of phthisis do not stand still. If there is no improvement it must be assumed that the disease is advancing.

The most chronic types of lesion, with fibrosis, are best served by surgical methods of collapse. **Phrenic paralysis** relaxes the lung in the vertical axis by allowing the diaphragm to rise into the thorax. This may be temporary, lasting for about six months following crushing of the nerve, or permanent, following evulsion or phrenicectomy. Though it is not an outstandingly effective method of collapse, it can help to turn the scale in chronic lesions of the upper lobe with thin-walled cavities and to relieve certain symptoms resulting from traction —the irritating cough or pain due to diaphragmatic adhesions, for example, or the stridor or dyspnœa arising from distortion of the trachea. Occasionally it has a place in supplementing artificial pneumothorax or pneumoperitoneum treatment.

In many patients, however, collapse of the lung and obliteration of cavities can only be obtained by allowing the chest wall to fall in after resection of portions of the ribs (**thoracoplasty**).

This can be total or partial, according to the amount of collapse required.

Thoracoplasty is the most effective method of dealing with cavities which cannot be obliterated by pneumothorax, alone or associated with the intrapleural division of adhesions. Its object is to abolish tubercle bacilli from the sputum by relaxing tension and approximating the walls of the cavities and so allowing them a better chance of healing. In this way the patient is made less dangerous to himself and to his fellows. In a patient suffering from chronic ulcerative phthisis, if tubercle bacilli are persistently present in the sputum, it is almost certain that cavitation is present, even though an ordinary X-ray film does not show it. Tomographic X-ray films should then be taken ; they will usually reveal it.

The operation is a major one, undertaken in patients who are far from healthy. It carries serious risks unless the patient has a fair margin of resistance ; the lesion should therefore be at the stage when it is undergoing fibrosis. Another reason for not doing a thoracoplasty in the acute exudative stage is that the operation causes rapid diminution in the volume of the lung, with serious danger of disseminating infection into other parts of the lungs. The lesion must be unilateral, for after operation the respiratory work is thrown on the contralateral lung and the strain is such that even an old healed lesion there may be reactivated. Large cavities or cavities near the hilum or at the base of the lung are not easy to obliterate ; the smaller the cavity the better the chance of success after operation. As a general rule the operation is suitable only for persons in the middle years. In children under 15 years of age a tuberculous lesion is usually exudative. Moreover, it may be (though I am not convinced that it is always so) that the plastic operation has a serious effect upon subsequent growth. In persons older than 45, cardiovascular, bronchitic and emphysematous changes are likely to diminish the vital capacity sufficiently to make the operation inadvisable.

There are other methods of collapsing the lung, of which extrapleural pneumothorax, extrapleural apicolysis with plombage, oleothorax, and pneumoperitoneum may be mentioned ; but the three already described are by far the most important. Once treatment becomes " surgical," student and doctor must realise that the problem has become a choice between two evils, for the word "cure" can be used only in a limited sense.

To sum up : in the acute or subacute phase of the disease absolute rest in bed is indicated, with or without pneumothorax. Rest remains the fundamental principle in the treatment of pulmonary tuberculosis, and collapse therapy must always be regarded as accessory to and not a substitute for it. If collapse therapy is indicated, the least serious and most suitable method applicable to the particular patient will then be chosen ; other methods may become necessary, depending on the effect obtained by the first. As the patient improves, as shown by subsidence of the toxæmia and pyrexia and by the X-ray appearances of the lung, he can be allowed out of bed for gradually increasing periods, until he becomes ready for "sanatorium regime." The sanatorium is the place where the patient's capacity to lead a gradually more active life can be observed under close medical control, and where he can also be taught the careful routine of the regular life which he must henceforward lead. As he continues to improve, more exercise can be allowed ; if he fails to improve, more rest or some form of collapse therapy may be needed. Finally, the disease may be arrested ; or it may advance, with the patient on the defensive perhaps for some years, until finally he dies of tuberculosis ; or it may pass into the chronic fibroid stage. The possibilities of collapse therapy for the second of the above groups have already been discussed ; for various reasons many of these patients leave the sanatorium, however, still with progressing disease and a positive sputum. They may "have their ups and downs," but are never free from symptoms, and even if they are able to work it is often difficult for them to find suitable occupation. Patients in the late fibroid stage (often they have survived long enough to be labelled "senile phthisis") have often surprisingly little toxæmia but much dyspnœa, which forces upon them a life of restricted activity. Many of them may easily pass for "chronic bronchitics" unless the sputum is examined. Bronchiectatic dilatations may determine repeated hæmoptyses or recurrent attacks of pyrexia. They are often too old or have too little vital capacity for collapse therapy, and they are likely to be dangerous, especially in the family circle, because of the tubercle bacilli in their sputum. They need careful supervision, therefore, rather than active treatment.

20

Certain new methods are available of assessing the progress and severity of the disease, though they are of little or no value in diagnosis. The *erythrocyte sedimentation rate* repeated at regular intervals is a useful guide to activity, immediate outlook and response to treatment. The *monocyte-lymphocyte ratio* in the blood is based on the belief that the " epithelioid " cell of the tubercle is derived from the monocyte, so that when tuberculosis is advancing the increase of monocytes in the tissues is reflected in the blood stream at the expense of the lymphocytes. The *von Bonsdorf count* is a modification of the Arneth index and consists in a count of the total number of separate nuclei in the first 100 polymorphs counted in a blood film. A good deal more research needs to be done on the significance of these tests, but enough is already known about them to show that they hold good promise of prognostic value.

Many drugs have been tried in the treatment of pulmonary tuberculosis, but none of them has established itself. Gold is the most popular, and is used in exudative or fibrocaseous types of the disease where there is little toxæmia. It has undoubted dangers, yet there is no convincing evidence of its value, or even of its advisability. The same can be said of tuberculin. In such a tedious disease as tuberculosis it must be remembered that a course of injections may have a psychologically beneficial effect, provided that they do no harm ; if such psychological encouragement were called for, however, I should prefer to administer some less risky medicament such as colloidal calcium.

SYMPTOMATIC AND PALLIATIVE TREATMENT

There are many distressing symptoms and complications which may do harm and which need treatment. An ineffective *cough* should be checked ; often the patient can be taught to restrain it. If it is due to pharyngeal irritation or some intranasal condition, it should be treated by the appropriate means. A painful laryngeal cough is helped by resting the voice and by antiseptic inhalations or sedative lozenges. Sticky sputum may be loosened by hot alkaline drinks, combined with an ephedrine-containing mixture if there is associated bronchial spasm. An effective cough should be checked only if and while it interferes with sleep ; a codein linctus will usually give sufficient temporary relief. *Night sweats* have become infinitely less common since the importance of proper hygienic management, sensible clothing, fresh air, and free ventilation has been appreciated. *Pain* is usually due to pleurisy, and some degree of it is so common that its treatment is primarily that of the disease as a whole. Nevertheless, it often needs special measures of relief. Care must be exercised in giving morphia, lest the cough reflex is abolished. Strapping the side is apt to cause severe dyspnœa, but kaolin poultices may be comforting. *Hæmoptysis* frightens the patient, but is not as a rule serious. If there is only streaking of the sputum no special treatment is necessary. Moderate bleeding calls for rest in bed and reassurance. If the patient is very nervous a dose of chloral hydrate will help to quieten him. A severe hæmoptysis demands rest in bed and competent nursing. An initial small dose of morphia (gr. $\frac{1}{6}$) may be needed to allay anxiety and lessen restlessness. The patient should be partially propped up in bed. He should be allowed to move his position and should be encouraged to cough up any clots and sputum, otherwise these may accumulate in the bronchi and produce either collapse of the lung or bronchopneumonic spread of the disease. For this reason, any further morphia which may have to be given must be small enough in amount to allow of retention of the cough reflex. It must not be forgotten that a hæmoptysis is a hæmorrhage, and that plenty of fluids or even blood transfusion may therefore be necessary. An important part of the after-treatment should be directed to any resulting anæmia. The various specific drugs which have been suggested for the control of the bleeding appear to me to have no value whatever. If the hæmoptysis is profuse, and if it is known from which lung the bleeding arises, collapse of that lung by means of an artificial pneumothorax is rational. The occasions on which this is possible are, however, exceedingly rare, if only because a patient with a breaking-down lesion who has been under treatment for some time has probably already had an unsuccessful attempt at pneumothorax collapse made on him.

Gastro-intestinal disturbances are very common. Anorexia and dyspepsia are often due to toxæmia and improve with the general improvement which follows rest and fresh air. It should be remembered that occasionally phthisis and peptic ulcer may be present in the same patient. A history suggestive of peptic ulcer should call, therefore, for the appropriate investigations. Injudicious attempts at "feeding up the patient" must be avoided. Constipation is common and should be treated on the usual lines. Diarrhœa may be due to toxæmic hypochlorhydria, in which case dilute hydrochloric acid will often help ; to tuberculous ulceration of the intestine, usually accompanied by occult blood and albumin in the fæces ; or in long-standing cases to amyloid disease. Tuberculous enteritis is a most serious complication, the more so because its treatment is disappointing in the extreme. The patient with phthisis must realise from the first the importance of not swallowing infected sputum, lest he encourage direct infection of the bowel. The proper diet for this condition is one with a low residue and a high vitamin content, similar to that given for ulcerative colitis. A wholly lacto-vegetarian diet is, as a rule, badly tolerated. Sooner or later, unfortunately, the aim of treatment becomes one of comfort rather than cure, and " drowsie Syrrup " the only feasible drug ; tincture of opium, ♏ 10, or if necessary more, should be given three times a day to ease the pain. Sometimes the intravenous injection of calcium chloride (5 c.c. of a 5 per cent. solution) will give temporary relief not only of the diarrhœa but also of the accompanying painful intestinal spasm. Surgical interference usually does more harm than good.

Tuberculous laryngitis is always secondary to pulmonary tuberculosis, and is caused by the direct and persistent impact of infected sputum, or by infection carried thither by the blood stream. Effective treatment of the underlying lung condition, directed towards reducing the amount and frequency of the infective sputum, is an essential part of treatment of the laryngitis. Control, if possible, of the pulmonary lesion by artificial pneumothorax is by far the most helpful method of achieving this ; tuberculous laryngitis is therefore an important addition to the indications for attempting this form of collapse.

Here again rest is the fundamental basis of the local treatment. It is achieved by not using the larynx for vocalisation for many months (*complete silence*), and also by reducing excessive cough. Sometimes the laryngologist can help to reduce local swelling by means of the galvanocautery, but this must never be regarded as a substitute for rest. If the laryngeal lesion is advanced, palliative treatment is all that can be

done. The widespread ulceration, particularly of the epiglottis, exposes nerve endings in the raw area and causes great
pain, especially on swallowing. The patient's comfort is the
prime consideration in what is now an incurable condition.
Cocaine, in the form of pastilles for sucking, or as a 5 per cent.
spray (in aqueous solution), is the best drug for the relief of
the pain. It is usually best used before meals. Orthocain, a
cocaine-containing powder, applied by means of a special in-
sufflator, is also of help. In desperate cases the laryngologist
may try coagulation by diathermy of the ulcerated areas, or
injection of alcohol into the superior laryngeal nerve. Sometimes the sufferer finds it less painful to swallow if he lies on
his face and sucks his semi-solid food through a tube. Whether
the local lesion is early or advanced, the guidance and co-
operation of a laryngological expert are essential.

SPECIAL PROBLEMS

Tuberculosis and marriage—From time to time the family
doctor or the consultant will be asked whether an individual
with pulmonary tuberculosis should marry. The problem can
never be settled by rule of thumb. Right advice depends on
the merits of the particular case, and the doctor can only base
his opinion on certain general principles. Moreover, the question is not merely a medical one, for it involves the wider issue
of the individual's life in the *milieu* of the family and of the
community.

The Elizabethan compilers of *The Book of Common Prayer*
were wise in pointing out that matrimony " was ordained for
the procreation of children " as well as " for the mutual society,
help and comfort that the one ought to have of the other,
both in prosperity and adversity." When two persons wish
to marry, and one or both has suffered, or is suffering, from
pulmonary tuberculosis, it is only right that they should know
what they are undertaking. Even though the tuberculous
lesion may be healed, a man may later break down again and
be unable to provide for his wife and family ; * a woman may
relapse under the strain of domestic work or of pregnancy and
become a heavy responsibility which her husband may be

* The Ministry of Health has recently provided for maintenance grants (Circular
266/T), which will go some way to meet this catastrophe.

unable financially to meet. On the other hand, life together may be easier for both if their financial position enables them to have sufficient help and if there is no need for undue strain or anxiety. The danger of contact infection of children has already been made clear. If the parents are intelligent and scrupulously careful, however, it is possible to avoid this, as has been shown by the experience of colonies such as Papworth.

If it is clear that a tuberculous woman dare not risk pregnancy the wisdom of marriage, whatever the material comforts, becomes much more dubious. A marriage which is conditioned by the need to avoid pregnancy can hardly be ideal, certainly if the partners are young. Two people in love may for a time be content to enjoy a unity of body, even though it must not result in the birth of a child. In the long run, however, the constant fear of pregnancy and the need to deny the natural fulfilment of sexual relationships are almost certain to exact too high a price from both parties. They may at length take the chance of pregnancy, with catastrophic results. On the other hand, if they frustrate the natural consequences of marriage husband and wife will miss its fundamental satisfaction, namely, the making of a family ; a lack which so often leads to subtle and devastating psychological effects and to great unhappiness.

As a rule, it is unwise for the family doctor to *dictate* to two young people in love. Nevertheless, when they or their parents come to him for counsel he has a duty to assess the position, as far as possible, without fear or favour, and to try to make the issues clear to them, so that they have the facts on which to base their own decision. They may refuse to face these facts, as their problem is often a tragic one. In any case it calls not only for the truth but for sympathy and understanding.

Tuberculosis and pregnancy—It seems to be agreed that pregnancy, together with the period of puerperium and lactation, has an unfavourable influence upon the pulmonary lesion. It must be confessed that the conclusion is based on rather vague premises, for it is not always easy to separate the possible evil effect of pregnancy from aggravation natural to the disease. Certainly pregnancy is a strain even upon the healthy person, and the tuberculous woman needs a considerable margin of resistance if she is to meet it successfully. Many patients with chronic fibrotic disease have withstood even multiple pregnancies without coming to harm ; but if the lesion is recent and exudative the outlook is serious in any case, and the scales should not be weighted against recovery by the demands of pregnancy. This is true even if it is possible to establish an effective therapeutic pneumothorax.

Sometimes the patient improves as the pregnancy proceeds. The reason for this may be that in the later months the uterus progressively pushes up the diaphragm. X-ray films show that, on the right side at least, the fissure between the upper and the lower lobes is displaced upwards. A certain degree of collapse of the upper lobe is thus indirectly produced—the upper lobe being the usual site of the tuberculous lesion. When the uterus empties at term the diaphragm descends again, allowing the upper lobe to re-expand comparatively rapidly. This may easily cause exacerbation of the disease, and in the more acute forms may determine rapid and even fulminating spread. It is helpful to bear these various guiding principles in mind, for if therapeutic abortion is to be done, it should be done before the fourteenth week ; yet at this date it is still impossible to detect any specific deterioration or (apart from general principles) to forecast what effect the continuance of pregnancy will have. Once again the problem is one of " seed " and " soil," of the activity of the disease and the resistance of the patient. Active disease and tubercle bacilli in the sputum contraindicate the added strain of pregnancy. Even with arrested disease it is a risk, the extent of which depends not only on the resistance of the patient but on the facilities available to her of medical supervision, adequate rest, proper food, and the absence of economic or psychological strain.

Trauma and tuberculosis—An injury to the chest may bruise or lacerate the lung and thereby reactivate a healed focus or cause the spread of a lesion already active. Moreover, any injury (not necessarily of the chest) which puts a man out of work and leaves him drawing small compensation money, unable to buy adequate nourishment, worried about his family, his future capacity for work and the immediate litigation, can so reduce a man's resistance as to allow the " breakdown " of an old focus or the exacerbation of an active lesion.

" HOMO SUM : NIHIL HUMANI A ME ALIENUM PUTO "

The time has now come to correct a half-truth enunciated earlier. The treatment of tuberculosis of the lungs is not, after all, mainly the treatment of cavities ; it is the management of a human individual. A patient with even a relatively benign manifestation of tuberculosis, such as tuberculous pleurisy with effusion, is liable eventually to develop serious phthisis unless he is properly treated at an early stage, and thereafter continues to live sensibly so that his resistance is not undermined. Those with caseous lesions which have led to the breaking down of lung tissue and the appearance of tubercle bacilli in the sputum must hope and think in terms of *arrest* of the disease rather than of cure. Resistance may be overwhelmed once again, given the requisite unfavourable conditions.

Of the patients with minimal lesions most are able to leave the sanatorium with their lesion quiescent and to continue under the supervision of their own doctor and the tuberculosis officer. Soon they are well enough to return to work without harm, provided that they lead a well-regulated life. At the other extreme are the advanced cases, unfit for any work at any time. In between, and in a majority, are the " middle cases," just able to hold their own while life is sheltered, but quite unfit to withstand the strains and stresses of ordinary competitive existence.

Such a patient must work and earn if he is to live and keep himself and his family.* As things are at present, " light work " is not a feasible solution, for it is almost impossible to obtain it. " Crocks " are a nuisance in competitive industry, and even if light work can be found the wages are poor. He is compelled, therefore, to attempt to live a normal working life, competing with the fit and healthy. A heavy day's work, the tiring effort of travelling to and fro, the impossibility of taking rest when he needs it, the worry lest he should not be able to carry on with his job and so cease to be the mainstay of his family all contribute to the undermining of his small resistance. If he is not fit for a full-day's work, he will be supervised at home by his own doctor and the tuberculosis officer, and the

* The recent Ministry of Health Circular 266/T provides for grants for tuber-culous patients who are getting back to work, but they are not available where " treatment cannot do more than alleviate a chronic condition."

local " Care Committee " may be able to grant him extra nourishment and other help. If he has already been ill for more than six months his National Health Insurance benefit will have fallen to 10s. 6d. a week. Yet he needs to spend something like 18s. a week on food if he is to be adequately fed as a tuberculous person, besides meeting his own and his family's further needs of rent, food and other unavoidable expenses. The gap is far too wide to be covered by the Care Committee. He may apply for public assistance, a humiliating matter for many self-respecting patients ; here also the gap is seldom covered. What usually happens is that his wife goes out to work in order to earn some money for the household while he stays at home to mind (and perhaps infect) the some- what underfed children, and to grow bitter, hopeless and de- moralised. Both these types—the man who goes back to his job though he is not really fit for full-time work, and the man who is unable to go back to his job, and who perhaps has tubercle bacilli in his sputum—could do a certain amount of work under special conditions if only they could get it.

Clearly, to the great majority of our fellows, the diagnosis of pulmonary tuberculosis is a social and economic catastrophe. The student, trained in a narrow " medical " view of disease, tends to think that the sanatorium is the beginning and end of treatment. He is apt to regard it vaguely as a place of segregation for those who otherwise would be spreading in- fection, where sufferers from what is regarded as a rather hopeless disease can be treated by those specialising in it. If they are lucky to come out " cured " the family doctor knows only too well that it is primarily money (the Atlantic Charter's " freedom from want ") and not advice or bottles of medicine which is needed if they are not to relapse. The thoughtful doctor feels helpless, therefore, against what he knows is a hard economic and sociological problem. It may be argued that medicine, like the cobbler and the Church, should stick to its own last and not dabble in politics or economics. Yet it is the duty of our profession, knowing the facts, to press home the magnitude of the evil and to emphasise the data on which any adequate solution of it must be based. If men desire a tubercle-free community there are two alterna- tives open to them. They might follow certain veterinarians and strive to establish a tubercle-free herd by killing off all human reactors to tuberculin or (if this is too drastic) all those with tubercle bacilli in their sputum—a measure hardly likely to find favour either with our profession or with the majority of the people. The alternative is a major war on the disease, for which the people must pay in hard work, money, brains, organisation and all the other things necessary for waging a total war. At present, diagnosis and treatment are moderately well provided for, but with serious gaps ; little is done to follow up and consolidate the initial treatment so as to ensure permanent results. " Too little and too late," so that the enemy is able to wrest ground gained previously at considerable cost, can be said of this campaign also. What is needed is to seek out the disease before lung tissue breaks down and infection is spread : to treat it early and well : to guard and foster resistance not only of the patient but also of the community : to do everything possible to prevent relapses : and to prevent the spread of infection when caseation does occur.

For the " middle case" who, on leaving the sanatorium is not fit to take his chance in the open market, there are various schemes already in being, but they touch only a very tiny proportion of the patients concerned. The gain of working capacity which has been achieved in the sanatorium can but rarely be converted into wages. Unsatisfactory palliatives are adopted because there is insufficient zeal on the part of the community to resolve the economic and sociological factors which make up the hard core of the difficulty. Here **rehabilitation,** followed by work under conditions appropriate to the patient's capacity and to the avoiding of the spread of infection, are what are needed. One method of achieving this is by colonies such as the Papworth village settlement, Preston Hall and a few others (all voluntary organisations), and a couple of colonies maintained by local authorities in Cheshire and in Nottinghamshire. These institutions fit the environment to the patient rather than allow him to take his chance with the environment. Light work is ensured by up-to-date mechanisation. The machine does the heavy work, the man minds the machine and earns a living wage, and hope and morale are safeguarded.*

* The student should make himself familiar with the principles and details of these schemes by consulting the writings of the late Sir Pendrill Varrier-Jones, who founded Papworth ; the report on " After-Care and Rehabilitation " by E. Brieger, published by the *British Journal of Tuberculosis* as a special supple-

In 1944, following the Tomlinson report on Rehabilitation of the previous year, the Disabled Persons (Employment) Act became law. It provides for the voluntary registration of the disabled, and enables them to undergo vocational training, to be placed in ordinary employment, and if need be to obtain employment under sheltered conditions. It offers an opportunity to the Tuberculosis Officer and the Ministry of Labour to build up machinary which will enable tuberculous patients who are fit for a measure of employment to achieve some degree of economic independence. The Act can only work, however, if all the persons intimately concerned—employers, fellow workmen and the disabled—wish it to succeed.

The U.S.S.R. have undertaken a series of industrial experiments which are of great importance. Tuberculous patients able to work part time only have the balance of their wages made up by subsidy from social insurance funds. Special workshops are set aside for " sputum-positive " patients. Sometimes a special room is provided in the factory where the conveyer belt moves more slowly to suit the pace of those who are not fit enough to work at the normal rate. Night sanatoria are available for those who still require some degree of active care and treatment. Care is taken to safeguard the interests not only of tuberculous workers but also of the healthy who might otherwise be exposed to infection.*

Rehabilitation and the means of converting partial working capacity into the opportunity to earn wages has obviously a much wider application than merely to tuberculosis. It would save an enormous amount of wastage both in money and in human work, and its cost would be offset by the saving of much unproductive expenditure on unemployment and health benefits, compensation payments and the like. Insurance companies, friendly societies, trade unions, local authorities and the State are all dispensing money which could be used to better purpose. Above all, rehabilitation would save much human misery.

The war, as was expected, brought a disturbing increase

ment in October 1937 ; and various reports, articles and editorials which he can find in medical journals such as the *Lancet*, the *British Medical Journal* and *Tubercle*. He will find an article by Roberts on " The After-Care of Pulmonary Tuberculosis " in the *Practitioner* of August 1942 interesting and thought-provoking.

* More details can be read in Sigerist's *Socialised Medicine in the Soviet Union*, Gollancz, 1937.

in the incidence and mortality of tuberculosis. There can be no shallow optimism about the future. It will need a tremendous effort to reverse the position and eradicate the disease. Much more must be done to ferret out patients with minimal disease. If they are to be given prompt and efficient treatment far more accommodation for them in hospitals or sanatoria will be necessary. Later, the treatment of the patient must be continued in the form of rehabilitation and after-care. The earlier proper treatment can be instituted the less need there will be for major surgery, or for the more complex arrangements to restore the sufferer to productive work.

CHAPTER XXI

UNCOMMON PULMONARY INFECTIONS AND OTHER LESIONS

THERE are certain inflammatory and other lesions which, though uncommon, are liable on clinical or X-ray grounds to give rise at times to difficulties of diagnosis. For this reason they are brought to the student's attention in this chapter, though their relative infrequency calls for a less detailed description.

VIRUS PNEUMONIAS

In recent years small epidemics of " atypical pneumonia " have been prevalent, especially in America. These pneumonias are " atypical " in that they differ importantly, in certain of their clinical and pathological features, from the usual types. Some of them have been shown to be caused by various viruses.

The exact nature of viruses is not yet fully known. They are considerably smaller than ordinary bacteria, and cannot be cultivated save in the presence of living cells. They can thus be regarded as " obligatory parasites," intimately associated with the cells which they injure, and in which they multiply.

They directly damage the tissue cells of the host. If the infection is severe the result is tissue necrosis, whereas if it is mild a hyperplastic reaction occurs, accompanied by mononuclear infiltration.* As a response to tissue destruction, inflammation follows. In the lungs, further secondary inflammation may take place as the result of the inhalation of pyogenic organisms such as the pneumococcus or streptococcus.

Most virus diseases are followed by permanent immunity, though the common cold and influenza are notable exceptions. The production of immune bodies determines precipitation,

---

* This is true of injurious inorganic substances also, such as HCl, and certain gases.

agglutination, and complement fixation reactions. The viruses are intracellular, and damage the associated tissue cell from within. In this situation they cannot be affected by antibodies, and once the disease is established, specific serum therapy is of no value.

The broad clinical features of virus pneumonia are as follow : the incubation period is about two to three weeks ; after a period of malaise, the acute phase is ushered in with pyrexia, headache, and generalised aches and pains. At this stage influenza or tuberculosis may be suspected. The development of a distressing unproductive cough directs attention to the chest, but the physical signs which are discovered are usually indecisive. An X-ray film of the chest reveals shadowing of greater or less extent, usually near the root of the lung or in the lower lobes, caused by patches of bronchopneumonic consolidation. Provided that there is no secondary pyogenic infection, the leucocyte count is either diminished or approximately normal.

In *mild* infections the pyrexia falls after three or four days by lysis. In *severer* infections the acute stage lasts for a week or more, and patches of bronchopneumonia may be obvious to physical examination. The pyrexia may not fall for two or three weeks, and as the spleen may be obviously enlarged, enteric fever is often suspected. *Intense* infections cause a grave illness, with hæmorrhagic bronchopneumonia which in many instances passes on to necrosis. If the patient survives, the fever may persist for a month or more, and secondary invasion of the lungs by pyogenic organisms is common. In all these types of the disease, mononuclear and not polymorphonuclear cells are found in the alveolar walls and spaces, save when secondary infection has supervened.

In some of the epidemics the virus of psittacosis was found to be the cause : in others, that of " Q " fever (a Rickettsial infection) : in others, cytoplasmic inclusion bodies were found in the alveolar epithelium, though the exact nature of the virus was not identified.

These diseases are highly contagious, and call for strict isolation of the patient. The pathological diagnosis involves expert investigations by those familiar with virus problems. Treatment is symptomatic, for (except when secondary pyogenic infection has taken place) chemotherapy and serum treatment are both ineffective. As yet knowledge of these diseases is very incomplete, and much pathological and epidemiological research is still necessary for their elucidation.

PSITTACOSIS

Psittacosis (or ornithosis) is an infectious disease which especially attacks members of the parrot family, though it may also be found among domestic fowls, pigeons, cats, mice and other animals. It is caused by a filterable virus, which can be isolated from the nasal discharges and droppings of infected birds. It is highly infectious for human beings, the virus entering through the mucous membrane of the upper respiratory tract.

In birds the lungs are rarely involved, but both liver and spleen are enlarged, and contain areas of focal necrosis. In man (and in experimental monkeys) the lungs suffer a patchy bronchopneumonia ; the alveolar walls show marked cellular infiltration together with active proliferation of the epithelium, and the alveolar spaces are filled with mononuclear cells and fibrinous exudate. There is much congestion and thrombosis of the capillaries, and if the infection is severe, extensive necrosis of lung tissue. Secondary infection by pneumococci or streptococci alters the pathological picture accordingly (see Chap. XVIII). In gravely toxic cases the liver is damaged and areas of necrosis are found.

The incubation period is about eight to fourteen days. Instances of the disease occur as a rule among isolated families exposed to infection from a sick parrot or budgerigar or canary. The onset of the illness is sudden, with malaise, severe headache, photophobia and maybe shivering attacks. Epistaxis is common. The temperature rises rapidly, becomes continuous or remittent, and falls by lysis during the second or third week. The pulse is relatively slow, a feature which together with the pyrexia, headache and severe toxæmia may lead the doctor to suspect one of the enteric fevers. Cough develops, but it is usually unproductive. Unless the patches of bronchopneumonia become confluent, the physical signs of consolidation may not be found, but a radiogram shows the shadows of the pulmonary lesion.

Diagnosis—In a patient known to be associated with parrots, or with poultry, an unusual type of pneumonia, with a slow pulse rate, a normal or subnormal leucocyte count, intense headache and a clinical picture suggestive of either influenza or typhoid fever, should suggest the possibility of psittacosis. The possibility is more readily thought of when other reported cases indicate the presence of an epidemic of the disease. Enteric fever is excluded by negative blood and fæces cultures, and by negative agglutination tests (Widal reaction). Proof of the disease is established by special tests for the presence of psittacosis virus in the sputum, white mice being used for the experiments.

The *outlook* in severe infections is poor, especially in older persons. The death rate is put at something of the order of 40 per cent., but this is almost certainly too high, for many mild examples of the disease are probably unrecognised. *Treatment* is entirely symptomatic. If secondary pyogenic infection supervenes, the treatment must be modified accordingly (see Chap. XVIII).

PNEUMONIC PLAGUE

Plague is an infectious disease of man caused by *Pasteurella pestis*, and transmitted from diseased rats which frequent dwellings, ships and warehouses. It is found in India, China and other parts of the Far East, in certain parts of Africa and in South America. Very rarely cases have occurred in England and America, brought to the seaports. Bubonic plague is transmitted to humans by the rat flea. *Pneumonic plague*, on the other hand, is spread by droplets of sputum which are loaded with *P. pestis* in almost pure culture : a form of transmission favoured by lack of ventilation and overcrowding (such as occurred in the great Manchurian epidemic in 1910-11 during exceedingly cold weather).

In primary pneumonic plague the inflammation spreads from the bronchial mucous membranes to the peribronchial tissues, and thence to the alveoli. Patches of hæmorrhagic bronchopneumonia result, which rapidly become confluent. The sputum is watery, and stained with blood. The incubation period is from one to three days ; and within a few days of the onset of the pneumonia the patient inevitably dies.

The disease is obviously highly dangerous to those attending

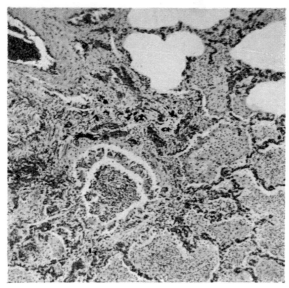

FIG. 106.

Acute Bronchopneumonia—the bronchiole below and to left of centre and the alveoli related to it are congested and filled with inflammatory exudate, while the alveoli situated top right are free of exudate. Hæmatoxylin and Eosin. (See Text, p. 232)

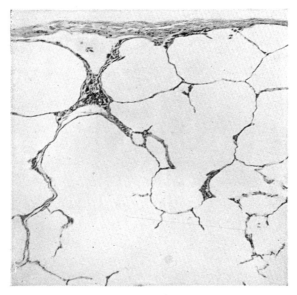

FIG. 107.

Emphysema—the alveoli are distended. The walls of the alveoli, the interlobular septum toward top left, and the pleura are abnormally thin. In several places rupture of their walls has thrown adjacent alveoli into communication with formation of large, irregular spaces. Hæmatoxylin and Eosin. (See Text, p. 196)

to face page 320

sufferers from the disease, and even the wearing of masks may fail to give protection.

Pneumonia may also result from metastatic infection carried by the blood from a primary bubo. Here, recovery is possible, and large doses of antiplague serum (up to 200 c.c.) should be given daily as soon as the initial diagnosis of bubonic plague is made.

Tularæmia, an infectious disease met with largely in America, and caused by *Bacterium tularense,* may cause pulmonary lesions. The main source of infection in man is wild rabbits and hares. The disease does not spread directly from one human being to another.

The primary lesion is a papule of the skin, which later ulcerates and is accompanied by enlargement of the corresponding lymph nodes. Hæmatogenous spread to the lungs is indicated by the development of severe cough, pain in the chest, cyanosis and dyspnœa. The course may be fulminating, death occurring in a few days, or a very slowly progressing bronchopneumonia may occur. The clinical picture may therefore simulate suffocative bronchiolitis, lung abscess, acute pneumonia, chronic bronchopneumonia or a mild bronchitis. Occasionally, pleural effusion occurs. Diagnosis is clinched by agglutination tests, which become positive in nearly all cases by the second or third week of the illness. The recognition of tularæmic pulmonary lesions depends, therefore, on the recognition of primary tularæmic infection in a patient showing symptoms and signs of pulmonary disease. Treatment is symptomatic. Recently an antiserum has been prepared, but its value is as yet undecided. Prevention is by thorough cooking of rabbits used for food, and by the wearing of rubber gloves by those who have to skin and dress wild rabbits.

Undulant fever (brucellosis) very rarely manifests itself by predominantly pulmonary symptoms and signs. When it does, a mild general illness persists for some weeks, due to the brucella infection, and then pneumonia supervenes. Whether this is due to the brucellosis or whether it is always secondary, and caused by the lowered resistance of the patient, is not as yet determined.

21

FUSOSPIRILLAL BRONCHITIS

This form of bronchitis is characterised by the presence in the sputum of large numbers of spirilla and fusiform organisms. Originally thought to attack only dwellers in the tropics, the disease has more recently been found to be fairly prevalent in America and France. The causal organisms are found in the mouth, and are associated with dental caries or pyorrhœa. They gain access to the bronchi by inhalation, sometimes after inhalation anæsthesia. As has been described in Chapter XIX, they may penetrate further into the lungs, to produce putrid lung abscess.

The affected bronchi show necrosis of the mucosa, with destruction also of elastic tissue in the bronchial wall. The necrotic tissue sloughs away, leaving deep ragged ulcers which can be seen through the bronchoscope, and from which the causal organisms can be isolated. Erosion of blood vessels results in bleeding and hæmoptysis. As the destruction of elastic tissue progresses, the bronchi dilate. Unless the advance of the organisms is arrested, they eventually spread into adjacent lung tissue. The resulting pulmonary lesions vary according to the resistance of the body to the invasion. They may consist of fibrosis, or of necrosing bronchopneumonia, or of putrid abscess with cavitation. Pleural effusion may sooner or later complicate the picture.

The disease may be acute or chronic. In the acute form the onset is sudden, with shivering and marked malaise. An irregular fever develops, while cough, expectoration of blood-stained offensive sputum, and coarse crepitations heard over the chest indicate the presence of the bronchitis. After two or three weeks the patient's condition may improve, but relapses are frequent, and the disease may settle down to a chronic course which may last for months or even years. Sometimes the onset is insidious, and no acute phase is obvious. The sputum is abundant, mucopurulent, offensive, and frequently is streaked with blood. From time to time more copious hæmoptyses may occur. As the illness develops, loss of weight and asthenia result from the prolonged toxæmia. The physical signs of bronchitis are found predominantly over the lower lobes. Extension to the lungs is characterised by an increase in the toxæmia and the obvious development of bronchopneumonia. If lung abscess develops, the clinical picture becomes similar to that of putrid abscess due to the inhalation into the finer bronchi of infected particulate matter (see Chap. XIX).

The *diagnosis* is established by the finding of bronchitis, associated with large numbers of fusiform organisms and spirilla in the sputum. In chronic cases X-ray films of the chest reveal a picture which may be mistaken for that of pulmonary tuberculosis, for at this stage the pulmonary parenchyma is liable to be involved by extension of infection from the affected bronchi. Tubercle bacilli, however, are not found in the sputum.

Treatment is by organic arsenic given intravenously, as, for example, neoarsphenamine in 0·6 gm. doses, or novarsenobillon in doses of 0·3 gm. In patients who receive treatment at an early stage, before necrosis or fibrosis of the lungs supervenes, the symptoms, signs and radiological evidence of the disease diminish after the first one or two injections, and in favourable cases disappear completely after four or five injections. As a rule, the injections are given at intervals of four days for a few weeks. In more chronic lesions, when there is destruction of lung tissue, the arsenical injections may arrest the progress of the infection, even though they cannot influence the pulmonary destruction which has taken place. If the organisms in the sputum are found to be sensitive to penicillin, this drug may be a helpful addition to the treatment of both acute and chronic lesions.

In the absence of specific treatment spontaneous cure may occasionally occur, but if the disease progresses, extension to the lungs is liable sooner or later to cause grave complications which may prove fatal.

ALLERGIC INFILTRATIONS OF THE LUNGS

A condition which needs fuller elucidation has been described by Loeffler of Zurich, and by several other observers. It is characterised by the appearance of fleeting shadows seen in radiograms of the chest, in patients who suffer hardly any disturbance of the general health. The X-ray film may show dense shadows of varying size, single or multiple, similar to those of early tuberculous infiltration ; within three to eight days, however, these shadows disappear. The patient, usually a child (though adults may be affected), suffers from slight lassitude, but has no fever nor disturbing general symptoms. There may be a slight irritating cough, with a little sputum in which tubercle bacilli or elastic fibres are never discovered. *Eosinophilia* of the order of 10 to 30 per cent., though it may occasionally be as high as 60 per cent., is invariably found.

The lesion is almost certainly allergic in origin, and its transience is a characteristic feature. Some think that it is a response to tuberculo-protein, and therefore analogous to erythema nodosum. Others have described instances where it might possibly be due to the migration of ascaris larvæ through the lungs, or to sensitivity to drugs such as the sulphonamides. It is probable that, as with erythema nodosum, the fleeting infiltration is an allergic response which may occur to a variety of causative factors. In India, a largely similar picture of disease is given the name of *tropical eosinophilia* ; here the lung infiltrations appear to persist considerably longer than those in the patients described by Loeffler.

SYPHILIS OF THE RESPIRATORY TRACT

Syphilis of the larynx, trachea, bronchi or lungs is uncommon. **Syphilitic laryngitis** may arise during the secondary or tertiary stages of the disease. In the secondary stage it usually takes the form of subacute laryngitis, without ulceration. In the tertiary stage, gummatous inflammation occurs, followed as a rule by fibrosis, sometimes by deep ulceration. The lesion begins at the base of the epiglottis. The fibrosis may cause stenosis of the larynx, with resulting stridor and dyspnœa.

Syphilitic inflammation of the **trachea** or **bronchi** may similarly be followed by stenosis. Secondary inflammatory changes in the lungs result from the interference with the mucociliary defensive mechanism, or from obstruction (which leads to pulmonary collapse, if the block is complete) of a main or segmental bronchus.

Syphilis of the lung may be met with in three forms. The *white pneumonia* of infants, a manifestation of congenital syphilis, is of pathological rather than of clinical interest, for these children are either stillborn or they survive only for a few days. The lungs are solid, greyish white, and smooth on section. They are neither friable nor granular in appearance. Microscopically there is diffuse cellular infiltration and thickening of the alveolar connective tissue, and the alveoli are filled with solid exudate. By suitable staining methods spirochætes may be found in the diseased tissue in enormous numbers.

In the adult the lesion may appear as one or more gummata, situated in the middle or lower zones of the lungs, and accompanied by dense scar tissue which may extend outwards to the pleura. Alternatively, it may take the form of diffuse pulmonary fibrosis. The clinical picture is one of cough, expectoration, dyspnœa, pleural pain and maybe hæmoptysis, thus resembling tuberculosis. The physical signs are those of local induration and catarrh. The X-ray film shows local or generalised fibrosis of the lungs.

The diagnosis is never easy. It must be remembered that syphilitic disease of the respiratory system is rare, and that a positive Wassermann reaction, or even signs of syphilis elsewhere in the body, do not of themselves justify the diagnosis. Bronchial obstruction in a syphilitic, for example, is more likely to be due to carcinoma than to a gummatous granuloma. If, however, the lesion responds rapidly to the usual antisyphilitic measures, and no other cause can be found for it, it may then be regarded as likely to be due to syphilis. To be successful, treatment must be undertaken early, before the establishment of extensive fibrosis.

ACTINOMYCOSIS

The term " actinomycosis " is used in human and veterinary medicine to describe infection by a group of different, but related, organisms which results in a particular type of chronic, localised suppurative process or granuloma. The lesions may take the form of nodules, abscesses or fistulæ.

In man the disease is most commonly caused by a grampositive anaerobic hyphomycete, the *actinomyces bovis*, which is also the cause of a considerable proportion of the actinomycotic infections in cattle. This invades the tissues and forms small granules which are found in any softened focus, and are composed of an aggregated mass or colony of the fungus, usually surrounded by a radiating series of gramnegative club-like processes.

Distinct from actinomyces bovis, there are other mycelial organisms. One of these causes " Madura foot " (mycetoma), seen in Africa and Asia. An actinobacillus which may take on a filamentous habit of growth, but which is not a true mycelial organism, causes " woody tongue " in cattle, but hardly ever attacks man. There are also certain streptothrix infections both of man and cattle in which the organism is mycelial, but does not produce club-like processes.

Actinomycosis is therefore a disease primarily of cattle, which is communicable to man, probably by infected straw or dust. It attacks particularly those who are associated with cattle. In the last war infection sometimes attacked men who had to sleep on straw, in barns or other farm buildings : and there is some evidence that the fungus may gain access to the mouth and reside for a considerable time in carious teeth.

The organism causes a granuloma, with local necrosis and a surrounding zone of polymorphonuclear reaction. Later, the central portion of the lesion breaks down, and pus forms. The pus contains the characteristic pale yellow (" sulphur ") granules. As a rule the area of chronic suppuration slowly but inevitably extends, though attempts at healing are shown by the presence of fibrosis. The histological appearances are noteworthy—clusters of pure polymorphonuclear abscesses (typical, that is, of acute inflammation), surrounded by intense fibrosis (typical of a chronic lesion). At times the lesion may appear to have become arrested, only to break down again later.

This infection spreads through the tissues by direct contiguity. It may recede in one place and advance in another. Sometimes it spreads to distant organs by the blood stream, as, for example, in infection of the liver from the appendix, by the portal vein. The lymph nodes are not affected—a curious and characteristic feature. The reaction of the connective tissue is also remarkable, in that fibrosis occurs at a considerable distance from the site of the fungus. This fibrosis is obviously an attempt on the part of the body to establish a barrier to the advance of the disease. In organs such as the lungs or the liver, where the connective tissue is relatively scanty as compared with the epithelial tissue, arrest is much less likely, and the prognosis is correspondingly grave.

The jaw is the most common site of the initial lesion. The alimentary tract may become involved from swallowed portions of the mycelium. These lodge most often in the region of the appendix and cæcum ; the disease usually spreads from an infected appendix, following perforation or operative removal. **Thoracic actinomycosis** may arise from infected particulate matter inhaled into the lungs, or by metastatic spread (as, for example, from the appendix). More frequently, however, it appears to gain access to the mediastinum through small abrasions of the lower œsophagus, and later spreads to the pleura and lungs, and thence to the chest wall. Finally, a subcutaneous abscess is formed, which discharges pus from which the typical pale yellow sulphur granules can be obtained.

The onset of pulmonary actinomycosis is insidious, and the disease follows a chronic course. Bronchopneumonic infiltration of the lungs is followed by the development of abscess cavities. Irregular fever, cough, hæmoptysis and wasting are the main symptoms, and the physical signs are those of the corresponding lesion. Symptoms, signs, and radiological appearances may suggest tuberculosis, or (because tubercle bacilli are not found in the sputum) chronic pulmonary suppuration. Diagnosis is unlikely until the organism is found in the sputum, or in the pus from a lung abscess which has been submitted to operation, or in the discharge from a sinus of the chest wall. When granules are found, they must be examined microscopically for the typical mycelium. This is necessary because granules of cell debris or of masses of leucocytes may occasionally simulate those of actinomycosis.

When the lungs or the mediastinum are involved, the prognosis is grave, and in most instances death occurs within a year or two. There is no specific treatment which has proved consistently successful, in the sense in which arsenicals can favourably influence the course of syphilis. Some strains of the organism are sensitive to penicillin, others are not. For the former, high and prolonged systemic dosage is necessary (*e.g.* 200,000 units daily for 2 to 3 weeks). Full doses of iodides (sodium iodide 30 gr. three times a day) sometimes appear to have good results. X-ray therapy, sulphonamides, and vaccines may also be tried. Otherwise, attention to the general health and the opening of abscesses or the scraping of sinuses is all that can be done. Other fungus infections of the lungs are described in Chapter XXII.

RETICULOSIS

Reticulosis (Hodgkin's disease) of the mediastinal lymph nodes has already been described in Chapter X, p. 150. The enlarged glands are typically seen on the X-ray film as a dense mediastinal shadow, spreading outwards for some distance into the pulmonary areas. They may or may not be associated with enlargement of the lymph nodes elsewhere in the body. They produce symptoms and signs of mediastinal pressure, or of pressure on the bronchi and lungs.

Very rarely the intrapulmonary lymph nodes are the only intrathoracic structures involved. In the absence of more obvious manifestations of the disease in other parts of the body, diagnosis of such isolated pulmonary foci (revealed by radiograms) is hardly possible. If these lesions are accompanied by a pyrexia of the Pel-Ebstein type, the diagnosis can be made with reasonable confidence.

BOECK'S SARCOIDOSIS

It is only recently that a number of apparently isolated diseases have been recognised as manifestations of a single generalised disease. Boeck's sarcoid, Besnier and Schaumann's lupus pernio, uveoparotid fever, Mickulicz's syndrome, certain bone lesions termed "osteitis multiplex cystica," and various other syndromes are all facets of this single disease. It is characterised by "sarcoid" (lymphogranulomatous) deposits in the skin, lymph nodes, spleen, bones of the hands and feet, eyes, salivary glands, lungs and other organs. Some think it an atypical manifestation of tuberculosis, others a systematised disease of the reticulo-endothelial system.

In the thorax the mediastinal and bronchial lymph nodes may be involved, and there may be extensive infiltration of both lungs. As a rule there are few symptoms or physical signs, and instances have been described of pulmonary involvement recognised only on routine X-ray examination. Some patients show weakness, undue fatigue, loss of weight, cough and pain in the chest, and as radiograms reveal glandular enlargement and pulmonary infiltration, tuberculosis is suspected. Tubercle bacilli are not found in the sputum, and the tuberculin reaction may be negative. Reticulosis of the

Hodgkin type and silicosis have also to be considered in the differential diagnosis. The course of sarcoidosis is, however, prolonged and benign, and tends towards spontaneous recovery. The diagnosis is less difficult when lesions are present in other organs—painless tiny papules in the skin, granulations on the conjunctiva and iris, enlargement of the phalanges, adenopathy or parotid swelling. It is of interest to note that many of the instances of so-called chronic miliary tuberculosis of the lungs, which run a comparatively benign course, are in reality examples of sarcoidosis.

CHAPTER XXII

DISEASES DUE TO THE INHALATION OF DUSTS, FUMES AND GASES

THE student who frequents the post-mortem room is well aware that the dusty, smoky atmosphere breathed over a long period of years by the town-dweller results in a patchy dark pigmentation of the lungs which is absent in the young child or the countryman. The lungs of old coal-miners may be jet black with carbon deposit. These dusts are relatively harmless ; but certain dusts are exceedingly harmful, and if inhaled over a long period can cause disabling and maybe fatal damage to the lungs.

Within some twenty years of the establishment of gold-mining in the Rand, the inhalation of silica dust caused by the drilling of the rock in the mines caused such a spectacular incidence of grave and often fatal respiratory illness that special measures of prevention had to be taken in hand and the provision of compensation instituted for disablement or death. After the Boer War, when the mines began to work again, it was found almost impossible to get back experienced miners, for the majority had meanwhile died of what was then called " miner's phthisis." In Great Britain the first scheme of compensation for silicosis was put into force in 1919 (see p. 339), though for a long time before that it was common knowledge that certain dusty occupations were " dangerous trades."

The conditions under which miners engaged in rock-drilling had to work were once described by Sir Thomas Oliver after a visit to the Cornish tin-mines. " We crawled through an opening into a chamber from which a certain amount of ore had already been extracted. After we had squatted as best we could, the rock-drilling was begun. In a few minutes the atmosphere became so thick that breathing was, to those of the party unaccustomed to it, somewhat uncomfortable and difficult, and although we were squatting closely together, we could not see each other. Even the glare of our lights could not penetrate the dusty atmosphere."

SILICOSIS

Silicosis is by far the most important of the group of dust-inhalation diseases which have been given the collective name of the **pneumoconioses.** It results from prolonged exposure to certain kinds of dust encountered in the course of various occupations. *Sand-blasting* is perhaps the simplest example of such an occupation ; it involves the projection of sand or other grit, by means of compressed air, for the cleaning or polishing of a metal surface. Nowadays, metal grit is much more commonly used for the purpose, but silica dust may still be produced when the more modern process is used on metal castings, to which much of the sand used for the moulding adheres. *Flint and pebble crushing* is an allied industry, providing grit for sand-blasting, brake sand for tramcars, abrasive papers and chicken grit. The *refractories industry* is occupied with the mining, crushing and binding together of ganister and other sandstones to use as refractories (that is, substances resistant to heat) ; silica bricks, silica cement and various silica compositions are thus made for the construction of gas retorts and for use in the manufacture of metals. The *sandstone industry* brings danger to the workers who quarry and dress the stone, and to the masons who use it. Tunnel miners and grave-diggers who excavate in sandstone may develop silicosis. The *grinding of metals* is dangerous if grindstones of natural sandstone are used, the more so if the grinding is done dry and stringent preventive measures are not adopted. The *pottery industry* is dangerous, especially in its branches of earthenware and china manufacture ; the silica-containing raw material is harmless while it is moist, but when fragments dry and form dust, or when powdered flint is used for polishing, the incidence of silicosis becomes high. The manufacture of *scouring powders* and *abrasive soaps* involves the use of quartz-powder which is almost pure silica ; before it was realised how dangerous was exposure to this siliceous dust, the death rate was appalling. *Mining for gold, tin, lead, hæmatite iron ore* and other ores is hazardous as the result of drilling, by compressed air, in hard

rock headings. In *coal-mining* typical silicosis undoubtedly
follows the drilling of headings and the " ripping " of road-
ways in mines where the rock is hard and highly siliceous ;
the special problem of coal-miners' pneumoconiosis will be
discussed later.

THE PRODUCTION OF SILICOSIS

For the development of silicosis, silica (silicon dioxide,
SiO_2) must reach the lungs in sufficient amount and over a
sufficient period of time. The more silica the dust contains,
the more rapid is likely to be the development of the damage
to the lungs. The almost pure silica used, for example, in the
making of abrasive soaps caused a rapid development of the
disease ; whereas in a certain colliery where the hard rock of
the headings contains about 28 per cent. of free silica, some
fifteen to twenty years of exposure was necessary before the
miners began to complain of symptoms which led to the diagnosis of silicosis. Moreover, the more silica dust there is to
inhale, the greater the hazard. In the granite industry, for
example, where the dust is composed of about 33 per cent. of
silica, the disease was not generally found among the workers so
long as hammer and chisel alone were used. The introduction of
pneumatic machinery for carving and cutting, however, resulted
in the generating of very large quantities of dust. As a consequence, the mortality among granite cutters has been steadily
increasing, until it is now very disturbing. Again, it is clear
that, other things being equal, the longer the exposure to a
particular siliceous dust, the more serious will be the pulmonary
damage.

The size of the dust particles is important ; particles of
greater diameter than 10 microns rarely reach the pulmonary
alveoli. The most dangerous are those below 5 microns in
diameter. Water-spraying clears dusty air by allaying coarse
dust, but it does not cope equally well with very fine particles
of under 2 microns. These dangerous invisible dusts can be
removed, however, by adequate exhaust ventilation.

Dusts inhaled into the alveoli act as foreign bodies with
different capacities for mischief. They are dealt with by the
alveolar macrophages (" dust cells "), which ingest the particles,
carrying some towards the ciliated epithelium of the bronchi,

whence the mucociliary blanket carries them towards the mouth, there to be expectorated or swallowed : and carrying others into the lymphatics and peribronchial lymphatic nodes.

Silica particles do not injure the lung by " microscopical trauma " caused by their sharp-pointedness and hardness. They are harmful only after they have passed into solution in the body fluids. Alkali increases the solubility of silica, an important factor in the rapid, progressive (" acute ") type of silicosis, met with among abrasive soap workers. On the other hand, it is claimed that adulterant dusts, for example coal dust, clays and iron-ore dust, may reduce the solubility of silica ; the evidence for this is not convincing, however, and the diminished harmfulness in these instances may well be due to the " dilution " of the silica, so reducing its percentage content rather than its solubility.*

PATHOLOGY

Silica dust from the alveoli is carried into the lung after ingestion by macrophages. These enter the lymphatic channels, and many are arrested and die in the tiny peribronchial and perivascular lymph nodes on their way to the glands at the hilum. Within these nodes the silica slowly dissolves in the tissue fluids. In solution, or in colloidal form, it is a protoplasmic poison, giving rise to necrosis or to a fibrous reaction, according to the intensity of its action. If it dissolves comparatively freely and rapidly, the resulting lesion is necrotic. As a rule, however, solution is so slow that the irritative reaction is predominantly fibrotic ; around the silica deposit, concentric layers or whorls of fibroblasts are laid down, with the result that small nodules of dense, avascular, non-cellular fibrous tissue are formed (Fig. 108). These nodules in the moderately severe case are typically about $\frac{1}{8}$ to $\frac{1}{4}$ in. in diameter, pigmented by fine brownish granules of foreign material, much of which is true silica, though there is usually some carbon as well. Thus the silicotic nodules appear darker than the healthy parts of the lung ; this is especially well seen just under the pleural surfaces.

As the disease progresses the fibrous tissue matures, and

* Nevertheless, recent experiments on animals suggest that a small percentage of aluminium in a siliceous dust may greatly modify the capacity to damage the lungs.

the central part of the nodule undergoes hyaline change, so that the nodule shows a pale centre with a halo of pigmented tissue round it. Adjacent nodules coalesce, until eventually large areas of normal lung are replaced by dense, leathery fibrous tissue, within which shotty material is imprisoned. Normal areas of the lung undergo compensatory emphysema. The fibrosis extends to the pleural surfaces and the lungs become adherent to the chest wall. The glands at the hilum are stony hard with enclosed, finely shotty material, and the abdominal para-aortic glands become likewise involved. Whereas the normal town-dweller's lungs contain less than 0·2 gm. of silica per 100 gm. of dry weight, the silicotic lung may contain up to as much as 7 gm. per cent. As might be expected, the extent of the fibrosis bears no constant relationship to the percentage of silica found ; it is not the actual amount of free silica, but the extent and rate of its solution in the body fluids which determine the irritative pulmonary reaction.

The fibrous nodules formed round the slowly dissolving silica particles are thus the essential and characteristic lesion of uncomplicated silicosis. It is these which render the lung so hard, give it a shotty feel and cause the same shotty sensation when the lungs are cut with a knife. They give X-ray shadows indicative of nodulation, or denser opacities when the nodules become confluent.

Tuberculosis is a frequent complication, altering the anatomical picture by its own typical lesions—tuberculous bronchopneumonia, fibrocaseous tuberculosis or fibroid tuberculosis. At the same time it alters the clinical and radiological picture and the course of the disease. Many victims of silicosis die of pulmonary tuberculosis ; others, in the absence of superadded tuberculous infection, die of the end results of the fibrosis. Fibrosis, chronic bronchitis and emphysema lead eventually to right heart failure ; or the grossly impaired vital capacity is unable to withstand the impact of an acute respiratory infection.

There is some reason to believe that syphilitic infection increases the rapidity of the fibrotic change. Men with a positive Wassermann reaction are found to develop silicosis more rapidly than those in whom the Wassermann reaction was negative ; moreover, the disease runs a more rapid course.

CLINICAL MANIFESTATIONS

The symptoms and signs depend mainly on the fibrosis, which progresses at the expense of normal functioning lung. The inhalation of silica dust by itself is not immediately irritating, and for this reason workers and employers have in the past been lulled into a false sense of security.

" Acute " forms of the disease are very uncommon ; as a rule, silicosis develops slowly and insidiously. The action of silica is pathologically cumulative ; moreover, the production of soluble silica from the dust which has become fixed in the lung is usually slow. Exposure to silica dust, therefore, is not followed immediately by symptoms of illness ; there is a *latent period* varying from something like two to twenty or more years, and depending on factors such as the amount of dust in the occupation, the percentage of silica in the dust, the presence of alkali and the condition of the patient. Once there has been a certain degree of exposure, the pathological changes will inevitably follow, even though the victim ceases to inhale more silica ; if he continues to be exposed to the dust the inevitable damage to the lungs will, of course, be greater still.

In the usual chronic forms of the disease the period of time between the first exposure and the onset of symptoms is something of the order of ten years or more. The first symptom is usually slight *dyspnœa on exertion*. There may be less expansion and elasticity of the chest than normal. Mild secondary respiratory infections are common—recurrent colds or mild bronchitis. An X-ray film at this stage shows increased linear markings radiating from the hilum in both lung fields, with more or less discrete mottling due to shadows cast by the individual silicotic nodules. Apart from the slight dyspnœa, the patient might seem to be in robust health. His occupation should, however, excite suspicion and lead to the taking of X-ray films.

Gradually the breathlessness on exertion increases, together with a noticeable decrease in the expansion of the chest. Pains in the chest may indicate pleural irritation, and a *dry, irritating cough* develops. Respiratory infections become more frequent —recurrent colds, bronchitis which results in the expectoration of mucopurulent sputum, or occasionally the development of bronchiectasis with hæmoptysis. The X-ray film now shows generalised, bilateral medium-sized mottling. Against the background of peribronchial linear fibrotic shadows, and the now larger individual nodules, there may be opacities due to confluence of the nodules, or to patches of pleural thickening. The patient still looks fairly robust at rest, but on exertion he is seen to be dyspnœic. Signs of generalised fibrosis of the lungs are now to be seen : the upper part of the chest is smoothly flattened, the percussion note is somewhat duller than normal and the weakened breath sounds reveal the impaired expansion of the chest. By this stage the patient suffers an appreciable impairment of his normal working capacity.

If the disease progresses further, with still more extensive fibrosis, the dyspnœa becomes noticeable even at rest, and is distressing on even slight exertion. Cough is more frequent, and secondary bronchitis and emphysema are clearly established. Capacity for work is seriously and permanently impaired. By now the patient is an obviously ill man ; appetite is often poor and loss of weight obvious. The pulse rate is quickened, the heart may be dilated and cyanosis of the ears and mucous membranes indicates the chronic oxygen lack. Expansion of the chest is greatly reduced, even with forced inspiration ; the percussion note is dull over the localised areas of pleural thickening, and the breathing rapid, with short inspiration and high-pitched, prolonged expiration. X-ray films reveal that the mottling has become more intense ; the nodules larger and confluent, so that extensive shadows of dense fibrosis are seen ; there is a greater or less degree of emphysema. At this stage secondary respiratory infection is the rule.

The " acute form " of silicosis is rare. It occurred especially in the early days of abrasive soap manufacture, and the admixture with the silica dust of an alkali which greatly increased its solubility was probably the determining factor. The onset of symptoms was comparatively rapid, occurring within months, rather than years, after the first exposure to the dust. The lesions produced in the lungs were predominantly necrotic rather than fibrotic. The symptoms began with dyspnœa : then there was a rapid development of general constitutional disturbance, high fever, cyanosis and an acute illness which in a few weeks ended in death.

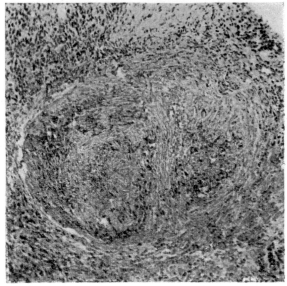

Fig. 108.

Silicotic Nodule—the dense fibrous laminæ of which the nodule is composed are concentrically arranged and infiltrated with quantities of brown pigment. Hæmatoxylin and Eosin. (See Text, p. 333)

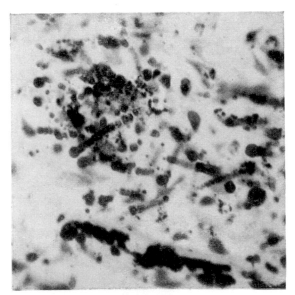

Fig. 109.

Asbestosis—the field contains an accumulation of yellowish brown pigment in the form of granules and "asbestosis-bodies." Variable in length these bodies consist of a series of closely arranged discs and may be swollen at one or both ends. Hæmatoxylin and Eosin. (See Text, p. 343)

to face page 337

SILICOSIS COMPLICATED BY PULMONARY TUBERCULOSIS

" Simple bronchitis is a recognised complication of dusty trades, and there is evidence that other respiratory infections may be increased by silica," wrote E. H. Kettle ; " but the one infection which stands out above all others is tuberculosis, and the great problem in the pneumoconioses is the relation of the dust to the tubercle bacillus." Kettle, himself a distinguished worker in this field, thought that in the development of secondary tuberculosis neither silicotic fibrosis nor necrosis had any special significance, but that the active growth of tubercle bacilli was encouraged by the presence of the silica itself. His own experiments and those of others are very suggestive that silica favours the proliferation of tuberculous bacilli by altering the environment ; but the exact mechanism of this action is not yet known.

The supervention of active tuberculosis of the lungs has long been known as a grave hazard to the patient suffering from silicosis. The infection may occur at any stage in the disease and modify the pathological and clinical picture accordingly. Clinically, the onset of tuberculosis is marked by a deterioration in the patient's condition. Dyspnœa is enhanced, pyrexia develops, cough and sputum are increased, tubercle bacilli may be found in the sputum, hæmoptysis may occur, and there is progressive weakness and loss of weight. The tuberculous infection, however, may itself be of the very chronic fibrotic type. The recognition of the superadded pulmonary tuberculosis then becomes a matter of great difficulty, especially if tubercle bacilli are not found in the sputum. In the more acute fibrocaseous types the presence of tubercle bacilli in the sputum and the recognition of cavitation in the silicotic lungs establish the diagnosis.

DIAGNOSIS

A satisfactory and final diagnosis of silicosis can be established by a consideration of three factors. The **occupational history** is important in that a comparatively brief exposure to the inhalation of silica dust may determine the onset of the disease, perhaps years later. Obviously there must have been exposure to the dust before silicosis can develop. The worker,

22

therefore, must be known to have been employed in a trade subjected to the silica hazard, and no period of his employment must escape notice.

The **clinical examination** of the patient provides the history not only of exposure but also of the symptoms and course of the disease. Though physical signs may be few, they may be valuable if they are integrated with the whole clinical picture. Examination of the sputum for tubercle bacilli should never be neglected.

Radiology of the chest is crucial, for it alone can provide a picture of the typical bilateral fan-like shadows made by the linear fibrosis, punctuated by those of macroscopically visible nodules. It can help also in the sometimes difficult problem of the detection of superadded tuberculosis infection ; and also in the diagnosis of chronic tuberculosis without silicosis, in a patient who gives a history of mild exposure to the dust.

With the knowledge that a patient has been a stone-mason, or employed in some dangerous dusty trade, symptoms of respiratory disability must always raise the suspicion of silicosis. The **differential diagnosis** then depends almost entirely on the history and the X-ray films. As for the occupational history, there is no easy criterion of what constitutes an effective degree of exposure to silica. The doctor has to make a rough-and-ready assessment in his mind, taking into account the nature and length of the employment, its accepted silica risk and the time relationship between the exposure and the development of symptoms. The X-ray picture in the various stages calls for expert assessment, and the differentiation, as far as it is possible, from passive congestion of the lungs, bilateral bronchiectasis, infiltrating malignant disease, pulmonary arteriosclerosis with resulting fibrosis of the lungs, mycotic infections, tuberculous bronchopneumonia and miliary tuberculosis. A massive area of fibrosis may be mistaken for a mediastinal or pulmonary neoplasm.

PROGNOSIS

As has already been seen, the prognosis depends on the amount of silica inhaled, on the length of exposure and on the occurrence of associated infective conditions, whether tuberculous or not. If the development of silicosis is recognised at an early stage, and the patient then removed from the risk of further exposure, the inevitable lesion which results from the silica already inhaled may not progress to a disabling stage. In any case, whatever the length of exposure, the victim should be removed from further silica hazard as soon as the disease is diagnosed, and put to other work within his capacity.

The longer the period of exposure before the onset of symptoms, the more chronic is the course of the disease and the slower its progress. The supervention of tuberculous infection is always serious. As the vital capacity becomes impaired, the greater is the hazard of coincidental respiratory infections.

TREATMENT

The first need in treatment is to remove the patient from further exposure to silica. There is no cure for the pulmonary damage and destruction once it is established. The danger of secondary infections is such that even with a simple cold the patient should retire immediately to bed and be carefully nursed. Bronchitis and emphysema are treated on the usual lines (see Chaps. XIV to XVI). The onset of tuberculous infection calls for the appropriate measures, including, if necessary, sanatorium treatment.

THE SOCIAL AND LEGISLATIVE ASPECT

Workers who are disabled by reason of their occupation cannot be thrown on the scrap heap ; they are part of the community, have worked and suffered for it, and are entitled to help. It is this acceptance of communal responsibility which lies behind the provisions for Workmen's Compensation. In Great Britain, the first Compensation Act for silicosis was passed in 1918, and the first scheme (for the refractories industries) came into force in February 1919. This was revised in 1924, and a Silicosis Medical Board of full-time experts was appointed by the Secretary of State. In 1927 a scheme was put into action for the metal grinding trade ; in 1929 a group of " various industries," including coal and metal mining, was brought in, and in the following year the sandstone industries were added. In 1931 new legislation was enacted to cover the existing schemes, and to include asbestos.

The effect of the schemes is to establish the right of compensation for compulsory suspension from employment, for disablement or for death. It is based on the discovery of silicosis, whether accompanied by tuberculosis or not. The certificate entitling the victim to compensation can be granted only by the Silicosis Medical Board, which, for legal purposes, makes or disallows the diagnosis. From their decision there is no appeal, though the right is allowed of re-examination after an interval. Certificates for fatal cases are, as a rule, given only after a post-mortem examination.

When a workman is found to be suffering from silicosis, and has been employed in the dangerous trade for at least five years, the disease is deemed to be due to the employment ; if the period is less than this, the onus of proof is on the workman or his dependants, and usually his trade union then takes the matter in hand and prepares his case for submission to the Silicosis Medical Board. Except in the refractories industries, his application must be made within five years of his leaving the dangerous employment.

Compensation for silicosis, insisted upon by the community, is based on the principle of employers' liability. In the refractories and sandstone industries, this liability is collective, and all employers subscribe to a general compensation fund. Under the other schemes the liability is individual, and the employer usually insures against it.

Meanwhile, research into the problems of industrial pulmonary disease is promoted by a special committee of the Medical Research Council, in co-operation with industrial and scientific bodies. An interesting illustration of this was a recent (1942) M.R.C. report on *Chronic Pulmonary Disease in South Wales Coal-miners,** which arose out of the routine work of the Silicosis Medical Board. An increasing number of claims for compensation, most of which arose in the South Wales coal-field, had resulted in an increasing number of refusals to grant certificates entitling to compensation for silicosis ; for although a disabling pulmonary disease (see the later section on Coal-miners' pneumoconiosis) undoubtedly existed among these miners, it did not fulfil the definition for silicosis which had been laid down by an international conference in 1930, and which was generally accepted. The Home Office and the

---

* Medical survey by P. D'Arcy Hart and E. A. Aslett : pathological report by T. A. Belt (with assistance from A. A. Ferris).

Mines Department therefore requested an investigation of the whole problem, and this was surveyed in its ætiological, clinical and radiological aspects.

PREVENTIVE MEASURES

In South Africa a marked decline in the attack rates for silicosis at each year of service has resulted from the activities of the Miners' Phthisis Medical Bureau, which was established in 1916, and the adoption of a policy of prevention. Measures of prevention should be twofold—engineering and medical. The former concern the prevention of the accumulation of dust by means of adequate ventilation and exhaust ventilation, both general and local. In mines, blasting is regulated as to its methods and times, and shifts and work are planned to avoid needless exposure to dust or fumes. The employment of water to lay the dust at its source, and remove it from the air when formed, is often adopted also ; it is not as effective as exhaust ventilation, however, for it does not remove the highly dangerous invisible dust, and too humid an atmosphere may have serious disadvantages.

The medical measures involve an initial examination of all new workers in the industry, in order to exclude any suffering from tuberculosis, or whose respiratory and general health makes them unsuitable, and periodical examinations of all workers, both clinically and radiologically, preferably at six-monthly intervals, in order to detect as early as possible the onset of silicosis or of tuberculosis.

Great advances have been made in recent years in preventive measures in surface industries in this country, with the result that silicosis can be said to be disappearing from some of the industries in which it was most frequently found. These measures can be summed up as follow : (i) Finding a safe substitute for a dangerous material, for example, the use of artificial abrasive wheels for sandstone wheels in metal grinding ; the use of alumina instead of flint in the pottery industry for placing china biscuit ware and for polishing ; the use, in sand-blasting, of metal grit or aluminous abrasive instead of quartz sand or flint. (ii) Suppression of dust at the point of origin, for example, by water in the machine drilling of rock. (iii) Localised exhaust ventilation to remove dust as near as possible

to the point of origin. (iv) Exclusion of persons not actually
engaged on the dusty process ; some dusty processes have
been made entirely mechanical. (v) Protection of individual
workmen by breathing apparatus specially adapted to the
conditions of their work. (vi) Medical supervision of personnel
by initial selection and periodic examination.

ASBESTOSIS

Asbestos is the commercial name given to certain complex
silicates of iron, magnesium and calcium which have a typically
finely fibrous structure ; the fine fibres can be spun into cord,
tape or sheeting, or can be woven into cloth. Being fire-
resistant, innumerable uses have been found for it ; for example,
in the making of insulating slabs and blankets, cement sheets
and asbestos textiles. The crude silicate is crushed and disintegrated ; the fibre is then opened, corded, spun and woven.
The operation is exceedingly dusty. The fibres are like frayed
cotton fluffs, and during the various processes the workroom
is cloudy with dust. The white fluff settles on the hair, the face
the hands and the clothing ; the casual visitor finds it difficult
to remove it by brushing. The industry has a comparatively
short history, and it is only in the last twenty years that the
disease arising from it has been extensively studied. In the
best type of factory today, an elaborate system of dust extraction and the introduction of " wet methods " of working have
entirely altered the outlook.

The **pathology** of asbestosis is essentially the same as that
of silicosis, but the distribution of the resulting fibrous tissue
is usually somewhat different, by reason of the physical form
of the asbestos fibres which form the greater part of the dust,
and the early fixation of these fibres in the lung. The disease
starts in the vicinity of the alveolar bronchioles, and a diffuse
network of fibrosis is the rule rather than the formation of
sharply defined nodules, though occasionally these may occur.
Consequently the pleural surfaces and the cut surface of the
lung removed at autopsy do not show the nodulation characteristic of silicosis. The fibrous condensation of the lung is
tough rather than shotty. Extensive, dense pleural adhesions
are common. The alveolar walls show diffuse thickening.
Fibres of apparently unaltered asbestos are seen scattered

through the lung tissue, together with the typical so-called "asbestos bodies," clumps of which may occur within the lung alveoli, and embedded in fibrous tissue. In the areas of lung least affected by the fibrotic change, patches of emphysema and of pulmonary collapse are common. The middle and lower zones of the lungs are most heavily damaged, in contrast to silicosis where the upper and middle zones show the most marked lesions.

The "*asbestosis bodies*" (Fig. 109) found in the sputum are golden-yellow structures, usually straight and with bulbous ends. It seems certain that they are produced from a central core of asbestos fibre, only after the fibre has gained access to living tissue and has remained there for some months. The golden-yellow coating of the fibre contains iron, which is probably derived from the body tissues.

The presence of "asbestosis bodies" in the sputum does not necessarily imply the development of fibrosis in the lungs. Singly, or in groups of two or three, they indicate merely that asbestos dust has been inhaled into the lungs and has remained there for a certain length of time. They should not lead to a diagnosis of asbestosis unless there is radiological evidence of the disease. On the other hand, the much rarer appearance in the sputum of a large clump or clumps of asbestosis bodies, similar to the aggregations seen in lung tissue (see Fig. 109), points to secondary disintegration of lung tissue, already affected by asbestosis there. Some complicating necrotic lesion, such as tuberculous caseation, or suppurating bronchopneumonia, or lung abscess, has allowed the escape into the sputum of these intrapulmonary formations. The interval between the first exposure to asbestos dust and the onset of symptoms is usually appreciably shorter than in silicosis. In a moderately severe example of the disease, for example, the period is something of the order of five to ten years.

As in silicosis, the striking symptom is breathlessness, which gradually increases as the disease progresses ; the other symptoms, signs and complications are the same as those described for silicosis. *Radiograms* show a fine type of pulmonary fibrosis over the whole of both lung fields, presenting what has been described as a ground-glass appearance. Adhesions about the pericardium and diaphragm produce a "shaggy" outline of the heart-shadow.

Other silicate dusts may produce fibrosis of the lungs ; among them the dust of mica (a silicate of aluminium with potassium) and sericite (a hydrous silicate of aluminium and potassium), found particularly in the South Wales coal-mines and the gold-bearing quartz rocks of South Africa, and met with in the production and manufacture of china-clay. Apart from mining, however, the effects produced by these silicates are not comparable either in frequency or in severity with those of silica or asbestos.

COAL-MINERS' PNEUMOCONIOSIS

The inhalation of carbon dust from the smoke of towns or the dust of coal (*anthracosis*) was considered until recently as a harmless matter, producing merely what might be called a " tattooing " of the lungs. Miners themselves, especially those who work in particular coal-fields, find that the dust hazard is not unimportant. Those who work in hard rock headings are exposed to the action of silica dust.

Workers in certain mines even without hard rock headings, however, appear unduly liable to develop a disabling form of chronic pulmonary disease, which does not fulfil the criteria laid down for the diagnosis of silicosis. As has already been said, the problem is disturbing in the South Wales coal-field, especially among workers in the anthracite mines.

The recent Medical Research Council report (see p. 340) shows that this chronic pulmonary disease is characterised in its earlier stage by a non-nodular type of reticular fibrosis (" dust reticulation ") associated with retention of an excessive amount of silica (mainly in the form of a silicate), as well as of carbon ; later there is nodulation and massive consolidation. The fibrosis gradually encroaches on the vital capacity, interferes with pulmonary elasticity and leads to emphysema. If phthisis supervenes, it usually is of the fibroid type, merging with the pneumoconiosis. The exact cause of the pathological and clinical changes is not known, apart from the fact that the dust at the coal-face is responsible. Other observers have described the same type of picture in dock workers who load anthracite or other types of coal on to ships. It is clear, therefore, that this is but one of many fascinating problems which still await complete solution in the field of the pneumoconioses.

Siderosis is a term which was formerly given to the dust-inhalation disease of knife-grinders, metal polishers and hæmatite iron-ore miners. It was thought that inhalation of iron dust was the chief pathological factor, but it is now clear that the condition is essentially a silicosis, due to the silica contained in the dust. The lungs of hæmatite miners may be coloured red with the dust, just as are the roads near the Cumberland mines ; rarely, the sputum is red also.*

ORGANIC DUSTS

Respiratory disease in the cotton industry—In 1863 Jesse Leach, who was a certifying surgeon under the Factories Act at Heywood Mills, wrote the first account of the respiratory disabilities special to cotton operatives. In those days dust in the workrooms was such that it was impossible to recognise a man at 12 yards' distance. Apart from cough and sneezing, due to direct irritation by very fine, short, cotton fibres, he noted that the workers " mostly suffer from a spasmodic cough, sore throat, expectoration of blood, pneumonia and confirmed asthma, with oppression of the chest."

The operatives affected by the disease are those employed in the blow-rooms and the card-rooms, where the new cotton is mixed and freed from dust, and prepared for the further manipulations of spinning and doubling. The carding machines are cleaned by " stripping " and " grinding," in order to remove fibre and debris which collects on them. Strippers and grinders of the carding machines were chiefly affected ; but the methods now used for cleaning these machines by local exhaust draught are removing the danger. The sufferers complain of mild cough in the early years of their employment ; eventually (after some ten to twenty years) they develop the typical respiratory syndrome, to which is given the name " byssinosis." The cough becomes exaggerated, and they suffer from attacks of breathlessness and tightness on the chest. At first this takes the form of " Monday fever " ; cough and breathlessness occur after the week-end break (or after any interval away

---

* The student interested in silicosis and allied conditions should read E. L. Middleton's Milroy Lectures (*Lancet*, 1936, ii, 1 and 59).

from work), and then subside for the rest of the week. Later, the symptoms become continuous, abating if the patient stays away from work, returning as soon as he is exposed again to the dust. Finally typical asthma becomes established, and the death rate from bronchitis and emphysema is high.

The determining cause of this industrial respiratory disease is a toxic agent in cotton dust * which produces irritation and inflammation of the upper respiratory tract, leading finally to chronic bronchitis, together with a protein which produces allergic hypersensitivity, demonstrable in these patients (but not, as a rule, in healthy operatives) by skin tests.

Prevention by proper general and local exhaust ventilation and humidifiers is the best form of treatment. Once the disease is established, it can be arrested if the victim is removed early from exposure to the dust. Otherwise the treatment becomes that of bronchitis and emphysema, or of asthma. Attempts at desensitisation against cotton dust have not been made on any large scale ; in any event, it could only abolish the specific hypersensitivity, not the irritative and inflammatory lesions caused by the dust.

Organic dusts may also be harmful because they carry with them toxic substances or pathogenic organisms. *Wool-sorters' disease* results from the introduction into the lungs of anthrax bacilli. *Weavers' cough* is caused by a contaminating mildew or mould ; a mould is probably the cause of *malthouse workers' cough*. *Aspergillosis* is a disease caused by the fungus Aspergillus fumigatus which contaminates grain and flour. It affects farmers, millers and workers concerned in the transport of grain. Another group of infections arise from a closely related family of fungi—moniliasis, blastomycosis and coccidiosis. *Moniliasis* is caused by the monilia fungus found on fruit, dead leaves, old straw or wood. The infection follows the inhalation of contaminated particles, and is found especially among workers in dusty straw, and in tea-tasters in Ceylon. *Blastomycosis* and *coccidiosis* affect not only the lungs but also the skin ; lesions in the lung arise either by inhalation or are carried by the blood stream from primary cutaneous lesions. These fungus infections may assume either an acute or a chronic form, varying from mild bronchitis, with or without fever, to bronchopneumonia and cavitation. The severer

* Recent research suggests that it may be bacterial.

examples may thus simulate pulmonary tuberculosis. Cough, expectoration and pyrexia are prominent, but tubercle bacilli are never found in the sputum unless, perchance, there is accompanying tuberculosis of the lungs. Diagnosis depends on the discovery of the yeast-like bodies in the sputum. In mild instances of fungus infection the outlook is fairly good, for many such cases recover spontaneously. Severer infections, especially those with cavitation, have a much graver prognosis. Treatment is by full doses of iodides, together with general hygienic measures. X-ray therapy is often tried, but the results cannot be regarded as convincing. *Streptothrix* infections by branching mycelial fungi are rare ; the most prominent of them, *actinomycosis*, is described in Chapter XXI.

Mill fever, *shoddy fever* (affecting workers engaged in the manufacture of shoddy) and *threshing fever* (suffered by farmers during the threshing of wheat and oats) are transient irritative disturbances caused by histamine-like bodies (or perhaps bacteria) contained in the dusty material ; in a few days immunity becomes established. *Fur-dust* treated by " carotting " (that is, by painting with nitrate of mercury) may cause mercurial poisoning, as in felt-hat makers ; the intention tremors characteristic of the disease are known in the trade as " hatters' shakes." New workers in *tobacco dust* suffer from the same symptoms which affect the boy smoking his first cigar, but usually immunity is established, and chronic nicotine poisoning is rare. Inhalation of *amido derivatives of benzene and its homologues* (for example, paraphenylene-diamine) used in dyeing or associated industries, may cause acute œdema of the bronchial tubes and asthma ; or when the substance is excreted persistently in the urine, from cancer of the bladder (chronic aniline poisoning : trinitrotoluene, which is excreted in the urine not as such but as an amido derivative).

The respiratory tract is also a portal of entry for the **dusts and fumes of metals and their salts.** *Chromic acid* and *chromates* (used in chromium plating, certain leather tanning methods, and in the manufacture of photographic materials) are caustic, causing " chrome holes," which are indolent chronic ulcers of mucous membranes and skin. Inhaled as a powder or as a spray, the chrome compound causes ulceration and finally perforation of the nasal septum. *Sulphur dioxide*, used in electric refrigerators, or produced in the sludge of certain tanning vats, is almost irrespirable to those unaccustomed to it, causing a violent reflex defensive laryngeal spasm. If it is inhaled by accident into the lungs, it may cause bronchitis, pulmonary œdema or bronchopneumonia. A certain degree of tolerance, however, is developed by repeated exposure. *Nitrous fumes* are not very soluble and are therefore all the more dangerous, because they do not set up a violent respiratory defensive reflex by way of warning. A workman may therefore breathe a fatal quantity without knowing the hazard he is running. In six to twenty-four hours, however, acute pulmonary congestion and œdema follows the caustic action on the alveoli, with intense dyspnœa and cyanosis ; finally the victim " drowns in his own fluids " within about thirty-six hours. Those who recover from the acute accident are apt to develop pneumonia later. Air contaminated by *lead fumes or lead salt dusts* is the most important source of industrial plumbism ; poisoning is far more rapid and intense than by other routes, because when it is absorbed into the respiratory tract it passes thence to the general circulation, instead of passing through the liver, as after gastro-intestinal absorption. The lungs are not themselves affected. The most striking example of this mechanism is the inhalation of tetra-ethyl lead, a volatile liquid used as an " anti-knock " compound for motor-car engines. Acute and rapidly fatal poisoning was very common in the industry, with many examples of fulminating lead encephalopathy. *Arsenical dusts* affect the mucous membrane of the respiratory tract, but not severely. Hoarseness, cough and a slowly progressing painless necrosis of the cartilaginous septum of the nose are the usual respiratory manifestations. Gaseous arsenic (*arseniuretted hydrogen*) may be accidentally produced in various industrial processes, often from arsenical impurities in other metals such as tin or zinc ; absorbed into the circulation through the lungs, it is a powerful hæmolytic poison. " *Metal fume fever*," caused by the fumes of zinc oxide in workers smelting zinc or in brass foundries, is a transient " chill " with sweating and some prostration ; it is a manifestation of a certain degree of necrosis of alveolar cells, due to the action of zinc oxide, with resulting absorption of the protein disintegration products into the circulation.

Inhaled *manganese dust or fumes*, produced in the grinding of manganese ore, or the manufacture of steel, dry batteries, chlorine gas, paints, enamel and linoleum, may (after an exposure of at least three months) produce a nervous syndrome almost identical with that of Parkinson's disease.   Instances of fibrosis of the lungs, with extensive pulmonary deposits of manganese, and death from pneumonia have also been described.

Cadmium, which is present in zinc ores, may in high concentration cause fibrotic thickening of the alveolar walls, or even acute œdema of the lungs.   The main hazard to workers is in the smelting of zinc ores.   *Nickel carbonyl* is a gaseous compound of nickel and carbon monoxide formed in the Mond process of producing pure nickel.   It is a highly dangerous process, for the substance is inhaled into the lung and deposited over the respiratory surface.   The nickel is then dissolved by the tissue fluids and absorbed into the blood.   It causes both local and general damage ; * in the lungs it causes congestion, œdema and pneumonia.

Of the **industrial solvents,** *petrol* and *benzine* aspirated into the lungs may produce immediate collapse, or an irritative inflammatory reaction, followed by patchy pneumonia or pleurisy.   *Carbon tetrachloride* may be breathed by the workers as a vapour in the air, and chronic poisoning results, with renal and hepatic injury.   *Tetrachlorethane* is the best solvent for cellulose acetate, but is highly dangerous ; chronic poisoning results from the fumes of this solvent, which are inhaled into the lungs, absorbed into the blood stream and eventually cause intense damage to liver, kidneys and red blood corpuscles. The solvent used to be used for aeroplane " dope " or coating, and many cases of toxic jaundice occurred during the First World War.   The fumes of *carbon bisulphide,* formerly used in rubber vulcanisation, and now extensively used in the manufacture of artificial silk, may after inhalation over a period cause various neurological symptoms.

WAR GASES

Chemical warfare began in earnest when in April 1915 the Germans employed chlorine gas on the Western Front. The modern development of air warfare greatly increases the

---

* Though nickel has been recovered from the tissues, some authorities think that the toxic action is due to the disintegration, by hydrolysis, of the carbonyl moiety, with resulting caustic action on the alveolar cells.

possibilities of disseminating war gases rapidly and over a wide range.

From the military point of view, the differentiation between "*persistent*" and "*non-persistent*" gases is important. In order to combine the military and medical aspects the following classification has been suggested * :—

    (i) Vesicants.

    (ii) Lethal : (*a*) lung irritants,
             (*b*) paralysants,
             (*c*) arseniuretted hydrogen.

    (iii) Harassing : (*a*) lachrymators,
              (*b*) sensory irritants.

    (iv) Accidental (*i.e.*, gases not used as weapons).

VESICANTS

The most important vesicants (or blister gases) are mustard gas and Lewisite. **Mustard gas** is an oily fluid, which has an odour of mustard or garlic. It vaporises slowly at ordinary temperatures and therefore it is "persistent," remaining as a dangerous liquid for many days if the weather conditions are suitable, and slowly giving off its vapour. Low concentrations of vapour are especially dangerous, for the smell may then be so faint as to escape notice, the gas remains undetected and inadvertent exposure may cause many casualties. Moreover, the liquid is not immediately irritating to the skin, nor the vapour to the respiratory tract or to the eyes ; the harmful action is delayed for some hours. It gives, therefore, no immediate pain or discomfort as a warning.

The severity of the damage caused by the vapour depends on its concentration and on the length of exposure to it. Apart from vesication of the skin and eyes the vapour may cause lesions of the respiratory tract, which vary from a slight inflammation to desquamation of the tracheal mucous membrane and fatal secondary bronchopneumonia. In the First World War the death rate was very high among victims whom the gas caught without respirators. Most deaths occurred three to four days after exposure, and were due, almost without exception, to secondary bronchopneumonia.

Inhalation of dilute mustard gas vapour for a short period

* *Medical Manual of Chemical Warfare.* H.M. Stationery Office (1940).

causes an early rhinitis (within five to forty-eight hours), with sneezing and running of the nose, and later, mucopurulent discharge, laryngitis with hoarseness and aphonia, and possibly tracheitis and bronchitis. Heavier concentrations, or more prolonged exposure, cause œdema of the larynx, intense tracheitis and bronchitis.

Sometimes the mucous membrane of the trachea is so badly damaged that sloughs form. Secondary bronchopneumonia follows, and is almost inevitably fatal. In any event, bronchopneumonia due to secondary invaders is very common, for the mucociliary defence is seriously hampered by any severe tracheitis or bronchitis.

A well-fitting respirator effectively protects the respiratory tract. If, however, mustard gas vapour is inhaled, treatment must be directed to the alleviation of symptoms and to the prevention of secondary pulmonary infection. If the *rhinitis* produces thick mucopurulent discharge, this should be washed away by warm nasal douches of 5 per cent. sodium bicarbonate solution. The discomfort produced by *laryngitis* and *tracheitis* is soothed by menthol-steam inhalations, and by the use of a linctus containing codein. Especial care must be taken not to expose these patients to extraneous infection which might determine bronchopneumonia ; segregation from other patients, and the wearing of masks by the medical and nursing attendants, are therefore advisable. If pneumonia develops, treatment follows the usual lines, including chemotherapy. At the earliest onset of cyanosis, oxygen therapy is essential.

If the patient recovers from the respiratory illness, after-effects are common. To be gassed is a dreadful experience, and may produce a persistent anxiety neurosis. Moreover, the original irritational reflexes may become persistent ; their organic cause is cured, but a neurosis perpetuates them. *Functional aphonia* or *cough* is common, and calls for reassurance, breathing exercises, and abstention from unnecessary treatment directed towards an organic lesion which no longer exists. The management of the convalescent patient is therefore very important ; as soon as possible, the convalescent should be transferred from hospital to a rehabilitation centre. During the last war tachycardia and effort syndrome were a frequent consequence of gassing ; the cause was usually a neurosis, and treatment should be directed accordingly.

There is no evidence that damage by mustard gas vapour causes any special liability to the later development of pulmonary tuberculosis. Patients who survive the initial illness but do not recover within a month or two are comparatively few. Those who continue to complain of symptoms referable to the chest have suffered more or less severe damage to the respiratory passages and lungs, with consequent peribronchial fibrosis, chronic bronchitis, fibrosis of the lung or bronchiectasis.

Lewisite, an arsenical compound (chlorovinyl-dichlorarsine), is both a vesicant and a lung irritant. Its action differs from mustard gas in the immediate irritation which it produces ; its pungent effect on the nose causes sneezing and nasal exudate, and great discomfort if it is inhaled farther. It has an easily recognisable smell, resembling that of geraniums. It is readily hydrolysed by water, with the production of highly toxic substances which, if absorbed into the system, produce acute arsenical poisoning.

The characters of the gas make its early detection likely ; it is thought, therefore, that if it is used in warfare it will be as a spray from aircraft, in order to gain the advantages of surprise. The immediate use of an adequate respirator protects the respiratory tract ; though, as with other arsenical gases, there is a short period of increased respiratory irritation after putting on the respirator, which may tempt the unwary to think that the respirator is useless.

If, however, the victim inhales an appreciable amount of gas before a respirator can be applied, serious pulmonary symptoms very rapidly supervene. Coryza and laryngitis are followed by acute bronchitis, which may lead to fatal bronchopneumonia. Treatment is that usually adopted for these various respiratory lesions.

LUNG IRRITANTS

The lung irritants (or *suffocating gases*) comprise a group of which the most important are **chlorine,** the gas initially used by the Germans in the First World War ; **chloropicrin,** a highly irritant liquid with a fairly high boiling point (and therefore " persistent ") ; **phosgene,** easily detectable by its smell of musty hay, least immediately irritant but most toxic of the group ; and **diphosgene,** an oily liquid, " persistent," and with an action similar to that of phosgene.

GENERAL PRINCIPLES OF THE ACTION OF LUNG IRRITANTS

Fundamentally the pathological effects of all lung irritants are the same, any difference in symptoms being due to differences in the localisation of their action. This localisation is determined almost entirely by their physical properties, *solubility* being by far the most important factor. Ammonia, for example, is very soluble in water and rapidly diffusible in solution ; ammonia vapour is readily extracted from inspired air, therefore by the first moist tissue which it reaches. Thus the upper respiratory passages take up most of any inhaled ammonia, and suffer the main impact of the toxic action. The lungs are relatively little affected, seeing that the concentration of gas which reaches them has already been greatly reduced. On the other hand, gases with a low solubility penetrate into the deeper parts of the lungs in concentration hardly diminished by their passage over the moist surfaces of the upper respiratory tract, with the result that toxic damage to the bronchioles and alveoli is severe.*

Ammonia, therefore, by reason of its high solubility, produces intense congestion of the upper respiratory passages, laryngeal spasm and œdema of the glottis. At the other end of the scale, phosgene and nitrous fumes cause irritation of the upper respiratory tract only if the exposure is severe. They do not provoke marked respiratory defensive reflexes, they may be fatal in concentrations which are insufficient to initiate these reflexes, and they induce œdema of the lungs by their action on the alveoli. A gas like chlorine, which comes intermediate in the scale of solubility, produces damage to the upper respiratory tract if it is present in small concentration, whereas greater concentration damages in addition the deeper parts of the lungs.

The importance of solubility (ammonia, chlorine) and of hydrolysis (phosgene, nitrous fumes) explains the vulnera-

---

* The approximate solubility in water of various irritant gases has been expressed in the following comparative figures :—

Ammonia	450·0
HCl vapour	385·0
Sulphur dioxide	20·0
Bromine	10·0
Chlorine	1·5
Phosgene : nitrous fumes .	These decompose, by hydrolysis, into toxic (acid) substances.

bility of moist, easily penetrated surfaces such as the mucous membranes of the respiratory tract and of the conjunctival epithelium. The damage is not due to gross corrosion, for phosgene may be fatal in concentrations which, after hydrolysis takes place in the alveoli, give an extreme dilution of hydrochloric acid. The pulmonary injury results rather from disturbances of the normal activities of cell protoplasm, as by dehydration or coagulation.

The protective respiratory reflexes already mentioned consist of coughing, constriction of the larynx, closure of the glottis, spasm of the bronchi and inhibition of respiration. They tend to prevent penetration of the irritant into the deeper parts of the lungs, and especially to the delicate alveolar cells. Coughing expels injurious material : stimulation of the nasal sensory fibres of the trigeminal nerve and of the superior laryngeal nerve results in the inhibition of respiration at the expiratory phase of the cycle : reflex closure of the glottis by the adductor muscles bars the passage of harmful vapours : constriction of the smaller bronchi helps to prevent penetration of the gas into at least some portions of the lungs. Intense stimulation of the glottic reflex may lead to acute asphyxia ; as a rule, however, respiratory inhibition is only temporary, being eventually overcome by the excitatory effect on the medullary respiratory centre of accumulating carbon dioxide.

As has already been seen in regard to bronchitis (see p. 178), the farther the penetration down the respiratory tract, the more serious the general systemic disturbance which arises from the lesion. This is true whether the damage is due to bacterial, physical or chemical agents.

Chlorine and chloropicrin are very irritating to the upper respiratory tract, causing smarting of the nose, throat and upper respiratory passages, and evoking severe laryngeal and bronchial spasm. Phosgene, on the other hand, is far less irritating, and in low concentrations provokes no protective respiratory reflex to prevent deep inhalation. In the presence of water (as in the moist alveoli) it hydrolyses to form hydrochloric acid. The liberation of this acid in the bronchioles and alveoli results in congestion and œdema, which usually take a little time to develop. The harmful action is similar, therefore, to that of nitrous fumes described earlier (see p. 348). If the concentration of gas inhaled is high, the lungs may become waterlogged within an hour or two ; the lower the concentration and the less the exposure, the longer it takes for the œdema to become established and the less intense its degree. While chlorine produces a severe irritative reaction in the upper respiratory passages, it will also cause pulmonary œdema if it is inhaled into the alveoli, owing to the production of HCl. With all these lung irritant gases, the damage to the respiratory passages and lungs is such that even if the victim survives the initial pulmonary œdema, secondary bacterial infection is a common sequel. The lungs of patients who die at an early stage of the poisoning are œdematous and congested ; frothy blood-stained fluid fills the bronchi, and areas of collapse and of acute emphysema may be seen. If the lung is cut across, sero-sanguineous fluid drips freely from the cut surfaces. If the patient dies at a later stage, bronchopneumonia and pleurisy complicate the picture.

The outpouring of serous exudate into the alveoli prevents proper oxygenation of the blood, with resulting anoxia and cyanosis. If the exudation is widespread and severe, its effect is suffocating. It also robs the blood of fluid, so concentrating it and increasing its viscosity ; the hæmoglobin rises well above 100 per cent., the erythrocyte count reveals a marked polycythæmia and there is a tendency for the development of thrombosis in the blood vessels of the lungs and elsewhere. The accumulation of œdematous fluid in the lungs, together with the anoxia, lead to a combination of circulatory obstruction in the lungs, and poorly oxygenated medullary centres and myocardium. The result is cardiac fatigue and circulatory failure.

SYMPTOMS

Certain instances have been recorded of men exposed to overwhelming concentrations of irritant gases who died almost immediately from asphyxia and heart failure. As a rule, however, even with heavy concentrations the patient survives for some hours. With **chlorine** and **chloropicrin** there is an initial irritation of the upper respiratory passages. The victim feels that his breath is suddenly taken away, and that his throat and thorax are gripped as in a vice. At the same time, the eyes smart and water, and the respiratory passages feel as though they are being stung with red-hot needles. The irritation brings on violent bouts of coughing, which are intensely painful and are accompanied by an agonising feeling of rawness behind the sternum. The sensation of suffocation is accompanied by great mental anguish. As the patient recovers his ability to breathe, he gulps and retches and often vomits. Soon he is prostrated, and passes into a semi-stupor, still coughing and retching painfully. Muscular fatigue is extreme, so that he hardly has the power to put on a respirator. Left in the poisonous atmosphere, he breathes more chlorine, becomes unconscious and dies. If, however, he is rescued and removed from further exposure, the breathing remains gasping, rapid and shallow, and is punctuated by frequent and painful spasms of coughing, with the bringing up of copious frothy sputum, which may be blood-stained. The accessory muscles of respiration are brought into use in order to overcome the obstruction to aeration of the lung. The chest is over-distended, with little respiratory excursion. The expression is anxious ; the face and extremities are bluish-red or deep blue, the pulse full and bounding with a rate of about 100, and the veins of the neck are distended. Headache is intense and epigastric pain is common.

Save for heavy exposures, the effects of **phosgene** are less immediately dramatic. The onset of serious symptoms may be delayed for some hours. After removal from the gas any initial discomfort may pass, and a deceptive period of apparently complete recovery ensue until hydrolysis produces the damaging effect of hydrochloric acid in the alveoli. This usually begins within a few hours ; if, therefore, pulmonary symptoms do not develop within twenty-four to forty-eight hours of exposure, they are unlikely to do so later.

The insidiousness of this development is highly dangerous. An officer, apparently slightly gassed, soon recovers and refuses to leave his post ; the next morning, on coming out of his dug-out, he quickly develops acute pulmonary œdema and dies. An industrial worker engaged in the manufacture of phosgene accidentally breathes " a whiff of the gas," carries on at work instead of reporting it, later begins to feel uncomfortable, walks to hospital on his way home and within a few hours is gravely ill with pulmonary œdema.

In phosgene poisoning the stage of deep-blue asphyxial

cyanosis without circulatory failure is often absent. The lungs fill with fluid and respiration is gravely obstructed ; but the poisoning may cause almost simultaneous profound circulatory collapse. The cyanosis is therefore livid, the pulse is feeble and thready, its rate over 120, and the skin is cold and clammy —a picture similar to that of the respiratory and circulatory failure seen in influenzal and other types of pneumonia (see p. 167).

In view of the danger of circulatory collapse, it is vital to remember that muscular exertion calls for a considerable increase of oxygen. This is often beyond the capacity of the damaged lungs to supply, even at a time when the symptoms do not appear serious. Hence the necessity to avoid all forms of exertion.

PHYSICAL SIGNS

The appearance and general condition of these patients have already been described. The chest expansion is poor, and the percussion note may be little affected, at least in the earlier stages. Breath sounds are diminished owing to the obstructed respiration and the accompanying lack of expansion of the chest. Fluid in the bronchi results in coarse or medium crepitations ; the typical finding, however, is of fine crepitations, determined by the pulmonary œdema and alveolar exudate. If, later, bronchitis, bronchopneumonia or pleurisy develop, the temperature rises, the character of the sputum changes and the physical signs typical of the complication are found.

PROGNOSIS

Patients with mild degrees of poisoning recover from the immediate effects in a few hours. Cough, vomiting and a feeling of rawness in the chest may persist for a few days, and during convalescence there may be some degree of brady-cardia, due to reflex vagal action. Those with moderately severe poisoning, with deep-blue cyanosis and no circulatory failure, who respond to oxygen therapy, begin to recover within forty-eight hours ; after this period the œdematous exudate is rapidly absorbed, disappearing usually in four or five days. Those with circulatory failure and livid cyanosis are in grave jeopardy, and the mortality among them is high. Even if they survive the initial poisoning, they are particularly liable to develop secondary bronchopneumonia later, which is nearly always fatal.

An important prognostic factor is the existence of previous pulmonary disease which has caused a diminished respiratory reserve. This will obviously lessen the chances of recovery from the effects of lung irritant gases. If, therefore, these gases are effectively used against civilians the mortality among older people is likely to be very high.

TREATMENT

In view of the delayed action of phosgene, any person who has suffered exposure to it should be put to bed and kept under strict observation for at least twenty-four hours, even though he may feel perfectly well. If no pulmonary symptoms have developed within forty-eight hours, he may be regarded as free from the danger of poisoning, and can return to his usual work. During the period of observation, muscular effort of any kind is forbidden, in order to reduce the call upon the cardio-respiratory apparatus for oxygen. He must not, for example, walk to a first-aid post. He must lie quietly, flat on his back, on a stretcher. Equipment and clothing should be removed or loosened wherever it might impede breathing. For the first twenty-four hours he must lie in a well-warmed bed, under conditions of *absolute* rest. Warmth not only combats shock but also prevents the muscular contractions involved in shivering. The call upon oxygen is also lessened if the digestive mechanism is required to deal only with bland drinks sweetened with glucose.

If pulmonary œdema develops, the principles of treatment are the same, whatever the degree of severity. Once the patient is removed from the gas-laden atmosphere the need is to tide him over the period during which the alveoli are choked with fluid exudate, until in three to four days it is mostly absorbed ; and to prevent, if possible, secondary bacterial infection.

In the acute stage the prime danger is that of anoxia, leading to circulatory failure. Not only must the needs of the body for oxygen be reduced to a minimum : as long as any degree of anoxia exists enough oxygen must be supplied to combat it.   Absolute rest, warmth, fluids with glucose and good nursing will ensure the first ; continuous oxygen administration by an effective technique (see Chap. XIII), begun at the very earliest appearance of cyanosis (and therefore applicable to the moderately severe as well as to the graver cases) is necessary to meet the second.

Atropine is ineffective in reducing the pulmonary œdema, which is a response to acute inflammation.   Vomiting is a constant feature of the illness, and is usually accompanied by the evacuation of considerable quantities of the fluid exudate from the lungs.   It should not, however, be deliberately induced.   As a rule, the patient freely expectorates the thin frothy fluid, unless he is too weak to do so ; in grave cases the fluid may be so copious that it wells out of the patient's nose and mouth.   Expectorants should not be given ; nor is it safe to ask the patient to adopt active measures of postural drainage, even if he is capable of them.   If the secretions are copious and threaten to drown the patient, however, it is worth while raising the foot of the bed or of the stretcher on to a chair so that the fluid will drain towards the mouth.   Moreover, an attempt should be made to control the coughing, so that it occurs periodically and deliberately, as a means of getting rid of as much of the œdematous fluid as possible.   Hot drinks and a codein linctus are therefore given to soothe ineffective and exhausting cough ; at intervals (the length of which will depend on the accumulation of intrapulmonary fluid) the foot of the bed is raised and the patient's head or even his whole body are turned by a nurse in order that he may have a period of coughing, during which she supports the chest firmly in order to minimise any pain.   If there is much bronchial spasm, as when, for example, chlorine has irritated the upper respiratory passages, ephedrine ($\frac{1}{4}$ gr.) will be helpful.   Morphia is dangerous in that it may abolish the cough reflex and depress the cardio-respiratory centres already threatened by anoxia. If there is great restlessness, oxygen administration is more likely to abolish it than any other measure.   In intractable cases, however, the medical attendant may feel that in spite of the danger morphia is essential.   If so, not more than $\frac{1}{6}$ gr. should be given.

Seeing that circulatory failure is so common a complication every precaution against it must be undertaken.   The first step is to prevent anoxia. If by continuous oxygen administration the patient's colour can be kept pink, the outlook for recovery is good. In a patient with pulmonary œdema and deep-blue cyanosis, without general circulatory failure but with venous engorgement and strain on the right side of the heart, venesection reduces the load on the myocardium. About a pint of blood should be removed by the first bleeding ; if it is necessary to repeat the venesection later, not more than 200 c.c. should then be withdrawn. The bleeding also brings about a dilution of the polycythæmic blood with tissue fluids. In patients with livid cyanosis and circulatory failure, venesection is contraindicated. Nikethamide (coramine) is a useful stimulant ; an adequate supply of oxygen, however, is by far the best cardiac tonic for these patients. As the general condition improves and the intrapulmonary fluid is absorbed, it becomes possible to reduce the amount of oxygen administered, until finally it can be withdrawn altogether.

If after recovery from the initial pulmonary œdema the temperature begins to rise, the onset of secondary bronchitis or bronchopneumonia must be suspected. At the first signs of this, full doses of sulphonamide should be given and other appropriate treatment instituted (see Chaps. XVII and XVIII).

In patients who have suffered from anoxia, convalescence is slow and prolonged. The pulse rate is a good criterion of the state of the myocardium. Patients with tachycardia or bradycardia should not be allowed out of bed too soon lest " effort syndrome " become established. As soon as the patient is fit to leave hospital, however, he should be transferred to a centre where rehabilitation can be carried out under medical supervision.

Of those who die from poisoning by irritant gases, 80 per cent. succumb in the first twenty-four hours. Of those who recover, the great majority regain full health. A few develop " effort syndrome," often because activity during convalescence is too hurriedly undertaken. Others develop spasmodic attacks of shallow rapid breathing which occur at night ; these have been called " nocturnal asthma," but are probably a form of neurosis. Some who have suffered from secondary bronchopneumonia may be left with permanent fibrotic, bronchiectatic or emphysematous changes in the lungs. There is no evidence that lung injury due to these gases predisposes to tuberculosis.

Of other forms of gassing, little need be said here. Phosgene is produced when carbon tetrachloride, used in certain types of fire extinguisher, is sprayed upon fire or burning objects ; thus, in addition to the dangers in its manufacture, it is occasionally a hazard in ordinary civilian life. The organic arsenicals used as *nose irritants* (harassing gases) produce effects which increase in severity for some time after withdrawal from exposure to the gas, or after the respirator has been put on. They are used, therefore, to induce men to take off the respirator and so to expose themselves to other more lethal gases. The irritation is characterised by severe pain in the nose and nasal sinuses, sneezing, a feeling that the head is bursting, tightness and pain in the chest, lachrymation, nausea and perhaps vomiting. The discomfort is great and leads to much apprehension, especially in the untrained and undisciplined.

Poisoning by *nitrous fumes* in industry has already been described (p. 348) ; it may also occur when nitro-explosives are incompletely detonated in confined spaces, as in mining and tunnelling operations, gun pits, armoured cars and tanks, and the burning of cordite in ships set on fire. As a rule, carbon monoxide is set free at the same time, adding to the danger, and often killing its victims immediately.

CHAPTER XXIII

PULMONARY FIBROSIS

FIBROSIS of the lungs is not a disease in itself. It is the expression of a pathological process which replaces dead tissue by fibrous tissue, and may therefore be a sequel of many pulmonary diseases, as has already been seen in earlier chapters. When it is extensive it produces a typical clinical picture by reason of its interference with the normal anatomical structure and physiological functions of the thoracic organs.

Destruction of lung tissue by bacterial or other agents is followed, if the patient recovers, by the process of repair. Many infections excite an inflammatory reaction without necessarily causing any great destruction of tissue. This is especially true of lobar pneumonia (see Chap. XVII), in which as a rule the repair of slightly damaged alveolar walls is made by the proliferation of neighbouring cells. Fibrosis is absent, save in the rare instances of organisation of unresolved intra-alveolar fibrinous exudate. When destruction of lung tissue is extensive, however, with accompanying destruction of normal pulmonary architecture, repair takes the form of an attempt at restoration of continuity. Macrophages invade the dead, coagulated debris in order to accomplish their scavenging work ; meanwhile, fixed connective-tissue cells (*fibroblasts*) grow into the area, following in particular the course of any threads of fibrin already deposited as a result of inflammation.

When bacteria or destructive chemical agents persist in the area after repair has begun, and repeat the injury to adjoining tissue, the fibrosing process extends peripherally, as in tuberculosis, syphilis or the development of the silicotic nodule. The original destruction is followed by the formation of a nodule of new fibroblastic tissue, which, if it matures, will become hard fibrous tissue. Owing to direct bacterial or chemical action this nodule may undergo necrosis, to be surrounded in

362

its turn by a wall of cells farther out from the central zone. Examples of this process have been given in the chapters on tuberculosis (Chap. XX) and silicosis (Chap. XXII).

The importance of fibrinous deposits in canalising the advancing growth of fibroblasts is seen in the pleural fibrosis which follows the deposition of fibrin on the pleural surface. While the pneumococcus, for example, may cause an extensive lesion of the lung without destruction or fibrosis, the same organisms may produce a fibrinous pleural exudate which bridges the pleural membranes and is invaded by fibroblasts and new blood capillaries (*organisation*). This leads finally to the formation of adhesions. The same mechanism may be seen in tuberculous infection, or following hæmothorax, especially when the blood has not been evacuated from the pleural cavity. The organisation of fibrinous exudate in the interstitial tissue of the lungs is a cardinal factor in the diffuse pulmonary fibrosis (so-called " indurative pneumonia ") which follows persistent pulmonary œdema (see Chap. XXXI).

The cicatrix which results from a pulmonary infarct is an outstanding example of the repair of continuity by the laying down of scar tissue. The dead cells are attacked by macrophages ; at the same time invasion by fibroblasts and new blood capillaries leads to organisation of the damaged area. A similar mechanism ensures the encapsulation (or, when possible, the permeation) of an inert foreign body by fibrous tissue.

Obviously the fibrosis may be limited and localised, or diffuse and extensive. Extensive fibrosis signifies the replacement of much respiratory tissue, and therefore a corresponding reduction of respiratory reserve. It makes the lungs more rigid, so that the Hering-Breuer reflex comes into play at an earlier stage of inspiration than in the normal individual, with resulting dyspnœa and shallow breathing. It is associated with diminution of the capillary bed, and therefore an increased resistance in the pulmonary circulation. This leads to hypertrophy and eventual failure of the right side of the heart. As the fibrous tissue contracts it produces mechanical changes in the thorax—shrinking of the lung, retraction of the chest wall with marked diminution of expansion, and drag upon the mediastinum.

The **symptoms** shown by a patient suffering from pulmonary fibrosis consist partly of those of the underlying primary disease, and partly of the dyspnœa caused by the fibrosis. Later, the symptoms of right heart failure may be added. The deficient aeration due to the diminution of normal respiratory tissue leads to cyanosis and polycythæmia, and if there is associated chronic infection, also to clubbing of the fingers. When one lung is mainly involved, the **physical signs** are particularly characteristic. The chest wall on the affected side is retracted, and expansion is greatly diminished. The shoulder is dropped, and there is compensatory scoliosis. The trachea and heart are pulled over towards the diseased side. Over the fibrotic area vocal fremitus is diminished, the percussion note is dull to a degree which is determined by the amount of fibrotic tissue present, and the vocal resonance is also diminished, unless there is associated consolidation or cavitation. Breath sounds are present, but owing to the poor expansion they are weak. The unaffected portions of the lungs show compensatory emphysema. Any adventitious sounds which are heard are due either to the primary disease or to associated complications. Radiograms confirm the presence of mechanical displacements, of pleural or pulmonary thickening, and maybe the lesions due to the primary disease. In the later stages they may also show obvious dilatation of the right side of the heart.

The **diagnosis** is usually easy, and is based largely on the evidence of mechanical traction. *Collapse of the lung* also causes mechanical tractions, but these depend fundamentally on the anatomical distribution of the bronchi affected (see Chap. VII) : moreover, breath sounds are absent over the affected area, save in those instances of aspiration of the occluding plug into the peripheral bronchioles. With a considerable *pleural effusion* the mediastinal structures are displaced away from the side of the lesion. When there is doubt, an exploratory puncture by needle and syringe should be made.

Prognosis and **treatment** depend largely upon the primary disease. As has been said, however, extensive fibrosis of the lungs is likely to lead sooner or later to right heart failure.

CHAPTER XXIV

PLEURISIES

THE ANATOMICAL BACKGROUND

THE parietal sheet of the pleural membrane lines the internal aspect of the chest wall ; a subserous layer of areolar tissue allows it to be easily separated from the parts which it covers, except over the heads of the ribs and vertebral column, over the diaphragm and over the pericardium.

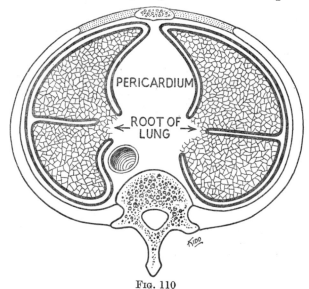

FIG. 110

The pleural membranes at the level of the root of the lung.

The visceral sheet invests the lungs, and as the subserous tissue is continuous with the areolar tissue of the lungs, the attachment is such that the pleura cannot be stripped off without tearing the lung surface. The visceral pleura dips down into the interlobar fissures, lining them for the whole depth. The two pleural layers become continuous only over the root of the lung (Fig. 110) and through the ligamentum latum pulmonis.

Inflammation of the parietal pleura arises especially from lesions of the thoracic wall (including the diaphragm and the mediastinum). Inflammation of the visceral pleura arises particularly by extension from the lungs ; later, it may implicate the parietal pleura also by contact infection.

The pleura is a typical serous membrane derived embryologically from the mesoderm. It consists of a single layer of flat endothelial cells, which cover a layer of tissue containing crossed bundles of connective tissue and fine elastic fibres arranged as a honeycombed elastic lamina. The *visceral pleura* is thin, its subserous areolar tissue and elastic fibres being continuous with the connective tissue and elastic fibres of the lung. Its blood supply is derived from the bronchial and pulmonary arteries. It is rich in lymphatics, which form a network beneath the surface endothelium, and which communicate with those surrounding the lobules on the surface of the lung. They are drained by the superficial collecting trunks which course over the surface of the lung and end in the hilar glands, or indirectly by the perivascular and peribronchial lymph channels and nodes of the lungs, which also drain into the hilar glands.

The *parietal pleura* is thicker, and, except for the areas already mentioned, is less firmly bound down to the underlying structures. Its blood supply is from the intercostal, internal mammary, phrenic, mediastinal and bronchial arteries. Its costal lymphatics drain by the deep intercostal lymphatics to the sternal and intercostal lymph nodes, and indirectly, via the fourth and fifth intercostal spaces, to the axillary glands ; the lymphatics of the mediastinal portion pass to the posterior mediastinal glands, and those of the diaphragmatic portion communicate with the lymph vessels of the abdominal surface of the diaphragm, though extension of inflammation along them is almost invariably in the direction of abdomen to thorax (see Chap. XXVI). In the thorax the diaphragmatic lymphatics drain into the sternal glands in front and the posterior mediastinal glands behind.

The parietal and visceral pleural membranes are separated by a thin film of serous fluid which acts as a lubricant between two sliding surfaces. Owing to the extent of the pleural surface, a large amount of fluid (transudate or exudate) may rapidly accumulate in the pleural cavity.

The normal pleura can quickly absorb water, substances in solution, toxins, and particles of dyes, both by the blood and the lymph vessels. It can also act as a membrane through which exchange of gases takes place (see p. 430). Absorption is diminished if the pleura is thickened or fibrosed, a factor which in all probability helps to determine the persistence of effusion in certain chronic lesions.

THE MORBID ANATOMY OF PLEURAL INFLAMMATION

Inflammation of the pleura may arise as the result of trauma, either mechanical (bruising or lacerating injuries) or chemical (the hæmoglobin of a hæmothorax). It may be caused also by infection, carried in through the chest wall to the parietal pleura by a penetrating wound or by spread from the mediastinum or the subdiaphragmatic area, or extending to the viscera pleura from a lesion in the lung.

The initial response is congestion of the pleural membrane, with desquamation of many of its endothelial cells. The pleura consequently loses its normal glistening appearance. When the cause of the inflammation is bacterial, both visceral and parietal membranes are soon affected, for the sliding of one on the other during respiration encourages dissemination of infection. The inflamed membrane is thickened and swollen by blood, œdema and leucocytic infiltration, and a varying amount of inflammatory exudate escapes into the pleural cavity. As a result, masses of fibrinous lymph are deposited on the pleural surfaces, which later may undergo change to firm fibrous tissue (see Chap. XXIII). When the fibrin forms a bridge between the two membranes, organisation of it results in pleural adhesions. When there is a considerable pleural exudate, the lung retracts as it accumulates ; if the visceral pleura is heavily invested with fibrin, and the pulmonary collapse is allowed to persist for a sufficient length of time, the eventual pleural fibrosis may encase the retracted lung in so rigid a shell that re-expansion becomes impossible.

The inflammatory exudate varies from a few cubic centimetres up to several pints. At first it is straw-coloured. It contains the proteins which are found in blood serum (albumin, globulin, fibrin). It may become turbid from the presence of cells, while the exudation of red blood corpuscles into it gives it a tinge which may vary from rose to dark brown, according to the amount and the condition of the hæmoglobin contained in it. The older the effusion the more likely is it to be opaque and of deeper colour. If the pleurisy is due to an acute infection the organisms responsible may be found in the fluid, together with polymorphonuclear leucocytes. If it is due to tuberculous infection it may be impossible to detect the organisms without highly specialised methods, and the predominant cells are likely to be lymphocytes. When a pleural exudate persists and becomes chronic, its contained fibrin is apt to be deposited in successive layers on the pleural surfaces, particularly on the posterior and basal surfaces, which are the most dependent parts when the patient is propped up in bed.

Pathologically, therefore, pleurisy takes the form, in the initial stage, of pleural inflammation accompanied by a sticky fibrinous exudate, but with no appreciable effusion of fluid. The lesion may not progress beyond this. On the other hand, it may progress to effusion, which may be serofibrinous or purulent, according to the severity or the nature of the pleurisy. Clinically the picture may be predominantly one of pleural irritation, with pain and a pleural rub, of " fluid on the chest," or of empyema. The fundamental unity of these varieties of pleurisy must always be borne in mind, although for convenience of clinical description pleurisy is usually divided into two main types—the " dry " (or " plastic "), corresponding to the initial stage : and serofibrinous, corresponding to the later stage of effusion. Empyema presents such important problems of its own that it is usually considered apart, almost as though it were an entirely separate clinical entity. In this book it will, for convenience, be discussed in a separate chapter, but its fundamental relationship to other types of pleurisy must be remembered. Any of the different varieties of pleural inflammation may result in pleural cicatrisation, which may vary from localised adhesions to complete symphysis of the two pleural membranes.

Fibrinous pleurisy may follow trauma of the chest wall, which results in bruising of the parietal pleura. Far more commonly, however, it is initially an inflammation of the visceral pleura, involved as a complication of disease in the underlying lung. It may be a response, for example, to the death of pulmonary tissue in an infarct or a lung abscess. In many instances tuberculosis is the determining cause. Sometimes the tuberculous lesion in the lung is obvious on clinical or radiological examination ; sometimes the lesions are small and subpleural, and diagnosis may only be possible by induction from general clinical and pathological evidence. Other important primary causes in the lungs are the pneumonias. Infection may also spread from neighbouring organs other than the lungs.

The symptoms vary greatly in intensity. It is clear from the frequent finding of pleural adhesions, and from other evidences of old pleurisy at autopsy, that many patients must have had mild attacks without arresting symptoms. In the unmistakable attack, however, the patient has a *pain in the side* which is very sharp, stabbing or tearing. It is made worse by coughing, by deep inspiration or by pressure from outside. He therefore breathes shallowly, with jerks and grunts, for he is frightened to take a deep breath. Usually he has a *cough*, slight, irritating and unproductive, which he tries to smother because it is so painful. It is salutary for the student or doctor to realise that pressure or percussion over the intercostal spaces on the affected side will hurt the patient, and he must therefore be as gentle as possible in his examination. The pain is due to stretching of the inflamed parietal pleura (see p. 55), and is most intense at the end of inspiration. Anything which lessens the tension in the pleura helps to reduce the pain—immobilisation of the ribs by strapping of the chest or by the accumulation of intrapleural fluid, or diminution of the œdematous swelling of the membrane itself. It is interesting to note that the pain goes as soon as the intrapleural fluid appears, long before the ribs are effectively immobilised by the effusion, a fact which indicates that the outpouring of fluid releases tension in the pleural membrane in much the same way as the opening of an abscess releases tension.

When the pleurisy is due to an acute infection such as pneumococcus lobar pneumonia the onset of the pain may appear as a bolt from the blue. When the origin is tuberculous, careful inquiry often elicits the fact that for some time past the patient has not been wholly well, and maybe that already he has had mild pains in the side which have been mistakenly regarded as muscular or rheumatic.

Chilly sensations may herald the onset, but rigors are rare,
24

save in the pleurisy associated with acute lobar pneumonia. In these latter instances the pleural symptoms are but part of those of the acute pulmonary disease, and are often overshadowed by them.

Dyspnœa, in the form of painful shallow breathing, is the rule: even in the mild cases with but moderate pain the breathing may increase considerably in frequency with any form of exertion.

Pyrexia is usually moderate, reaching perhaps 100° or 101° F., though in severe cases it may rise to 103° or 104° F., and it is more likely to be intermittent than continuous. It is always difficult to know whether the pyrexia is due to the pleural lesion alone or whether it is determined also by disease in the underlying lung.

Clinical examination reveals a marked diminution of movement on the affected side, with a consequent and corresponding weakness of the normal vesicular murmur. Sometimes fine crepitations are heard ; they are not *pleural* crepitations, but result from exudate into the subpleural alveoli which follows the extension of inflammation to or from the tissues of the visceral pleura. The conclusive physical sign is the *pleuritic friction rub*. Hippocrates described it as "creaking like leather." Hilton Fagge described it as follows : "In its most typical form it consists of an irregular succession of short, harsh sounds which give one exactly the impression of something catching or dragging against an obstruction and then slipping, but only to catch or drag once more. The patient himself is often conscious of a rough grating sensation each time he breathes ; and one may be able to *feel* the rub quite plainly by placing one's hand over the affected part of the chest." (See also p. 85.)

Diaphragmatic pleurisy—Pleurisy localised to the region of the diaphragm has certain particular features of its own. The diaphragm on the diseased side is kept immobilised in order to avoid the agonising pain brought on when the diaphragm contracts. The patient shrinks, therefore, from abdominal breathing, cough or swallowing. Respiration is hurried and grunting, and confined to the upper part of the chest. If the pleura over the central part of the diaphragm is inflamed, the pain may be referred along the phrenic nerve to the cutaneous area of the fourth cervical nerve, and be felt at the point of the shoulder. Inflammation at the periphery of the diaphragm gives rise to pain in the lower thorax, the lumbar region, or the abdomen, referred along the sensory fibres of the lower intercostal nerves to their segmental areas. (See also p. 55.)

This referred pain over the abdomen may lead to serious errors of diagnosis. Many patients have in consequence suffered an unnecessary laparotomy for an " acute abdomen " because their illness has been regarded as due to appendicitis, to inflammation of the gall bladder, or to other abdominal lesions.

In addition to the pain, there is on rare occasions a persistent, uncontrollable hiccough. Faced with a patient so obviously ill the doctor may be disconcerted to find so few physical signs to explain the condition. No friction rub is heard, but the nature of the pain, the character of the breathing and the unmistakable lack of movement of the affected side of the chest should lead to a right diagnosis.

If effusion follows, it is often limited by adhesions to the diaphragmatic surface, though occasionally the fluid finds its way to the costophrenic angle and then accumulates between the layers of the costal pleura. If the infection is pyogenic, whether from a lesion above the diaphragm or below it (see Chap. XXVI), an abscess may form between the pleural layers, eventually to burst into the lung and to be coughed up via the bronchi.

Pleurisy, then, is usually but an episode in injury or disease either of the thoracic wall or of the lungs. The underlying lesion will add its own particular symptoms and signs to those of the pleural inflammation. The manifestations of pneumonia, tuberculosis, lung abscess or infarct may soon overshadow the initial pleural pain. When the " dry " pleurisy does not progress to the formation of an appreciable accumulation of fluid, recovery takes place usually within a week or two, though occasionally it may be remarkably speedy, the acute pain subsiding in the course of a day or so, with the patient well enough to be about his business. Even so, it may leave behind varying degrees of pleural thickening and adhesions.

Serofibrinous pleurisy (" pleurisy with effusion ") is but a later stage of " dry pleurisy," following the outpouring of a clinically recognisable amount of inflammatory exudate. The same ætiological factors are therefore at work — injury, inflammation or neoplasm of the chest wall and parietal pleura : foreign material (especially blood) in the pleural cavity : and lesions of the lungs and visceral pleura. When the pleurisy is due to pus-producing organisms the effusion, as a rule, quickly becomes purulent ; nevertheless it is important to remember that in a few instances, at a particular stage of pulmonary infection (for example, in pneumococcal or streptococcal pneumonia or lung abscess), the exudate may, for a recognisable though short period, be non-purulent and sterile.

Non-inflammatory *transudation* of fluid into the pleural cavities may occur as a complication of heart or of renal disease, or by reason of a tumour compressing the pulmonary vein. It is usually bilateral, the physical and chemical characters of the fluid are different, and the term " hydrothorax " (see Chap. XXVIII), rather than " effusion," is applied to it.

Serofibrinous exudate which does not become purulent may result from bruising of the chest wall and parietal pleura ; it may develop in response to the irritation of the pleura by the hæmoglobin of a hæmothorax ; it may complicate non-purulent pleural or subpleural lesions such as tubercles or malignant nodules ; or it may follow blocking of the lymphatic drainage of the lung, by tuberculous or neoplastic lesions of the lymphatics, and of the lymph nodes into which the pleural lymphatics drain at the bottle-neck of the hilum.

In the majority of instances, however, it results from underlying **tuberculosis of the lung.*** Until comparatively recently, these examples of serofibrinous pleurisy were labelled " idiopathic." Their true nature was not recognised, as they presented no clinical or radiological evidence of tuberculous lesions in the lungs or pleura. In patients with obvious pulmonary tuberculosis it is not difficult to recognise that serofibrinous pleurisy is secondary to the disease in the underlying lung ; but the straw-coloured exudate which occurs in patients with no demonstrable tuberculous or other lesion was for a long time regarded as evidence of a primary pleural inflammation of unknown or uncertain origin.

Few patients with so-called " idiopathic " pleurisy die at this stage, and post-mortem evidence of the tuberculous nature of the disease is therefore not easy to obtain. In the rare instances when post-mortem material is available, the microscope reveals tuberculous lesions in both pleura and lung,

---

* " Under the effusion hides a localised tuberculous lesion " (Landouzy, the French physician, in 1881).

together with macroscopic subpleural tubercles, which can sometimes be seen through the thoracoscope during life.

The character of the exudate, with its high proportion of small lymphocytes, is very suggestive of tuberculous infection. It is rare to find tubercle bacilli in the fluid by direct microscopic examination, though they can more often be found in the clot which forms when the fluid has been allowed to stand, especially if the clot is digested and centrifugalised. Culture of the fluid on Loewenstein's egg medium is reported to give a fair proportion of positive results. Inoculation of adequate amounts of the fresh exudate into a guinea-pig provides the most impressive evidence of its nature, for it produces tuberculous lesions in some three-quarters of the cases.

More evidence of the tuberculous nature of these pleurisies comes from the study of the subsequent history of the patients. Since Fiedler in 1882 showed that 82 per cent. of his series had developed frank tuberculosis of the lung within ten years, and Barrs in 1890 reported nearly 60 per cent. within six to ten years, many others have analysed their own experience and given various but always considerable percentages. The differences in the reported figures can be explained largely by the economic status and after-treatment of the sufferers. The rich who could afford proper treatment and convalescence fared far better than the poor who had to go back to work as soon as they could. Moreover, with the coming of radiology of the chest, and therefore of more exact diagnosis of tuberculosis of the lung, the percentage of cases proved to be due to tuberculosis has been seen to be a good deal higher than was at first thought. The reports from the Scandinavian countries, for example, show this clearly. Finally, if these patients are not allowed to go back immediately to the stress and strain of ordinary life, but are given a few months of adequate sanatorium regime and treatment, over 90 per cent. return to work and remain well without any evidence of active clinical phthisis. From all this evidence it may be deduced that the patient who resumes normal living as soon as the exudate is absorbed is the one in whom pulmonary tuberculosis is likely to show itself after a period of years.

" Primary " pleurisy with serofibrinous effusion must, then, be regarded as tuberculous in origin. It is rare below the age of 10, and equally uncommon in old age. Its main incidence is in adolescence and young adult life. There is good evidence that these effusions often develop within a few months of the development of a primary lung focus (see p. 267), as the result either of tiny tuberculous foci in the lung parenchyma or in the hilar glands. These foci cause effusion either by the extension of inflammation from subpleural tubercles, or by mechanical obstruction at the hilar " bottle neck " by enlarged and inflamed glands, or by a specific sensitivity reaction. Certain characteristics of the exudate have already been mentioned. The specific gravity is about 1020, and it contains a good deal of fibrin, so that on standing a clot forms, varying in amount from one which is quite small to a large jelly-like mass. In addition to the small lymphocytes, it usually contains a small number of red blood corpuscles ; obvious staining by blood usually indicates a very acute lesion, with macroscopic tubercles present in the pleural membrane. The exudate differs from transudate such as occurs in cardiac failure and nephritis in that the transudate contains less protein (about 2 per cent. as contrasted with 4·5 per cent.) and has a lower specific gravity (1014 as against 1020). Moreover, in the transudate the cellular elements consist mainly of desquamated endothelial cells.

Onset and symptoms—Pleurisy with effusion has three characteristic modes of onset. It may come on acutely, either with a severe attack of pleuritic pain or as a " pyrexia of uncertain origin," which later is complicated by severe pleuritic pain : it may be subacute : or the illness may be insidious, with a prodromal period of undefined ill-health, vague aches and pains, and finally dyspnœa, so that when the patient comes to the doctor there is already an appreciable effusion, somewhat unexpected because there has been no clear history of a recent antecedent pleurisy.

It has already been shown that pleural effusion is so rarely primary in the absolute sense that it may be regarded as symptomatic of some pathological process, whether obvious to clinical examination or not, in the underlying lung or in the chest wall. The effusion is thus but an incident in the wider disease. Unless this is borne in mind, symptoms and signs may easily be mis-interpreted. Cyanosis, dyspnœa and distress, for example, may be due to the mechanical effects of a great bulk of fluid. They can also be caused by disease in the underlying lung.

If the effusion accumulates rapidly, dyspnœa may be severe.

On the other hand, even large effusions which have accumulated slowly enough to allow compensating mechanisms to come into play may produce surprisingly little disturbance of breathing, as long as the patient is at rest. Small effusions, the result presumably of comparatively few isolated foci only, may affect the patient's health so little at the time that he does not consult a doctor. The discovery, years later, of pleural adhesions or pleural thickening in an X-ray film may be the only clear evidence of the earlier disease.

Pyrexia may be remittent or intermittent, rising on the average to 102° or 103° F., and may persist for some weeks. Chills and drenching sweats occasionally occur, and the pulse rate is moderately increased. Pain in the side diminishes as the effusion of fluid releases the tension in the inflamed and swollen pleural membrane.

Usually absorption begins within two or three weeks and continues progressively, though in rare instances the effusion persists for a long time. After its absorption the physical signs do not alter appreciably for some little time, for the pleural membranes are still swollen and infiltrated and the collapsed lung re-expands but slowly. Thus dulness to percussion and feeble or absent breath sounds remain, and the doctor may be surprised not to find fluid if he explores the chest with a hollow needle and syringe. When persistent chronic effusion occurs, it usually follows a very acute tuberculous pleurisy which has finally resulted in great thickening of the pleural membranes, with numerous adhesions and " pocketing " of fluid in many places. The final result of a pleural effusion is usually the formation of adhesions between the two pleural layers.

DIAGNOSIS

1. **At the stage of pleural irritation**—Apart from the more general manifestations, the main feature is pain in the side, referred from the parietal pleura to the corresponding distribution in the skin. Pain in the side of the chest should make the student think of the various lesions which may give pain in that particular segmental area. Fig. 111 will remind him of the possibilities.

Perhaps one of the most difficult lesions to separate from true acute pleurisy is the simple one of a *tear of intercostal muscle fibres*, for here the pain can be severe and made worse by respiration, during which the torn muscle contracts. Palpation by the finger will, however, find a localised point of great tenderness where the muscle fibres are torn, and pyrexia and friction rub are absent.

The term " pleurodynia," meaning pain from fibrositis or myalgia of the intercostal muscles, should no longer be used. If indeed there is *intercostal fibrositis*, then it is better to use that term. There will probably be a history or some present

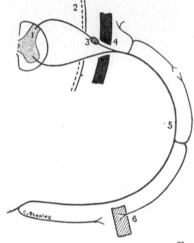

1. *Spinal cord:* tumour; inflammation (dorsal meningomyelitis).

2. *Meninges :* tumour ; dorsal meningitis.

3. *Posterior root ganglion :* herpes ; tabes.

4. *Vertebra and intervertebral foramen :* rheumatoid arthritis ; osteoarthritis ; spondylitis ; tuberculosis ; cancer ; pressure of aneurysm.

5. *Peripheral nerve :* neuritis.

6. *Muscle, fascia, skin :* myalgia ; fibrositis ; trauma ; diaphragmatic lesions.

Visceral referred pains : from lung, pleura, mediastinum, heart (anginal pains, left side).

FIG. 111

To show possible causes of pain in the side of the chest in relation to segmental nerves.

evidence of fibrositis elsewhere, and though the pain is increased by the local muscle contractions, there is no pyrexia nor friction rub. In *intercostal neuralgia* also there is no friction rub. Both these conditions are infrequent when compared with actual pleurisy. It must always be remembered, moreover, that in acute pleurisy a pleural friction rub is usually a fleeting thing, and so may never be heard by the doctor. A detailed history of the painful attack is then of cardinal importance.

It is very doubtful if there is a pleurisy of rheumatic origin, though the term " rheumatic pleurisy " is used. My own view is that it must be so rare that the student or doctor should not accept the diagnosis in the absence of other more convincing manifestations of acute rheumatism.

2. **The effect of effusion on the contents of the thorax**—Not until there is at least half a pint of fluid in the pleural cavity is it possible to detect its presence by clinical examination. Normally the heart and mediastinum are kept in their median position by the elastic traction of the two lungs. When effusion collects in the pleural cavity the corresponding lung relaxes to accommodate it. The traction of the lung on the sound side pulls the mediastinum over towards itself, provided that it is not fixed. With a moderate effusion at the base, the upper part of the mediastinum does not shift ; the base of the heart, together with the great vessels, remains in the middle line, and the apex of the heart swings either way along the arc of a circle, according to the side of the effusion. As the heart apex points downwards, forwards and to the left, it is clear that the greater shift is to the right, consequent upon a left-sided effusion. This particular movement is never big enough to cause any kinking of the large vessels at the base of the heart.

The displacement of the heart is thus not an actual pushing over by the positive pressure of the fluid. When fluid accumulates in the pleural cavity the intrapleural pressure on that side becomes less negative, with the result that the equilibrium of pressures on the two sides is disturbed, and the now relatively larger negative pressure on the sound side draws the mediastinum over towards itself.

With large effusions, the whole mediastinum goes over, giving rise to appreciable displacement of the heart and trachea. Now not only is there the elastic traction of the lung on the sound side, but in addition the weight of the fluid becomes an important factor. The force of gravity comes into the picture, and the fluid exerts a pressure which is a function of its weight.

It takes an accumulation of about a pint at least of effusion before displacement of the heart can be detected by clinical examination. Such an effusion reaches nearly up to the hilum of the lung. Fig. 112 shows schematically the evolution of a progressively increasing pleural effusion. The lung itself progressively relaxes, until with the largest effusions it becomes wholly collapsed and airless. It is compressed by the weight of the fluid, and in addition there is absorption of air, associated with the lack of normal functioning. Seen post-mortem, such a lung is blackish-grey or reddish-grey, does not crepitate under the fingers, and sinks in water. Insufflation may succeed in re-

expanding it, provided that it has not become encased in a fibrotic shell, consequent upon long-standing pleurisy with fibrosis.

3. **Physical signs of effusion**—The cardinal sign is the

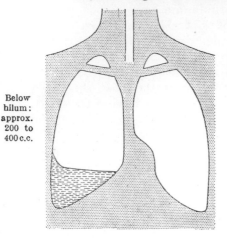
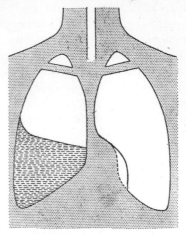

Below
hilum:
approx.
200 to
400 c.c.

Up to
hilum:
approx.
500 to
800 c.c.

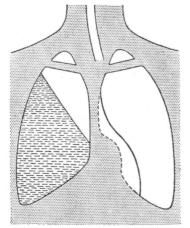
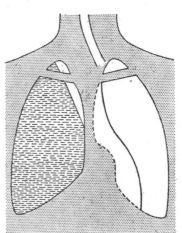

Above
hilum:
approx.
1000 to
2000 c.c.

Towards
apex:
approx.
2000 to
4000 c.c.

Fig. 112

Evolution of a pleural effusion (schematic).
(The figures of amounts are those of Barjeon and Courmont.)

" stony dulness " on percussion, to which are added displacement of the apex beat when the effusion is of sufficient amount
and (in most cases) absence of the normal vesicular breath
sound. The patient usually lies on the affected side, in order

to get the fullest expansion of the healthy lung ; with large effusions he may be most comfortable sitting up in bed. Movement of the affected side of the chest is impaired or abolished, according to the size of the effusion ; displacement of the mediastinum has already been mentioned. With large effusions there may be obliteration of the normal intercostal depressions on the diseased side. The fluid damps down vibrations both in the lung and chest wall, so that vocal fremitus is absent, and the percussion note is as dull as that of the finger placed against a thick board or a brick wall. The dulness is not only heard but felt. There must, of course, be enough fluid present to cause a retraction of the lung far enough away from the chest wall to ensure that any vibrations even of a partially collapsed lung are fully damped down. As has already been said, this involves an accumulation of at least some 300 to 400 c.c. of fluid. Percussion should be light ; there is no need here for a heavy fist, especially in marking out the upper level of the fluid.

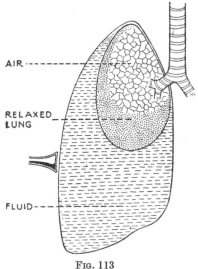

Fig. 113
Pleural effusion : relaxed lung.

The voice sounds and the breath sounds are absent over the effusion. Why are they not conducted to the surface of the chest ? Under certain circumstances, indeed, they *are* conducted, a point which will be discussed in a moment. It is not that fluid is a poor conductor of sound vibrations ; it is an excellent conductor, as submarine detectors know full well.

The student can find illumination of these points by a few simple experiments in his bath. If he allows the tap to drip water gently on to the surface of the bath water, he will hear a certain intensity of sound. If he then immerses his head under the water, the sound is heard much more loudly, for the splash of the drop is conducted far better from fluid to fluid to ear than from water to air to ear. If he strikes two stones together under the water, he will for the same reason hear the sound better if his ear is under the water than if it is above it. In the latter instance much of the sound is lost in its passage to the ear through two different media instead of one. Finally, if while he is still in the bath a collaborator makes a noise such as clapping the hands, he will hear it much better if his head is above water. Indeed, if the head is below the surface of the water, he may not hear the sound at all. The passage of sound from air to water is difficult, because so much of it is reflected by the denser watery

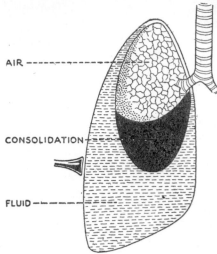

AIR

CONSOLIDATION

FLUID

FIG. 114
Pleural effusion : consolidation of lung.

medium instead of being absorbed and transmitted. The same principle applies to fluid in the pleural cavity, and is the main factor in conditioning this particular physical sign ; but there is also a subsidiary factor, for the ease with which sounds are transmitted through the lung to the air-fluid surface will depend on the condition of that underlying lung. When it is retracted and relaxed it will not vibrate and transmit sounds so readily as will the normal lung (Fig. 113). Thus in pleural effusion neither the voice nor the breath sounds traverse the lung with the normal intensity, and then these feeble vibrations have to " jump " the change from one medium to another—alveolar air to fluid. It is hardly surprising that they are lost to the examiner's sense of touch and hearing.

There are conditions, however, in which they are not lost. If there is not much fluid and not much relaxation of the lung, the vibrations may " jump the gap " between lung and fluid, and whatever vibrations do get through into the fluid will then be well conducted. This often occurs in the child's small chest ; the relatively loud puerile breath sounds may get through into the fluid and to the listening ear, and many a collection of fluid (usually empyema) in a child has been missed by letting diagnosis wait upon the discovery of absent breath sounds over an area of dulness. Another example is the occasional instance of lobar pneumonia complicated by semipurulent effusion or empyema in the adult, in which the consolidated lung conducts the sound of the voice or the breathing to its own periphery, and the sound vibrations succeed in passing into and through the fluid (Fig. 114). If it were possible to put the stethoscope at the periphery of the lung instead of on the chest wall, loud bronchial breathing would be heard. Sometimes the sound does " jump the gap," and the vibrations which get through are well conducted through the effusion to the chest wall. If many of these do so, then the empyema is accompanied by the signs of dulness to percussion, of pectoriloquy and bronchial breath sounds over the area of dulness, and the condition may be mistaken for pure consolidation of the lung. More often, however, even if vibrations get through to the fluid, only a small quota do so, so that although bronchial breathing is heard, it is faint, as though heard at a distance.

Thus the condition of the underlying lung is an important factor in the physical signs of effusion, and not all examples of empyema or effusion complicating underlying consolidation of the lung show absence of the vesicular murmur. Under the appropriate conditions, bronchial breathing may come through to the ear. In actual fact this is relatively uncommon, but its possibility underlines the fact that the cardinal sign is the "stony dulness," and where that is unmistakable the doctor or student must not be turned aside from diagnosing effusion because he hears breath sounds over it. It is clear that in the apparently primary pleurisy with effusion, with no underlying consolidation of the lung, it is extremely unlikely for breath sounds to " jump the gap " and be transmitted to the stethoscope. Here there is not only dulness but also abolition of the normal voice and breath sounds.

Sometimes at the upper limit of the fluid the voice sound comes through to the ear with a " nasal " or bleating character. The sound can be imitated to a certain extent by pinching the nose and saying " ninety-nine." There is only a thin layer of fluid here, between the lung and the chest wall, which is sufficient to cut off the lower fundamental tone while allowing the higher pitched overtones to get through. This *ægophony* is not by any means an invariable accompaniment of fluid in the chest, and it would seem, therefore, to require a combination of favourable physical conditions, probably in the lung as well as in the pleural cavity, to produce it ; but what these conditions are, in their full detail, no one seems to know.*

4. **X-ray examination**—Apart from helping to confirm suspicions based on clinical examination, radiograms often reveal small effusions which cannot easily be detected otherwise. They are also useful in demonstrating encysted collections of fluid above the diaphragm, in the interlobar fissures, or between the mediastinum and the pulmonary pleura. In the last type of lesion the patient may suffer severe pain behind the sternum, made worse by coughing, breathing or swallowing ; and cyanosis may result from pressure on the great veins in the mediastinum.

5. **Differential diagnosis**—When effusion is suspected, an exploratory puncture with a 5 or 10 c.c. syringe † and a moderately bored needle should be done, after preliminary anæsthetisation down to the pleura with a cubic centimetre of 2 per cent. novocain. The nature of any fluid withdrawn can then be determined by the appearance, and by bacteriological, cytological and, if need be, chemical investigation. This will determine particularly whether pyogenic organisms are present or not. The decision to " put in a needle " will be made whenever the possibility of intrapleural fluid is suspected. Where the history and clinical features point to lung abscess, however, needling of the chest in the absence of fluid may result in puncture of the lung and consequent infection of the pleural space.

Differential diagnosis must be made from *chronic fibrinous pleurisy* (" thickened pleura "), in which there may be dulness and feeble or absent breath sounds but no displacement of the heart away from the side of the lesion : from *consolidation of the lung* due to pneumonia or tuberculosis, in which percussion is impaired, but without the added " stony " feel, and there is no appreciable mediastinal displacement : and from *collapse*

---

* As was pointed out on page 73, Skodaic resonance may be found over the upper part of the chest : and the upper limit of dulness is highest in the axilla.

† It is much easier to aspirate some effusions with a 2 c.c. syringe and a wide-bored needle. If, therefore, the 10 c.c. syringe fails, a 2 c.c. syringe should be tried.

and *fibrosis of the lung*, in both of which conditions the media-stinum is displaced towards the side of the lesion. A massive new growth infiltrating the pleura itself may cause much difficulty in diagnosis, especially as it may be also complicated by an effusion ; here the fluid is apt to be blood-stained, and to contain a large number of endothelial cells.

The sterile " reactionary effusion " of *lung abscess* (see p. 247) may simulate acute tuberculous pleurisy, with high pyrexia and grave illness. A carefully studied history of the course of the illness frequently gives the cardinal clue. Perhaps the patient has had a recent anæsthetic, or teeth extracted : or the sudden coughing up of a copious amount of purulent sputum (perhaps following an initial hæmoptysis) draws attention to the likelihood of lung abscess. Even before the expectoration of the pus the patient may have noticed a foul taste in his mouth or an unpleasant smell in his breath. As a rule, the effusion does not remain sterile for long. It is soon infected from the lung lesion, with resulting empyema or pyopneumothorax.

PROGNOSIS

At the initial " dry " stage the outlook for the patient is obviously conditioned by the nature of the lesion giving rise to the pleurisy—an underlying pneumonia, for example, or a lung abscess, or a bronchial carcinoma. When there is no obvious disease in the lungs, and particularly if the condition does not progress to effusion, the immediate outlook is good. Many cases, however, are tuberculous in origin, and unless the patient is properly advised and cared for, active tuberculous lesions in the lung may eventually develop. In any event, full clinical and radiological investigations should be made to determine, if possible, the cause of the pleurisy, and the patient should be kept under medical supervision for some considerable time after his illness.

The prognosis in serofibrinous pleurisy depends largely on the condition of the underlying lung. An effusion due to a bronchial carcinoma with involvement of the hilar glands, for example, will soon end in the death of the patient. In the tuberculous effusions, which form the great majority, the future depends largely on how far the lung is affected. In the apparently primary cases *the outlook is good provided that the patient has proper treatment.* Indeed, pleurisy with effusion supervening in a patient with only microscopic or minimal tuberculous lesions in the lung is to be regarded as a fortunate illness, for it takes him to the doctor at a stage when treatment of the underlying condition is likely to be successful.

TREATMENT

1. **In the " dry " stage** the patient must be kept strictly in bed, irrespective of the mildness or severity of the attack. His diet should be light and mainly fluid. The pain in the side and the irritating cough are the salient features which distress him. Three ways of relieving the pain are open to the doctor—analgesics, especially opiates : poulticing : and immobilisation of the painful side of the thorax. If the pain is very severe, $\frac{1}{4}$ gr. of morphia should be given at once, and repeated, if necessary, the same evening (after a lapse of at least four hours), in order to give him a good night's rest. If the pain is only moderate, 10 gr. of Dover's powder with 5 gr. of aspirin may be sufficient. Morphia, by relieving the pain, actually improves the respiration. The doctor need not be afraid of giving it at this stage, when there is no danger of poisoning the respiratory centre. It may also quieten the cough, though often some form of linctus is more helpful, such as

> ℞ Syr. codeinæ
> Syr. tolu.
> Tr. opii camphorat.   Partes æquales,
> in teaspoonful doses, four-hourly.

For most patients a poultice of linseed or kaolin to the affected side will be comforting (see p. 183).

If a combination of these methods is not effective, immobilisation of the painful side must be tried. This can be done by means of surgical strapping applied along the direction of the ribs, in overlapping strips 2 or 3 in. wide, and extending from a point 2 in. beyond the spine on the sound side behind to 2 in. beyond the sternum in front. It is put on from below upwards, and each strip is secured during full expiration. Unless strapping is really necessary, however, its inconveniences outweigh its advantages, for it prevents easy examination of the chest, it may work havoc with a tender skin if left on too long, and it is usually painful to take off. In any case, it should not be left on after its task is accomplished and the pain has subsided. Moreover, not all patients find relief from strapping of the chest ; sometimes it increases the dyspnœa and the local discomfort. A rough-and-ready test of its likely effect is to support the diseased side of the chest with firm pressure of the hand. If this gives a considerable degree of relief, strapping will probably do so also ; if it produces more pain or dyspnœa, so in all likelihood will strapping.

Sometimes the pleural pain is so severe as to be uncontrollable with any of these methods, even morphia. On the theory that the pain is due to the friction of the two inflamed pleural surfaces, it has been argued that separation of these surfaces by the establishment of a small pneumothorax of about 200 c.c. must abolish the pain ; while there are those who, knowing that the pain originates in the parietal pleura, seek to relieve it by infiltrating the painful inflamed spot with some form of local anæsthetic. I have not enough experience of either of these manœuvres to be able to judge their worth fairly. Reports of the effectiveness or otherwise of a small pneumothorax are contradictory, but in acute inflammation of the lung and pleura the real dangers are clear enough. If there is underlying pyogenic infection, a pneumothorax makes it likely that any subsequent pleural infection becomes widespread throughout the pleural cavity, instead of being localised. Again, the infiltration of an inflamed area by local anæsthetic solution is not usually accepted as good surgical practice, though it is possible to infiltrate the intercostal nerves without touching the pleura.

Once the patient has recovered from the acute illness of a " dry " pleurisy, convalescence is usually rapid. As most of the apparently primary cases are due to tuberculosis, the doctor owes the patient the duty of sound advice about the future. If effusion does not develop, it may seem an excessive precaution to ask the patient to sacrifice some months to sanatorium regime if there is no obvious parenchymatous disease of the lung. Nevertheless, the situation should be frankly explained to him. If he can afford to do so, a long restful holiday, or even a stay at a sanatorium for two or three months, is the soundest advice. If he cannot, he should not be allowed to go back to work until he is fully fit. He should be kept under regular medical supervision, and radiograms of the chest should be taken at intervals of three months. He should be asked to report again without delay if untoward symptoms such as excessive tiredness, " feverish attacks " or persistent cough develop. More will be said about this problem when the management of patients suffering from pleurisy with effusion is discussed.

2. **At the stage of effusion**—If the effusion is the result of a pyogenic lesion of the lung or chest wall (pneumonia, lung abscess, chest wound), or of a hæmothorax, the treatment is primarily conditioned by the underlying disease, and is discussed in the appropriate chapters. Tuberculous effusions raise problems of the greatest importance, and the treatment of the sterile variety will be dealt with in this chapter in some detail. When the effusion forms, there is no point in giving the patient drastic hydragogue purgatives in the hope of promoting absorption of the fluid. Nor are drugs such as iodides, or diuretics like caffeine, theobromine, or the mercurial diuretics, likely to be effective for this purpose.

Ought the fluid to be removed ? If by its mechanical effects it is causing respiratory or cardiac distress (either because it is very copious or because it has accumulated rapidly), enough should be withdrawn to relieve the urgent symptoms. Otherwise it will usually be absorbed naturally and in its own good time. The important question is not what to do with the fluid, but how to deal with the primary disease in the lung. If the fluid is evacuated, the lung expands again, there will be a change from lymphatic stasis to flooding of the tissue spaces with fluid, and a real danger of dissemination of the lesions, whether they are microscopical or macroscopical. Pleural effusion has often been called " Nature's splint," and with justice ; though where there is an obvious tuberculous focus in the lung it is not the best splint, for the lesion is nearly always at the apex and the effusion at the base. For this reason there are some who advocate withdrawal of the fluid in all cases and replacement by air, a manœuvre which also helps the doctor to see more easily in the X-ray picture whether or not there is an obvious tuberculous or other lesion in the lung. If there is, however, it is commonly in the upper lobe, and can be seen in any case on the X-ray film in all but the huge effusions. In the less common instances where the lesion is confined to the lower lobe and hidden by the fluid, frequent

X-ray examinations as the fluid absorbs will reveal it in time, and careful examination of the sputum for tubercle bacilli will indicate an open lesion in the lungs.

It would be wise to substitute for the term " air replacement " that of **" replacement pneumothorax."** The latter phrase gives the right emphasis. For the proper question to ask when considering this form of treatment is " Does the condition of the underlying lung call for the establishment of an artificial pneumothorax ? " If the pleurisy is apparently primary, the answer is " No " ; this is a lung with minimal microscopic lesions, highly suitable for sanatorium regime, akin to the " early case " of good prognosis. On the other hand, there is the effusion secondary to an obvious tuberculous lesion in the lung, revealed by an X-ray film and perhaps by the finding of tubercle bacilli in the sputum. Here, too, the doctor must make his decision by largely forgetting the fluid, and considering on its merits whether that particular lung is suitable for pneumothorax treatment. If so, then he must remove fluid in order to provide space for the air.

The persistence of pyrexia does not in itself necessarily call for evacuation of the effusion. In a severe case, with high temperature and general toxæmia, the pyrexia may persist for weeks ; but the effusion is the result and not the cause of the condition, and unless mechanical distress from a rapid accumulation of fluid is present, aspiration will often do harm. Indeed, aspiration before the pyrexia has subsided is nearly always followed by re-accumulation of the fluid, because the pyrexia indicates the continuing activity of the fundamental lesion.

To sum up, then, the doctor should let the fluid be, unless he has very good reason to interfere. This does not mean that he is forbidden to draw off about 5 c.c. of the fluid at intervals for diagnostic purposes or to see if there is any alteration in its character. If there is mechanical distress, he should withdraw enough to relieve symptoms, considering at the same time whether a replacement pneumothorax is advisable or not.

There remains the difficult problem of the effusion which does not absorb. Usually this means that the pleural membranes are markedly thickened after an acute pleurisy, and that now a low-grade but active inflammation is continuing, perhaps in spite of a fall of temperature to normal. Sometimes, but by no means always, the fluid will be absorbed even after an interval of six months. The best procedure for such a patient is to transfer him to a good sanatorium, where he can have all the advantages of regime and treatment. If there is no sign of absorption within some two or three months, the fluid can then be withdrawn and a replacement pneumothorax established, in the hope that re-expansion of the lung will occur, and with the safeguard that the lung can be observed radiologically during its expansion. If there is active pulmonary tuberculosis, the pneumothorax can be maintained, if this is seen to be the right treatment.

After the acute stage of a tuberculous effusion is over, these patients must not go back immediately to the rough and tumble of ordinary life. Their illness is tuberculous, part of the story of a primary infection of the lung. If they are to recover, they need time, rest and careful treatment. When there is little or no obvious infiltration in the lungs, they can expect to do astonishingly well with a proper sanatorium regime for a few months. If they are not properly treated, many of them will develop parenchymatous lesions in the lungs within a period which varies roughly from three to ten years. The doctor must have the courage, therefore, to be frank with the patient, informing him of the situation, and what he may expect of good or ill. Adolescence or early adult life is not an age which takes kindly to the necessity of several months' rest from activity, but it is the price of security in the years to come. No diffidence about committing himself to the unpleasant word " tuberculosis " should lead the doctor to agree to any inadequate compromise, such as a medically uncontrolled sea voyage or a holiday in the country. Most patients brought to face the serious issues involved will make their peace with events, and respond to the doctor's frankness. For at least three years after the illness an X-ray film of the chest should be taken at intervals of three months.

THE TECHNIQUE OF WITHDRAWAL OF EFFUSION

The fifth or sixth intercostal space in the mid-axillary line or the eighth space just below the angle of the scapula are the best spots for the puncture. The skin is sterilised and the tissues anæsthetised down to the pleura, as for diagnostic puncture.

The object is to make the manœuvre painless, except for the prick of the hypodermic needle. A moderately wide-bored needle is then inserted, attached either to a two-way syringe, a Potain's aspirator or a Burrell's aspirator. The ordinary trocars of the Potain's aspirator are too brutal for this purpose. Whatever method is used, the withdrawal should be slow, and the suction (negative pressure) of the aspirator or syringe only slight. The removal of a pint of fluid should take at least ten minutes. There are certain dangers in aspiration—faintness or sudden death from " pleural shock " or air embolism ; œdema of the lung, alarming dyspnœa, or hæmoptysis from too rapid a withdrawal of the fluid and too high a negative pressure in the pleural cavity ; reflex paroxysms of cough with severe pain in the side. Apart from air embolism, which is a rare accident, these dangers can usually be avoided by gentleness, care and the removal of only relatively small amounts of fluid at a time (at most a pint). If any of these symptoms show themselves, the operation must be stopped at once. Morphia should then be given for pain and distress.

CHAPTER XXV

EMPYEMA

PURULENT pleural effusions are, for practical purposes, always secondary. The infection may reach the pleura directly from a penetrating wound or from a ruptured lung abscess : it may travel by contiguity or via the lymphatics from lesions in neighbouring structures (such as pneumonia, phthisis, suppurative diseases of the lung, subdiaphragmatic abscess, osteomyelitis of the ribs or vertebræ, pericarditis) : or it may travel by the blood stream, as in pyæmia, though here it is often caused by the rupture of a tiny subpleural abscess. In the vast majority of instances empyema is a sequel to inflammation of the lung tissue ; those due to other causes are much less common. Of the pulmonary inflammations, those complicating pneumococcus lobar pneumonia and streptococcus bronchopneumonia are by far the most frequent.

There are two main types of empyemata. The *total empyema*, with no localising adhesions between the chest wall or diaphragm and the lung, is relatively uncommon, and is generally due to a fulminating infection by the streptococcus (Fig. 115).

The other type is the *encysted empyema*, of which the commonest is one where what is in effect an abscess of the pleural cavity is localised to a greater or less area by adhesions between the lung and the thoracic wall (Fig. 116). Much less common are the interlobar, diaphragmatic and mediastinal collections of pus (Figs. 117 and 118).

Seeing that the majority of instances result from pneumococcus or streptococcus pneumonia, the history of the illness as a rule takes one of two forms. On the one hand, the patient has usually suffered from a lobar pneumonia due to the pneumococcus, often but not always accompanied by a severe initial pleurisy. After about a week, he recovers from the acute phase of his illness, the temperature falls to normal or nearly so, and it seems that he is on the way to convalescence. Then, however, he is not so well. Perhaps he again has a pain in the chest and a recrudescence of cough. The temperature rises, once more he looks flushed and ill, and clinical examination reveals a persistent leucocytosis and an accumulation of

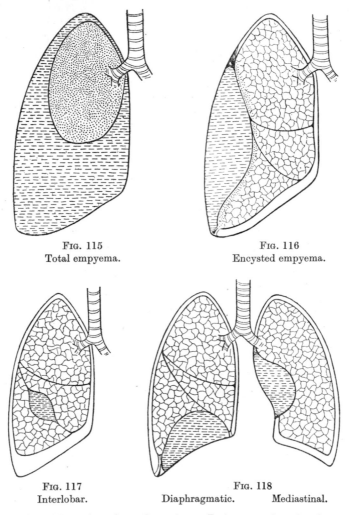

Fig. 115
Total empyema.

Fig. 116
Encysted empyema.

Fig. 117
Interlobar.

Fig. 118
Diaphragmatic.   Mediastinal.

purulent fluid in the pleural cavity. It is true that in the early stages of the pneumonia there was no doubt a fibrinous pleurisy with a small amount of thin seropurulent fluid ; but by the time enough fluid has collected to make diagnosis of empyema likely, the pneumonic lung is already resolving. The pus is thick and yellowish, with a heavy cellular and fibrinous content.

The story is vastly different in the streptococcus infections. The patient was, maybe, struck down by a sharp attack of influenza, or if he is a child, by measles. Secondary invaders, especially the hæmolytic streptococcus, broke through the defences of the lung, and a diffuse bronchopneumonia followed, with its widespread bronchiolitis, interstitial inflammation, areas of localised collapse and emphysema, alveolitis and grave toxæmia. The bronchopneumonia drags on unsatisfactorily as fresh patches develop, and the patient is dyspnœic, cyanosed and still critically ill. Finally it is recognised that in addition to the lesions in the lung there is an effusion into the pleural cavity, and thin greenish or greenish-brown turbid fluid is withdrawn by the exploring syringe.

In the **metapneumonic** pneumococcus empyema the affected lobe or lobes have appreciably recovered from the inflammation and are even regaining some of their respiratory function. The intensity of the infection is subsiding, and a deposit of fibrin from the pus has already caused the formation of adhesions. These have localised the pus, and are holding the lung to the chest wall along the outer edge of the walled-off abscess. In the **synpneumonic** streptococcus infection of the pleura, active and widespread inflammation of the lung is still present, and the added toxæmia is a further serious danger to the cardio-respiratory function. Pleural adhesions are as yet few and tenuous, and if the effusion is considerable it constitutes a total rather than a localised empyema.

The problem which empyema raises in these markedly different clinical conditions is essentially the same, namely, to remove the pus without unnecessary delay so as to prevent further absorption of toxins, to obtain re-expansion of the lung with as little damage to its functional capacity as possible, and to produce obliteration of the septic empyema cavity. Before the war of 1914-18, an ill-conceived " rule-of-thumb " application of these principles resulted in the immediate evacuation of pus discovered in the pleural cavity by rib resection and open drainage, whatever the character of the empyema. Far too many patients died after the operation. In the influenza epidemic of 1917-18, in which large numbers of patients suffered from streptococcus empyema, the death rate after open drainage was so appalling among American soldiers in camp (as much as 70 per cent. of the cases in some

army camps) that an Empyema Commission was set up to
find the cause. It was able to point out the fatal errors which
arose from neglect of principles based on the pathology of the
various types of empyema (especially the two main types) and
on the physiology of the open chest wound produced in this
instance by the surgeon's operation. The pathological differences have already been mentioned : the importance of the
open chest wound lies in its effect upon the vital capacity.

For the purposes of respiration under ordinary quiet conditions the 500 to 600 c.c. of tidal air is sufficient. This constitutes about one-twelfth to one-fifteenth of the total vital
capacity (see also Chap. I), so that normally there is a wide
reserve of safety. An **open chest wound,** however, makes serious
inroads into this reserve, unless the mediastinum happens to be
well fixed : for the mediastinum in a healthy person is mobile
and flexible, and not a rigid barrier between the two lungs.
If, therefore, an opening is made into the chest wall, air enters
the pleural space and the lung on that side collapses. The
mediastinum is pulled over by the elasticity of the opposite
lung, which in its turn is diminished in volume and therefore in
its capacity to fill with air. Even if (as actually happens) the
patient increases the amplitude of his respiration in order to
compensate for this disability, he cannot do more than produce
during inspiration an expansion of the lungs which is considerably less than normal. As, during expiration, the mediastinum
is swung back towards the affected side, there is a to-and-fro
swing of the displaced mediastinum which causes a great deal
of shock and cardiac disability. The consequent diminution
in the inspiratory negative pressure causes a loss of the normal
thoracic aspiration of venous blood towards the right side of
the heart ; this produces venous stasis and diminished cardiac
output. There is, moreover, a to-and-fro movement of air
between the " good " and the " bad " lung (Figs. 119 and 120).
The expired air from the " good " lung is driven into the " bad "
lung during expiration, there to lose still more of its oxygen
and gain CO_2. During inspiration the atmospheric air drawn
into the " good " lung is mixed with this deoxygenated air
from the " bad " one. Thus the pulmonary circulation picks
up air which is not only less in quantity but also is poorer in
quality than it should normally be. Finally, to make things
even worse, the exposure to atmospheric air of the large pleural

surface on the affected side helps to produce a loss of heat from the body. After operation this is not great, owing to the overlying dressings, but in an open wound on the battlefield, where dressings are not immediately available, the loss may be important.

For the patient submitted to open drainage of his empyema this is not the whole story. To it must be added the effect of the underlying disease. Fever, with its increased metabolism, increases the demand for oxygen. Toxæmia damages the heart and circulation, and lesions in the lung itself impair respiratory function and further diminish the vital capacity.

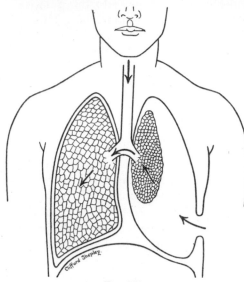

FIG. 119
Open chest wound (inspiration).

From what has already been said it is clear that by the time the presence of an empyema is diagnosed the patient suffering from a pneumococcus infection is likely on all grounds to be less severely ill, and in particular to have a better vital capacity than the patient with a streptococcus empyema ; for the underlying pneumonia is resolving, the pus is thick and creamy, the empyema is already walled off by adhesions, the mediastinum is fixed and the dangers of an open operation are small. The streptococcus bronchopneumonia, on the other hand, takes longer to subside ; the active inflammatory exudation persists longer and so the fluid remains thinly serous and cloudy ; and adhesions effective to fix the lung and also the mediastinum are late in appearing.

It is not surprising, therefore, that early open operation in the streptococcus cases has so often " evacuated pus by free incision " and killed the patient ; nor is it surprising that dilatoriness in dealing properly with an obvious pneumococcus empyema results often in a chronic empyema, a fibrotic visceral pleura, and a badly functioning lung. Doctor and student must keep in mind all the pathological principles enumerated and balance their judgment accordingly, since on these, as will be seen later, are based the principles of treatment.

The **symptoms** are those of the primary disease, together with those due to the mechanical and toxic results of a purulent pleural effusion. Something of the clinical picture has already been given, and it is clear that in streptococcus infections the gravity of the general illness may overshadow the pleural manifestations (see Chap. XVIII). Renewed fever after a pneumococcus pneumonia, slumber sweats, discomfort and pain in the chest, pallor, loss of appetite, wasting, and an irritating cough in spite of the diminution of expectoration are all symptoms which should lead the doctor to think of empyema

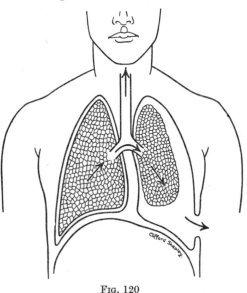

FIG. 120

Open chest wound (expiration).

as a possible explanation of them. The **physical signs** are those of fluid in the pleural cavity, but these may be modified by the pus becoming localised by adhesions and by the condition of the underlying lung. If the collection of pus is localised, the appropriate signs are localised too. If it is a small one, or if there are several pockets of pus, the signs may not be clear-cut, while in interlobar, diaphragmatic or mediastinal collections the usual signs of fluid may be difficult or impossible to elicit. Rarely there is œdema of the thoracic wall over the effusion, and occasionally enlarged glands are palpable in the axilla. On the left side an empyema may occasionally pulsate, because the localised pus and its containing wall are in contact with the heart and pericardium, so that the expansile cardiac impulse is transmitted through the collection to the chest wall (Fig. 121). Encysted collections in contact with an area of consolidation in the lung may similarly transmit whispered pectoriloquy and bronchial breathing to the surface of the thorax. The course of the disease has already been partly described. If the empyema is not discovered it may eventually kill the patient by toxæmia, extension to the pericardium, metastatic brain abscess, or amyloid disease. If he is less unlucky it may rupture into a bronchus, or discharge itself

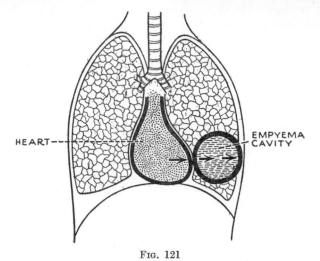

HEART

EMPYEMA CAVITY

FIG. 121

Diagrammatic representation of pulsating empyema.

through the chest wall as an " empyema necessitatis." If it is inadequately treated the patient will be left with a chronic empyema.

Diagnosis depends to a large extent on being on the *qui vive* for an empyema. Its manifestations are toxic and local. The persistence or recrudescence of toxæmic symptoms after an attack of pneumonia should always bring empyema to mind. The clinical picture of the two main types of empyema has already been described (p. 391). The local signs are those of fluid in the chest, though when the collection of pus is interlobar or diaphragmatic, the picture may be indefinite. Whenever there is a likelihood of empyema, it should be a rule to " put in a diagnostic needle " if there is an area of " stony " dulness, whatever the rest of the physical signs may be. The pus may not easily come through a small-bored needle, even though it is attached to a syringe of good capacity. If there is difficulty, a wide-bored needle attached to a 2-c.c. syringe should be used. Radiograms in both anterior and lateral positions are helpful, especially in showing the presence of collections of pus in unusual situations—interlobar, diaphragmatic or mediastinal empyemata, or encysted apical empyema which may clinically be very puzzling.

Differential diagnosis must be made especially from *delayed resolution* ("unresolved pneumonia") and from *lung abscess*. A diagnosis of unresolved pneumonia is much less likely to be correct than that of empyema. The finding of "stony" dulness and the wise use of X-rays and of the exploring needle will be of most help. A carefully taken history will in most instances prevent the doctor from needling a lung abscess in mistake for an empyema, a proceeding fraught with serious risk of infecting the pleural cavity. *Collapse of the lung*, especially if it is accompanied by secondary infection, may (by reason of the absence of breath sounds over the area of collapse) be mistaken for empyema : the dulness does not feel stony, however, and the mediastinum is displaced towards the side of the lesion.

When the persistence of pyrexia is the main clinical feature, without clear-cut local signs, it must be differentiated from other causes of pyrexia, especially *septicæmia* and *ulcerative endocarditis*. *Interlobar empyema* is very liable to perforate into the lung, because it is near the larger bronchi. *Diaphragmatic empyema* (see also Chap. XXVI) may do the same.

Enough has been said already to indicate the factors which condition *prognosis*. Empyema may be but an incident in a grave general illness. A child, for example, may have septicæmia with otitis media or pericarditis or meningitis, as well as empyema. Synpneumonic empyema is more serious than metapneumonic empyema, by reason of the added pulmonary lesion. Moreover, the appropriateness and the efficiency of the treatment adopted has an immense influence on the outlook for recovery. This has already been shown by the report of the Empyema Commission, referred to earlier, and it will find further illustration in the later section of this chapter devoted to chronic empyema.

TREATMENT

Up to the time of the discovery of the empyema the patient with pneumonia will have had the nursing and the sulphonamide, penicillin and other forms of therapy described in Chapters XVII and XVIII. Thereafter, the special problem is that presented by the collection of pus, a problem to be dealt with according to the pathological principles discussed in the early part of this chapter. No " rule of thumb," not even the useful guide of the thickness or thinness of the pus, can properly be substituted for the discipline of these principles, though certain broad general propositions do emerge from them :—

1. It is dangerous, and may be fatal, to drain by open operation any empyema when the patient is still very ill, and the pus is not walled off. In actual fact, by the time an empyema is usually recognised, this holds only for the streptococcus empyema.

2. As soon as the patient is improving, and the empyema is localised, procrastination is folly, because of the new danger of the establishment of a chronic empyema, with its evil effect upon the future function of the lung.

3. It is obvious that as the patient masters his infection, accumulation of thin serous inflammatory exudate ceases, and the pus becomes thick and creamy.

4. While the patient is very ill and inflammation in the lung is still intense, time can be gained by a series of aspirations through a needle. In many instances, penicillin will control the virulence of both pulmonary and pleural infection, and indeed the pleural cavity can often be sterilised by injections of penicillin after aspiration of the pus (e.g. 250,000 units every other day in the highly toxæmic stage). Even so, aspiration can in most cases be only a temporary and preliminary measure, for it seldom leads to a real cure. If the patient is not so ill, airtight intercostal drainage through a catheter is even better, for it affords continuous " closed " evacuation, the rate of which can be controlled by the surgeon. It is, moreover, less distressing to the patient than many repeated aspirations through the hollow needle.

5. To avoid the formation of false membranes and adhesions which result in the binding down of the lung by scar tissue, it is wise, as soon as it is safe, to resect a rib and evacuate not

only the pus but also the fibrin masses and sloughs on the surface of the lung and in the cavity. These masses of infected fibrinous lymph are the rule in pneumococcus empyema, less common in streptococcus ones. If they are allowed to remain they maintain the suppuration, and though they may sometimes resolve slowly they are more likely to result in pleural thickening, adhesions, and restriction of expansion of the lung. Adhesions consecutive to the deposition of fibrin may form very quickly.

6. To encourage healthy expansion of the lung and obliteration of the cavity the operation wound should not be left open. Some form of airtight drainage should be established, the outer end of the drainage tube being led under water or connected to a suction apparatus. Suction is unlikely *directly* to bring about the expansion of a lung which would not expand otherwise : it probably acts as a mild application of Bier's hyperæmia principle, helping to hasten recovery from the local infection.

Faced with a patient who is very ill with acute inflammation of the underlying lung, and an empyema in which the fluid is thin and largely serous, the doctor should carry out aspiration by needle and two-way syringe, followed by instillation of penicillin, every second or third day. The amount removed should be well short of the total fluid present. The evacuated pus should never be replaced by air,* because this may determine a pyopneumothorax, cause general infection of the pleural cavity, and slow down recovery very appreciably. At this stage, too, resection of part of a rib for open or even closed drainage must on no account be done.

If the patient is not so ill, continuous drainage through an intercostal catheter is advisable. In a few of the streptococcus infections, this in combination with the administration of sulphonamides or penicillin may even lead to cure. Usually, however, even though the patient is obviously improving and the pyrexia largely subsides, continued accumulation of pus shows that better drainage must be instituted. Masses of infected fibrinous lymph, or sloughs, are probably keeping up the suppuration, and they must as far as possible be removed. As soon, therefore, as the patient's general condition allows it

---

* Air replacement may be justifiable in *encysted* collections of pus, for the purposes of diagnosis and localisation.

(a time which roughly corresponds to the development of thick, creamy pus, and of adhesions between the lung and the chest wall), resection of a rib should be undertaken, to be followed by adequate closed suction-drainage until in the course of about a fortnight the discharge has practically ceased.

It is of the utmost importance to obtain dependent drainage, yet not too dependent so that the subsequent rise of the diaphragm will obstruct the opening of the drainage tube. The most suitable site for the removal of a piece of rib can be discovered by inserting needles into successive lower intercostal spaces and withdrawing pus. By this means the surgeon can gauge the most dependent part into which he can insert his drainage tube, while allowing sufficient room for it when the diaphragm rises. This procedure should be done preparatory to the operation itself, while the patient is under a general anæsthetic.

In children adequate drainage is ensured as a rule only by the removal of portions of two ribs, together with the intercostal bundle.

After the operation the patient is nursed comfortably in the sitting-up position, his thighs and knees flexed over a supporting bolster. If he can be nursed in the open air, all the better. Plenty of fluid is given, sweetened with glucose, together with as nutritious a diet as he can take. If a stimulant is needed, nikethamide (coramine) injected intramuscularly is of help. Later, especially in infections by the hæmolytic streptococcus, full doses of iron are needed to combat the resulting anæmia. Sometimes a blood transfusion will greatly hasten the convalescence. To aid the re-expansion of the lung, breathing exercises should be undertaken as soon as the patient is fit for and not fatigued by them. With the same end in view, he should not be kept in bed longer than is necessary.

Some surgeons advocate irrigation of the healing empyema cavity with eusol or other disinfectants. In the acuter phases of the disease it is bad practice, and if by any chance there is a pleuropulmonary fistula, irrigation is dangerous in that it is likely to wash septic material from the pleura into the opposite lung, and so cause a septic bronchopneumonia which may well prove fatal. It can never be a substitute for the natural curative effect of proper drainage and the building up of the general resistance of the patient ; though in specially selected patients it may be of help in getting rid of persistent intrapleural deposits of fibrin.

The doctor must not be satisfied with the results of treatment unless the patient has completely recovered, the lung is fully expanded, the empyema is obliterated and the wound in the chest wall is healed. The drainage tube must remain in position until re-expansion of the lung forces it out ; otherwise a residual empyema cavity is almost inevitable. If discharge from the empyema wound continues, it may be due to one of several possibilities. There may be a mild osteomyelitis in the cut surface of the rib, or a proliferative osteitis which prevents closure of the sinus. Usually, however, drainage has been incomplete because of wrong positioning of the tube, either too high and therefore not giving dependent drainage, or too low so that the opening of the tube becomes blocked by the rise of the diaphragm ; or the tube has been pushed too far into the pleural cavity so that the opening is above the level of the pus. The importance of periodic X-ray control of the position of the tube thus becomes manifest. A pleural abscess cavity persists, small or large according to the circumstances, and discharge from it will persist also. The size of the cavity— sometimes there is a long and tortuous sinus leading to it—can be defined by radiograms after lipiodol injection into it. Once it becomes clear that the residual cavity is unlikely to close, further surgical intervention is necessary.

Something has already been said of **interlobar empyema** and its tendency to open into a bronchus. Rarely it discharges itself at the outer end of the interlobar fissure and becomes a parietal empyema. It may be difficult to diagnose from an abscess of the lung, especially if it has perforated into a bronchus. As the general pleural cavity is not likely, as a rule, to be infected, its surgical treatment must be similar to that of a lung abscess, and exploratory needling through virgin uninfected pleura is to be avoided. The same principles hold for the treatment of diaphragmatic and mediastinal collections of pus, the latter of which usually occur below the level of the hilum, and may be anterior or posterior to the broad pulmonary ligament.

CHRONIC EMPYEMA

There are three main reasons why an empyema becomes chronic :—

1. The local causes of chronicity are : osteomyelitis of the divided rib ; inadequate drainage or a partly sealed-off pocket of pus inside the pleural cavity, due to a misplaced opening ; or too early removal of the drainage tube, before there is satisfactory obliteration of the cavity ; or foreign bodies such as a lost drainage tube, forgotten gauze, or fragments of rib. To these must be added the presence of a bronchial fistula, the existence of which may be unsuspected because its opening into the lung is often so small.

2. The infecting organism may be the tubercle bacillus or actinomyces, which in themselves cause suppuration of the chronic type.

3. Unfortunately the most frequent cause is failure to discover the empyema within reasonable time. In consequence, proper treatment is delayed, and the pleural membranes become thick and rigid owing to the proliferative and organisational changes which result from prolonged infection. As time goes on the membranes become thicker, harder and more inelastic ; the parietal pleura may be an inch thick, the visceral pleura somewhat less so. The wall of the chest then shrinks and becomes rigid, its contents distorted. There is secondary scoliosis, and ribs and muscles atrophy from disuse. Plaques of calcium or even of true bone may eventually form in the thick pleural layers, so that the affected lung is almost enclosed in a coat of armour. In addition to an examination of the pus, a piece of pleural membrane should be removed for section, for the discovery of tuberculous lesions in it may be the only convincing evidence of a tuberculous basis.

The patient with chronic pyogenic empyema has recurrent attacks of pyrexia. The fingers are clubbed, and he is usually so pale and wasted that he looks as though he is suffering from advanced phthisis.

Advanced disease may cause **hypertrophic pulmonary osteoarthropathy**—a symmetrical subperiosteal hyperplasia of the bones of the hands and feet, accompanied or not by involvement of the joints. The condition is beautifully revealed by radiograms, as well as by the obvious enlargement of, for example, the wrists and arms.

There may be a small sinus discharging copiously or inter-mittently. The affected side of the chest is shrunken, distorted and does not move with respiration. Radiograms show dense shadowing through which the fluid level of one or more pockets containing pus may be discerned ; or they may even show a forgotten drainage tube inside the cavity.

The first essential of treatment is an adequate opening to ensure free drainage and the removal of any foreign body. This alone may produce a surprising degree of recovery in the general and local condition. If the operation is inadequate to secure healing, it may at least enable the ill and toxic patient to be built up sufficiently to tolerate the more drastic surgical measures to obliterate the cavity should these be necessary. The surgeon has the choice, according to the circumstances of the case, of trying by decortication of the lung to allow it to re-expand to the chest wall, or of arranging that the chest wall shall collapse on to the shrunken lung. In these almost desperate cases the first (" mobilisation of the lung ") is rarely success-ful ; the second (thoracoplasty) has often to be accomplished in stages. This is not the place to set out the very specialised details of the possible operative methods either for closure of the chronic cavity or for obliterating a bronchial fistula. Enough has been said, however, to remind physicians, surgeons, practitioners and students alike how vitally important it is to discover and cure all empyemata before they have come to the stage when any " cure " can only mean that the patient survives as a cripple for the rest of his almost certainly shortened life.

The student has been counselled to look behind the empyema to the lung beneath it. He must remember that not only pneumonic lesions of the lung but also suppurations such as lung abscess, tuberculous or actinomycotic lesions, and new growths in the lung may produce empyema. He will especially bear in mind that empyema in a patient of the cancer age may perhaps be secondary to a bronchial carcinoma.

EMPYEMA IN CHILDREN

In older children the problem of empyema is very much the same as in the adult. In young infants, however, there are certain special points of diagnosis, prognosis and treatment which are largely conditioned by the type of infection and by their tiny chests. Over the first two years of life the mortality from empyema is very high—about 75 per cent. in the first year, and 50 per cent. in the second, to fall sharply to about 18 per cent. in the third year, and 6 per cent. thereafter. This high death rate in the first two years is almost certainly due mainly to the type of infection. The pneumococcus is the most common organism found in the empyemata of that particular age—roughly in up to 80 per cent. of the cases, the remaining 20 per cent. being evenly divided between the streptococcus and the staphylococcus. Pneumococcus pneumonia in young infancy is not the short, sharp illness of the adult; often it is a bronchopneumonia, often it is complicated by infection elsewhere (otitis media, pericarditis, peritonitis, or meningitis), and in any case it lasts weeks instead of the seven days or so of the adult type. Thus pneumococcus empyema in these young infants is usually synpneumonic and not metapneumonic ; and the prognosis shows a corresponding gravity.

Moreover, in the infant's chest a small collection of fluid such as 250 c.c. (less than half a pint) is relatively equivalent to a huge effusion of roughly $2\frac{3}{4}$ litres in the adult—a grave embarrassment to respiration. The smallness of the chest also influences the physical signs of empyema, for the vesicular murmur is often not abolished, the puerile breath sounds coming through to the examiner's ear, sometimes indeed being transmitted from the healthy side. Thus the breath sounds may be well heard over the front of the affected half of the chest, but be absent over a small area in the axilla—a finding, therefore, which does not signify that the collection of pus is necessarily limited to the area of dulness. The less rigid infantile thorax shows asymmetry from the presence of pleural effusion far more readily than does that of the adult ; intercostal depressions are likewise more easily abolished, and the intercostal spaces are not sucked in during inspiration if there is a moderate amount of fluid in the pleural cavity. The one convincing sign, however, remains that of " stony " dulness, obtained by light and gentle percussion. Heavy percussion on the child's tiny chest is crude and may be very misleading. If such dulness is present the student or doctor must not wait expectantly for absence of breath sounds before he thinks of the likelihood of empyema.

Here, more than ever, is a wise surgical judgment called for. The chances of fibrotic damage in the lung from the long-

·continued pneumonia and the complicating empyema are great, so that early recognition of the nature of the illness and the condition of both lung and pleural cavity is vital. Until the lung has recovered, open operation will almost certainly be fatal ; time must meanwhile be gained by aspiration or closed airtight drainage.* Once the empyema is " metapneumonic," an open operation with removal of fibrin masses and sloughs will go far to ensure restoration of the function of the lung and to avoid the fibrosis which may lead later to serious deformity of the chest. In children under 3 years of age the soft thorax may allow this to be done intercostally, without resection of a rib, though surgeons differ in their view of the adequacy of this technique. Closed suction drainage follows.

TUBERCULOUS EMPYEMA

Tuberculous empyema is but a purulent variety of tuberculous pleurisy with effusion. Serofibrinous effusion (especially the primary type) has already been discussed in the previous chapter. It must be considered once more in this section, perhaps from a somewhat different angle, as part of the whole picture of tuberculous pleurisy.

Thoracoscopic examination of patients undergoing artificial pneumothorax treatment for a tuberculous pulmonary lesion has thrown much light upon the problem of tuberculous pleurisy. In particular, it has established that tuberculous effusion secondary to a parenchymatous lung lesion is always determined by an inflammation of the pleural membranes. This pleuritis may often be detected in radiograms by the development of a characteristic haziness in the appearance of adhesions which run across the pneumothorax space—a lack of definition which is caused by œdema round the adhesions. With mild pleurisy a few odd tubercles may be dotted about the pleura, each one surrounded by a zone of hyperæmia. Effusion may or may not be present. If the pleural inflammation is severe, many tubercles can be seen, and effusion almost inevitably follows. The parenchyma of the underlying lung may contain active tuberculous lesions, and the pleurisy arises by extension from them. On the other hand, the lesion may be so small as not

* It must be noted that a great objection to closed drainage is that a child is so apt to pull the tube out.

to be obvious on the X-ray film, or previous tuberculous lesions in the lung may have become apparently inactive ; here the pleural infection may be blood-borne.

It is impossible in any individual patient to forecast what the course of an effusion will be—whether it will remain clear, or become turbid, or progress to frank pus. A serofibrinous effusion may be absorbed, it may remain unchanged for many months unless it is aspirated, or it may slowly or rapidly become purulent. In acute cases it may be purulent from the early days of the pleurisy.

The factors which determine the characters of the effusion are : (1) the virulence of the infection ; (2) intervention, in the sense of successive aspirations ; and (3) secondary infection, introduced either via a pleuropulmonary fistula or from without in the course of aspiration.

1. As has already been said, virulent infection may quickly produce a turbid or purulent effusion, especially if a caseous focus ruptures and discharges its contents into the pleural cavity. Sometimes removal of the turbid fluid results in clearing up the effusion : on the other hand, the pleural inflammation may continue active, fluid reaccumulates, and soon becomes frank pus. The more chronic tuberculous lesions of the pleural membranes cause great thickening, especially of the parietal pleura ; here an effusion may subside, it may remain serofibrinous for a long time, or it may slowly change to pus.

2. It has already been pointed out that successive aspirations result in thickening of the fluid. They may also determine the formation of tuberculous granulation tissue, which will bleed and render the effusion hæmorrhagic.

3. Secondary infection arises, as a rule, either as the result of spontaneous pneumothorax from a tuberculous lung, with accompanying pleuropulmonary fistula ; or by infection introduced during pneumothorax treatment or during aspiration of the effusion. It is a grave complication, the more so when a fistula is present.

The onset of a tuberculous effusion may be insidious, or it may be abrupt. The abrupt onset, followed in favourable cases by a slow decline in the severity of the symptoms, should lead the doctor to suspect pleurisy rather than an exacerbation of a lesion in the underlying lung, for in the latter the onset is usually much more gradual.

The symptoms vary greatly, and naturally depend to a great extent on the condition of the underlying lung, and on the severity of the infection. Some patients remain fairly well and can get about with really large and even purulent effusions, complaining only of a feeling of fulness in the chest, and some breathlessness on exertion. Others have a high temperature and all the manifestations of a profound toxæmia. The characters of a serofibrinous effusion have already been described (Chap. XXIV). If frank pus is found on diagnostic puncture, with clots of fibrin, but with no obvious organisms in the smear or culture, the empyema is almost certainly tuberculous, though rarely it may be actinomycotic. Sometimes tubercle bacilli can be demonstrated in the smear, but more often they are absent. If there is any doubt, guinea-pig inoculation or culture for tubercle bacilli by the usual special methods are called for. The physical signs are those of fluid in the pleural cavity.

The outlook for the majority of patients with serofibrinous effusion has been discussed in detail in Chapter XXIV. Nevertheless it must be emphasised that for any individual patient the future cannot be foreseen. When pus is present, the prognosis depends not only on whether the tuberculous empyema is secondarily infected or not but also on the condition of the underlying lung, which may show active tuberculosis of greater or less degree, or no obviously active tuberculous lesions at all.

TREATMENT

If there are active, progressive lesions in the lung, the idea treatment is clearly to keep the lung collapsed in order to give them a chance to heal. If there is no active lesion in the lung, expansion of the lung is not contraindicated, though (because of fibrosis and pleural thickening) it often happens that such a lung will not expand.

A serofibrinous effusion should be left alone, unless it is causing mechanical disability or is associated with long-continued pyrexia. Collapse by effusion is better than collapse by air. Such an effusion may subside " on its own," with resulting expansion of the lung. If there is obvious tuberculosis of the underlying lung, therefore, a replacement pneumothorax should be instituted as soon as it is obvious that the pleuritis

has subsided and the fluid is being absorbed.   If it is already
clear that a pneumothorax will not give effective control or
the disease in the lung, early thoracoplasty may be advisable
even though the effusion has not become purulent.

If the effusion is purulent, evacuation of the pus and obliteration of the empyema cavity are the aims of treatment, but the
appropriate method will depend largely on the condition of
the underlying lung.   If there is a tuberculous lesion in the
underlying lung which is not controlled by the effusion, perhaps
by reason of cavitation, then it is unlikely that it will be
controlled by air.   A replacement pneumothorax is then a
waste of time, and thoracoplasty at the earliest possible moment
is the operation of choice.   If the opposite lung is also extensively diseased, neither replacement pneumothorax nor thoracoplasty are advisable, and the only feasible intervention is to
relieve any mechanical symptoms caused by the accumulation
of pus.   Here, as happens so often in the treatment of tuberculous disease of the lungs, the ideal is not possible, and the
doctor has to choose the lesser evil.   *Primum non nocere*—the
first consideration is not to do harm.

If there is a pure (that is, not secondarily infected) tuberculous pleurisy, and the lesion in the underlying lung is
quiescent, the pus should be aspirated from time to time, and
replaced by a gradually decreasing amount of air to encourage
the lung gradually to re-expand.   If the patient does well,
nothing further need be done for the empyema.   If, however,
following aspiration the lung does not re-expand and obliterate
the pleural space, thoracoplasty will be necessary.

Even with such simple manœuvres as repeated aspiration
of the pus, there is great danger of secondary infection of a pure
tuberculous empyema.   Airtight drainage also is almost always
followed sooner or later by secondary infection.   It is clear,
therefore, that a pure tuberculous empyema must on no
account be submitted to open drainage.   Once the empyema
is secondarily infected the outlook is serious.   If the secondary
infection is detected at an early stage, and there is no pleuropulmonary fistula, it is occasionally possible to clear it up by
aspiration of the pus, lavage of the pleural cavity with azo-
chloramide, and the administration of sulphonamides and
penicillin, or (if it persists) by the use of an airtight drain.
Sooner or later, however, most of these patients will need

thoracoplasty of an extensive order. Is the patient's condition such that he is unlikely to endure this operation, even if it is done in small and careful stages ? If so, the surgeon may temporise, hoping that by means of pleural irrigations or intercostal airtight drainage the patient may improve sufficiently for the operation to be justifiable. On the other hand, if the general condition is good and the opposite lung is sound, time should not be wasted and operation deferred, once it is clear that drainage by aspiration or catheter, with or without irrigation, is unlikely to give a successful result.

The presence of a pleuropulmonary fistula as a rule, but not necessarily always, causes immediate mixed infection. In the presence of a fistula the empyema should be drained, and thoracoplasty should be undertaken at the earliest possible moment.

When in addition to a mixed infection empyema there is also active tuberculosis of the underlying lung, the outlook is very serious indeed. The diseased lung should not be allowed to expand. Replacement pneumothorax in a pleural cavity with a mixed infection is unwise. Thus the proper treatment to obliterate the pleural cavity and keep the lung collapsed is thoracoplasty at the earliest feasible moment. The patient, however, is usually very ill, and the risk of operation great. Yet if operation is not done, he is unlikely to recover. It needs wise judgment (and here two heads, one a physician's and the other a surgeon's, can perhaps be better than one, if they are sympathetic and honest) to decide if and when a carefully planned operation is possible without killing the patient.

By following these principles Alexander obtained a " cure " of tuberculous empyema in some 60 per cent. of patients, an encouraging result when the seriousness and the difficulties of the problem are appreciated.

Throughout the discussion of the various types of pleurisies and of empyema the student will have noted how vital to his right thinking is his picture of the condition of the lungs. It is worth reminding him once more that, apart from the comparatively infrequent lesions of the chest wall, the lungs (especially the underlying lung) are the key to their development, their symptoms and signs, their prognosis and their treatment.

CHAPTER XXVI

THORACIC COMPLICATIONS OF SUB-DIAPHRAGMATIC INFECTION

THE ANATOMICAL BACKGROUND

THE localisation of infection beneath the diaphragm is determined by the anatomical relationships of the upper abdominal structures, and particularly by the peritoneal reflexions. The falciform ligament divides the superior area of the liver into a right and left peritoneal portion. The lateral extensions of the falciform ligament (coronary ligament and the lateral ligaments) mark off an anterior from a posterior space, the anterior space being much the bigger of the two, seeing that the anterior portion of the coronary ligament lies well posterior to the dome of the liver. A " bare area " of the liver, uncovered by peritoneum, lies between the anterior and posterior folds of the coronary ligament, and is separated from the diaphragm merely by a little areolar tissue. This extraperitoneal area projects for a considerable distance over to the right of the middle line, so that the right superior space beyond it is limited to a lateral position well to the right side of the abdomen.

On the right side, therefore, there is a right posterior superior space, a larger right anterior superior space, and a " bare" retroperitoneal area (Fig. 122). On the left side there is a single superior space. Underneath the liver on the right side is the right inferior space, divided from the left side by the ligamentum teres, bounded above by the liver, behind by the kidney, and below by the transverse colon. On the left side there are two inferior spaces (see Fig. 123), the left posterior inferior space (the lesser sac of the peritoneum) and the left anterior inferior space, which has the liver above, the stomach below and the gastrohepatic omentum posteriorly.

While an appreciable proportion of infections below the diaphragm subside without the development of suppuration, subphrenic abscess may arise from almost any intra-abdominal inflammatory lesion. The commonest causes are perforation

410

of an ulcer of the stomach or duodenum, appendicitis, and suppuration in the liver (including amœbic abscess). Occasionally

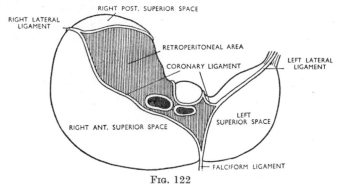

FIG. 122
Superior aspect of liver (which has been tilted forward a little).

it arises as an infective complication following operation on the stomach or duodenum.

Two-thirds of the subphrenic abscesses which follow appendicitis are situated either in the right posterior superior space or the right inferior space. More than two-thirds of those following gastric or duodenal lesions are left-sided. Half of those associated with hepatic suppuration are situated in the right anterior superior space. Eventually, however, more than one space may contain pus, either because separate columns of infection advance from the original abdominal lesion or because it is spread from one space to another.   The retroperitoneal space is but rarely infected.

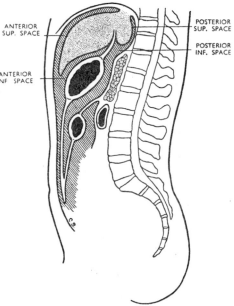

FIG. 123
Sagittal section to show the various spaces in relation to the liver.

While abscess underneath the liver has predominantly an abdominal symptomatology, abscess immediately beneath the diaphragm is liable to reveal itself by pleuropulmonary symptoms and signs. Extension of infection through the diaphragm into the thorax is common, raising problems of diagnosis and treatment not only of the acute inflammatory lesion but also of residual troubles, such as scarring of the lung or pleura, which may persist long after the acute inflammation has subsided.

The way in which subdiaphragmatic infection extends into the thorax has been greatly illuminated by studies of the course of the lymphatic vessels in that area. The diaphragm is traversed by a rich plexus of lymphatics which drains into the lymphatic nodes lying between the superior surface of the diaphragm and the pleura which lines it. The lymph flow is from below upwards. This has been shown experimentally by means of injection of Indian ink into the abdominal cavity. If the experimental animal is made to struggle by holding it head downwards by the hind legs, the resulting auto-massage of its abdominal contents produces a rapid staining of the thoracic surface of the diaphragm by ink particles. On the other hand, the diaphragm forms an efficient barrier to extension of infection from the thorax to the abdomen. In one series of over 300 instances of empyema, for example, only once was there extension of infection into the abdomen, and this was clearly due to injury of the diaphragm during operation for drainage of the empyema.

Organisms under the diaphragm can pass along the lymphatics into the thorax, just as do the particles of Indian ink. This may occur whether or not there is actual pus in the subphrenic area. Both above and below the diaphragm, these organisms may be exterminated by the defences of the body before they cause any appreciable damage. If, however, the defences are poor and the bacterial invasion makes headway above the diaphragm, the chest becomes the seat of inflammation. The organisms which penetrate into the thorax may cause a " dry " or plastic pleurisy, with adhesions between the under surface of the lung and the upper surface of the diaphragm ; or a localised effusion may result, which may remain sterile if the organisms are few in number or of relatively feeble virulence ; or an encysted empyema may form. The infection may pass into the lung, either via the area of plastic pleurisy or from the empyema, and result in pneumonia or lung abscess. The pus from the empyema or from the lung abscess may eventually find its way into a bronchus, whence it is coughed up. The serous or purulent exudate between the layers of the diaphragmatic pleural layers may remain localised, or it may extend laterally, finally reaching the costal intrapleural space.

Sometimes the supradiaphragmatic infection does not show itself until after the subphrenic infection has subsided, either naturally or as the result of surgical drainage. An occasional sequel of the surgical drainage of a subphrenic abscess, for example, is the breaking down of weak fibrinous adhesions in the thorax which have hitherto walled off an area of supradiaphragmatic infection. This is due to the descent of the diaphragm back to its normal position, and it carries considerable danger of the dissemination of active infection.

In long-standing cases there may be necrosis of the diaphragmatic tissue, with perforation of the diaphragm. The resulting hole may be minute, or it may be large enough to give the picture of an hour-glass type of abscess above and below the diaphragm.

The pathological process in any particular case, therefore, may be complex. The abscess may even communicate with a hollow viscus, so that eventually a fistula is established between some part of the gastro-intestinal tract and the lung : it may, for example, communicate with the duodenum or gall-bladder, with the result that the sputum is stained with bile.

Diagnosis—This is not the place to discuss in detail the symptoms and signs of the various types of subdiaphragmatic suppuration. What must be emphasised here is that the presence of subphrenic infection (or even the likelihood of its presence as a possible complication of perforation of a peptic ulcer or of abdominal or pelvic suppuration) should always bring to mind the danger of extension of the infection into the thorax. Although subphrenic abscess occurs far more often on the right side than on the left (84 per cent. of the total cases, as compared with 16 per cent.), the possibility of such a left-sided lesion must always be remembered, especially in the differential diagnosis of painful conditions at the base of the left lung or in the left hypochondrium.

Faced, then, with a patient who has a simple irritative effusion or empyema immediately above the diaphragm or a basal lung abscess, the doctor must always ask himself if there is a primary infection or suppuration under the diaphragm. The history of an abdominal operation, of an attack of appendicitis, of a possible perforation of the stomach or duodenum, or of pelvic lesions such as post-partum infection, pelvic abscess, or inflammation of a pelvic appendix, will call his attention to what may be a primary cause of the intrathoracic lesion. As a rule, the thoracic manifestations are late, arising because of delay in diagnosis or treatment, though they have been known to develop as early as the tenth day of the disease. Hence the importance of detecting subphrenic infection or suppuration early, in order to minimise the danger of these intrathoracic complications.

When subphrenic infection extends above the diaphragm, dyspnœa is added to the general symptoms of infection, to the phrenic nerve pain, and to the attacks of hiccough which occasionally accompany diaphragmatic irritation. Expansion of the chest on the affected side is much diminished, and there may be tenderness over the lower intercostal spaces. The signs of a basal pleural effusion may be elicited. If the infecting organisms produce gas as well as effusion, the signs are similar to those of a pyopneumothorax.

Radiology is of cardinal importance. If there is little or no effusion above the diaphragm, it is possible to detect the presence of a high fixed diaphragm, sometimes with a characteristic bubble of gas and a fluid level just beneath it on the affected side. It must be remembered, however, that after any abdominal operation air may be seen for at least two weeks. X-ray screening will help to differentiate a high diaphragm, with pus below it, from a paralysed one with paradoxical movement. If there is an extensive pleural effusion, it is impossible to detect the underlying shadow of a raised diaphragmatic dome. In the absence of effusion, radiograms may show the presence of basal pneumonia or, at a later stage, of lung abscess with cavitation. When there is difficulty in visualising the diaphragm, some surgeons introduce 300 to 400 c.c. of air into the peritoneal cavity : if there is a subphrenic abscess, no air gets to the space on the affected side.

Left-sided lesions (they form about one in five of subphrenic abscesses) present special difficulties. There is more space for the pus on that side, and the tension of the pus is therefore less, as a rule, than on the right side. There is consequently less pain, less diminution of expansion of the lower thorax, and less elevation of the diaphragm, though there is an appreciable degree, even if it is not complete, of fixation of the diaphragm. Pain may be referred to the shoulder and neck. Many of these left-sided abscesses are due to the tracking up, on either side of the descending colon, of infection which originally arose in the pelvis. Others are due to perforation either into the anterior space or into the lesser sac of the peritoneum. They are apt to be diagnosed late, and thoracic manifestations are therefore frequent. One of the most useful diagnostic features in these patients is that the stomach is pushed away from the diaphragm and displaced downwards and medially ; this may be seen after the administration of a barium meal.

It is always important to remember that thoracic complications may show themselves even after the adequate drainage of a subphrenic abscess. In such a patient the persistence of fever and leucocytosis may then be set down erroneously to inadequate drainage of the abscess under the diaphragm rather than to the development of inflammation above it.

The most difficult type of case is that in which a subphrenic abscess is present but not suspected. Here, indeed, the thoracic complication may be the first clear sign of a hitherto unrecognised subphrenic infection—revealing itself, for example, by the sudden coughing up of blood-stained pus after an attack of acute appendicitis, whether operated upon or not. In these patients, however, important clues have often been overlooked. The appendix attack perhaps did not subside normally, but was followed by a long convalescence during which the patient presented symptoms of sepsis, such as drenching sweats, loss of weight and fever. Any form of putrid empyema or putrid lung abscess, therefore, should bring to mind the possibility not only of infection from above via the respiratory passages but also from below the diaphragm.

Diagnosis will thus depend on the obtaining of a careful and suggestive history of the illness : on the symptoms and signs appropriate to whatever type of thoracic complication is present—plastic pleurisy, effusion, empyema, pneumonia, lung abscess, bronchial fistula, and (as later results of damaged and scarred tissues) thickened pleura, adhesions to the diaphragm, pulmonary fibrosis, or bronchiectasis; and on first-class radiograms of the chest and diaphragmatic areas.

If there is an obvious effusion, diagnostic needling of the chest should be performed. The finding of *Bacilli coli communis* in the fluid is very suggestive of a primary abdominal lesion, though sometimes the effusion is a simple sterile irritative one. Needling of the subdiaphragmatic space through virgin pleura carries with it the danger of grave pleural infection, and exploration of the space for pus should be a matter for open operation. Once it has been recognised that there is a subphrenic collection of pus, it must be evacuated. The technical problem of surgical approach is often difficult. The surgeon has to bear in mind that the contamination of an uninvolved serous cavity during the drainage of a subphrenic abscess more than doubles the mortality. The logical approach, therefore, is retroperitoneal, but seeing that the pleura is often involved, or alternatively that the general pleural cavity may be sutured off from the track of the wound, a transpleural approach is often justifiable. When the left inferior spaces are the site of an abscess, a transperitoneal approach is the only feasible one.

For the thoracic complications the usual appropriate treatment is adopted. The patient may cough up a diaphragmatic empyema or a basal lung abscess : if he survives the dangers of flooding of the lungs with pus (causing immediate asphyxia, or later, septic bronchopneumonia), he may then recover. Spontaneous recovery, however, is rare. Usually the suppuration persists, even though intermittent drainage via the bronchi may give periods of comparative relief. If so, operative drainage is called for on the same principle as that for any lung abscess (see Chap. XIX).

Sometimes it is exceedingly difficult to differentiate a septic infarct, followed by abscess of the lung and pleural effusion, from a subdiaphragmatic abscess, basal empyema and eventual pleuropulmonary fistula. It is in these cases that a diagnostic pneumoperitoneum would appear to be of special help, in order to obtain evidence of a collection of pus below the diaphragm. The end result of the thoracic complications is the same, as are the principles of treatment.

Long after drainage has ceased or a lung abscess has become healed the scar tissue which has formed in the basal part of the lung and pleura may cause a drag on the lung or diaphragm, with resulting pain and persistent cough. Relaxation of this tension by means of phrenic paralysis may then be advisable.

CHAPTER XXVII

PNEUMOTHORAX

UNTIL comparatively recently, pneumothorax was regarded as almost always the result of the rupture of an active tuberculous focus underlying the pleural covering of the lung ; with the result that an exaggerated idea of the seriousness of its prognosis was widespread. It might occur as a dramatic and maybe fatal complication of extensive phthisis ; if, on the other hand, it was not immediately serious, it was still looked upon as a mark of tuberculosis in the underlying lung. Nowadays, however, it has become clear that many patients who suffer a spontaneous pneumothorax are healthy enough ; they neither have active tuberculosis of the lung, nor do they develop it later. Kjaergaard's monograph,* published in 1932, did much to call attention to the apparently healthy patient who develops a spontaneous pneumothorax and usually quickly recovers from it ; it crystallised certain earlier conceptions of a benign type of pneumothorax, especially Galliard's (1888) "simple pneumothorax without effusion," and his description in 1892 of what he called the "pneumothorax of conscripts."

The various forms of pneumothorax may therefore be classified as follows :—

1. Benign spontaneous pneumothorax (pneumothorax simplex, "the pneumothorax of scarred lung").
2. Pneumothorax from rupture of an emphysematous bulla in generalised emphysema of the lung.
3. Pneumothorax complicating active pulmonary tuberculosis.
4. Pneumothorax from other causes.

Pneumothorax caused by injuries and wounds will be dealt with separately (see Chap. XXXII).

* Hans Kjaergaard of Copenhagen, 1932, *Acta medica Scandinavica*. Supplement 43. Written in English, and a classical contribution to the subject.

BENIGN SPONTANEOUS PNEUMOTHORAX

Benign spontaneous pneumothorax is usually due to the rupture of a small subpleural bulla or " bleb." These bullæ are formed by the rupture or splitting of the subserous connective tissue layer in an area where the lung tissue is fibrotic and scarred, poorly developed, or of lowered resistance by reason of some other form of damage. In a local patch of cicatricial tissue, for example, the connective tissue layer may lose its elasticity and may be split because of interruption to its blood supply. The fibrosis is usually the result of previous bronchopneumonia, or of healed tuberculosis in which the fibrous tissue is all that remains of the original infection.*

Usually there are multiple air blebs, their size about that of a cherry or walnut ; they lie immediately underneath the visceral pleura. At times it is impossible to find any actual bullæ, yet the damage to the connective tissue allows air to collect just under the pleura and to seep through what must be regarded as a " leaky area " rather than an obvious tear.

In general, it may be said that while the lung is thus locally scarred it is otherwise healthy. The patient in whom the rupture of an air bleb occurs is usually comparatively young, in contrast to the older emphysematous patients who develop large emphysematous bullæ. It is obvious on pathological grounds that benign pneumothorax may occur at any age, for neither infancy nor old age is immune from fibrotic damage to the lungs ; but most instances of spontaneous pneumothorax of this type occur between the ages of 15 and 35 years.

As there are often several small blebs in the scarred area, the accident of spontaneous pneumothorax may be repeated at intervals as one bleb after another bursts and allows the escape of air from the lung into the pleural space. Since the local lesion is healed, there is no discharge of infected material into the pleural cavity, no infected pleural effusion, no continued pyrexia and no signs of toxic absorption such as occurs in patients suffering from active tuberculosis. If fluid does occur

---

* Similarly, occasional cases of asthma which have an underlying basis of fibrosis but no generalised emphysema of the lung may suddenly and unexpectedly be complicated by a spontaneous pneumothorax. Cases have been described following damage to the lung by poison gas. The same mechanism explains the pneumothorax which may complicate fibrosis of the lung associated with bronchiectasis or silicosis.

in the pleural space, it is usually very small in amount and due to pleural reaction to slight bleeding from the tear of the lung.

Benign pneumothorax occurs much more frequently in males than in females, and it does not appear to involve one side of the thorax more than the other. If a careful history is taken, the story may emerge of some earlier illness which at the time probably initiated scarring of the lung : for example, measles or whooping-cough complicated by bronchopneumonia in childhood ; or there may have been a " pneumonia " or even a vaguely recollected " chest illness " which kept the patient in bed for some weeks, and was perhaps accompanied by pain in the chest or by " pleurisy." Sometimes, however, no history of such an illness is obtained. It may have been insidious, as in a mild tuberculous or other infection which has run its course and become healed, though the patient has not been aware of it. It may have occurred so early in his life that it has been forgotten. Perhaps he has felt in good health for so long that only direct questioning of him or of his parents will bring to light the illness which in all reasonable likelihood damaged and weakened the peripheral tissue of the lung.

PNEUMOTHORAX DUE TO THE RUPTURE OF AN EMPHYSEMATOUS BULLA

Here the bulla is part of the picture of generalised emphysema, and is therefore found to occur mainly in older people. At the stage of clinical recognition these bullæ are apt to be quite large—sometimes so large as to be mistaken for a partial pneumothorax. Often they are solitary, or perhaps there are two or three of them at the apices or the margins of the lungs where the support of the thoracic wall is least effective. As the patient is already ill, with loss of respiratory tissue and a diminished vital capacity, rupture of such a bulla with the resulting pneumothorax is always serious.

PNEUMOTHORAX COMPLICATING ACTIVE PULMONARY TUBERCULOSIS

Here again the escape of air into the pleural space is, as a rule, serious ; it may on occasion be fatal, by its sudden curtailment of the already impaired respiratory reserve of a patient with more or less gravely damaged lungs.* The breakdown and rupture of an active tuberculous focus near the surface of the lung throws infective material into the pleural cavity, with resulting serous effusion, perhaps even a pure tuberculous pyopneumothorax, or a mixed infection pyopneumothorax. A similar pathological process, or maybe the tearing of a pleural adhesion containing a tongue of lung tissue, may cause a spontaneous pneumothorax during artificial pneumothorax treatment. Such a tear is not necessarily followed by pleural complications ; it may, however, result in tuberculous infection of the pleural cavity, or even a pyogenic infection if there is a persistent communication with a bronchus.

PNEUMOTHORAX FROM OTHER CAUSES

In this group are the instances of rupture of a congenital cyst of the lung, occurring usually in infants and young children ; of the rupture of a superficial pyæmic abscess of the lung, such as a staphylococcus abscess complicating osteomyelitis ; of traumatic laceration of the lung with or without a penetrating wound ; of the rare complication of rupture of an acute emphysematous patch in bronchopneumonia or other acute infective lesions ; and of rupture of the œsophagus, with consequent escape of air into the mediastinum and thence to the pleural space, either through a penetrating wound, or through a fistulous opening due to malignant growth, ulceration or abscess around a foreign body.

THE PRODUCTION OF SPONTANEOUS PNEUMOTHORAX

The accident may be dramatically sudden, gradual, or so insidious as not to be noticed. The immediate cause may often be obvious to the patient himself—some effort or heavy work (cranking a car, moving furniture, an unwonted mowing of the lawn, some athletic episode) or a sudden awkward twist of the body. Coughing, sneezing, crying, yawning, laughing or straining at stool precipitate the accident in a small number of instances, and sometimes it comes on when the patient is

---

* Another illustration of the grave influence of a diminished respiratory reserve is seen when spontaneous pneumothorax occurs in a patient with bilateral artificial pneumothorax. A common story is that " she was doing very well, but we found one morning that she had died in her sleep."

walking ordinarily. In a fair proportion, however (perhaps as many as a third), no precipitating cause is obvious.

What takes place when rupture of the pleuropulmonary tissue occurs depends on the size and nature of the tear ; on whether or not the lung is held to the wall of the thorax by adhesions ; and on the extent of those adhesions. Adhesions control the extent of lung collapse, so determining *partial pneumothorax*. As the air escapes into the pleural cavity, the lung retracts by reason of its elasticity. The elastic tension of the lung on the sound side will then pull the mediastinum over towards itself, provided that the mediastinum is not

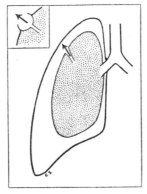 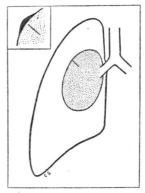

FIG. 124	FIG. 125
Pneumothorax due to rupture of subpleural bleb.	Rupture sealed : " closed pneumothorax."

fixed, and the apex beat of the heart will be displaced towards the sound side. It is clear that this may occur even though the intrapleural pressure on the side of the pneumothorax is not positive.

As the torn lung retracts, the edges of the tear may easily become tightly pressed together, so obliterating the hole in the lung (Figs. 124 and 125). The small amount of sticky effusion consequent on the trauma helps this obliteration. No more air can then escape into the pleural cavity; the margins of the tear in the retracted lung have a chance to unite and heal, and the partial, or it may even be complete, **closed pneumothorax** gradually disappears as the air is reabsorbed and the lung re-expands. On the other hand, the edges of the tear may be drawn apart when the tear is near the base of an adhesion ; one edge is held out by the adhesion, while the other (usually the lower) is drawn away by the collapsing lung (Fig. 126). The tear may also remain open when surrounded by indurated tissue which is so rigid that the retraction of the lung cannot close it (Fig. 127). In these instances of **open pneumothorax** there is free passage of air to and fro between a bronchus and the pleural space, through a **bronchopleural fistula,** and the intrapleural pressure will be found then to approximate to that of the atmosphere.

Another possibility is that, while the hole may close as the lung collapses, it may nevertheless be possible under certain conditions for air to be forced through it into the pleural space.

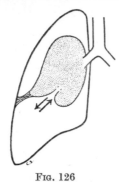

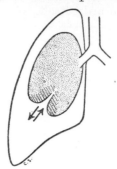

Fig. 126

Open pneumothorax :
fistula held open by
pleural adhesion.

Fig. 127

Open pneumothorax :
fistula surrounded by
rigid indurated tissue.

In the initial stages, before the intrapleural pressure becomes positive, deep inspiration may perhaps draw a small amount of air through the tear, which then closes again. Coughing, however, is by far the most important factor in separating the margins of the tear, and so forcing a passage through what is, in effect, a valvular opening. The glottis is temporarily closed during one of the phases of coughing (see p. 41) : the expiratory muscles are tensed for a forced expiration, and the intra-pulmonary pressure becomes considerably raised. The air which is under tension in the intact lung during this period cannot escape via the glottis ; provided the valve-like opening will yield, therefore, air is driven into the pleural cavity. The damaged lung behaves like a bicycle tyre from which air is forced through a tiny puncture with each stroke of the pump.

As the intrapulmonary pressure falls, owing to the opening of the glottis, the hole again closes. With every bout of coughing, more and more air is trapped inside the pleural cavity ; the longer it is possible to force air through the valvular opening the more positive becomes the intrapleural pressure, the more the lung will be compressed, and the farther the mediastinum will be displaced away from the side of the pneumothorax. Using the simile of the bicycle tyre in a different way, the pleural cavity may be regarded as the inner tube, inflated by periodic jets of air from the lungs, which act as a pressure pump during the forced expiration of coughing.

This **tension or " valvular " pneumothorax** is serious because of its effects on the cardio-respiratory mechanism. By the positive pressure of the air in the pleural space, the affected lung is compressed against the mediastinum and its blood vessels. As the right heart and the great caval veins are more easily embarrassed by this compression than are the left heart and the great arterial trunks, a right-sided tension pneumo-thorax is more dangerous than a left-sided one of the same degree. Nevertheless, a left-sided one which displaces the mediastinum will finally cause kinking of the great veins with consequent obstruction of the return of blood to the heart. Add to this the diminished oxygenating power of the collapsed lung, and of the opposite lung, reduced in volume by the displaced mediastinum, and it is easy to see that a tension pneumothorax may end in cardiac failure, asphyxia and death —in very truth a *pneumothorax suffocant*. It should, of course, be remembered that not every positive-pressure pneumothorax necessarily progresses this far, for the hole in the lung may become closed even to forced expiration against a closed glottis at any stage before this grave degree of intrapleural tension is attained.

With the excessive tension the diaphragm may be displaced downwards. With very high tension, actual herniation of the pleural space may occur ; a pocket of air bounded by pleural membrane, rather like an inflated thin-walled balloon, pushes its way across to the other side—occupying the anterior mediastinum above, in front of the arch of the aorta, and below, insinuating itself between the descending aorta and the œsophagus, behind the heart. It may then rupture into the mediastinum or, very rarely, even into the opposite pleural space.

Bilateral pneumothorax is rare, and unless it is but partial on one side at least, the patient will not recover. It must already be clear that patients with scarred lungs and multiple pleural blebs may suffer attacks of *recurrent pneumothorax* at intervals, on one or both sides of the chest ; an instance has been recorded of a patient who suffered fourteen separate attacks on the two sides, with, on one occasion, a simultaneous bilateral, though fortunately partial, collapse.

If the **intrapleural pressures** are taken by means of an artificial pneumothorax apparatus, the *tension pneumothorax* will show a mean pressure which is positive, the amount of which depends on the degree of tension. Serial readings may indicate the progressive accumulation of air trapped in the pleural cavity ; a reading of, say, – 2 c. of water (inspiration), + 8 (expiration), may later change to one of, say, + 4, + 18. An *open pneumothorax* with a bronchopleural fistulous opening shows a mean reading of zero, with little excursion either way : – 2, + 2, for example. A *closed pneumothorax* (not under tension) shows a mean pressure which is negative, as, for example, – 10, – 4. It is thus of cardinal importance, in assessing the nature of the pneumothorax, to take pressure readings and to plan the treatment accordingly. To evacuate a large amount of air from the pleural cavity without the control of intrapleural pressure readings may lead to the tearing open again, as the lung rapidly re-expands, of a hole which has become sealed. Irreparable damage may be done by such clumsiness.

EFFUSIONS COMPLICATING SPONTANEOUS PNEUMOTHORAX

In simple benign pneumothorax there is usually no effusion of fluid ; if it does occur it is small in quantity and due to slight bleeding, with consequent pleural reaction. A tear with a large hæmorrhage is rare, and gives the picture of **spontaneous hæmopneumothorax,** to be mentioned later (Chap. XXVIII). In patients who have underlying tuberculosis of the lung, the pleura may become infected with tuberculous material, and so a clear serous effusion forms (**hydropneumothorax**), or maybe a **pyopneumothorax,** with tuberculous pus, pure or secondarily infected with septic organisms (see Chap. XXV).

SYMPTOMS

The symptoms vary greatly, depending upon the amount of air in the pleural space, the rapidity of its accumulation, and the condition of the lungs, especially the unaffected lung. These all affect the amount of respiratory reserve, besides conditioning the degree of pain from stretching of the pleura. Moreover, while in some patients the pneumothorax may at first produce but few symptoms, yet as the air accumulates the clinical picture may change to one of alarming seriousness. At the one extreme, therefore, is the man who, apart perhaps from a vague discomfort in the chest, does not know that anything has happened ; later, in the course of exercise such as swimming or walking up a hill, he finds himself a little short of breath. He then consults his doctor, who discovers a partial or even a complete pneumothorax. If there happens to be a hitherto undiscovered tuberculous basis for his trouble, the splash of fluid in his chest which he is surprised to feel and hear when he jumps off a tramcar may be the first intimation to him that something is grossly amiss.

On the other hand the onset may be very sudden. He feels something give or snap in his chest ; he is seized with a stabbing, tearing and agonising pain in his side, upper abdomen or back. It may counterfeit the pain of coronary thrombosis, or of an acute abdominal disaster such as a perforated peptic ulcer, gall-stone colic or impacted renal stone. He is severely shocked, his face grey and covered with beads of perspiration, his temperature low and his pulse rapid. Accompanying the pain is an ever-increasing shortness of breath as the intrapleural tension rises. He becomes anxious and distressed, and feels that he is suffocating and about to die. If air ceases to escape into the pleural space, the pain may gradually subside as the chest adapts itself to the altered conditions—for example, by the depression of the level of the diaphragm. If, on the other hand, the tension continues to increase and the return of blood to the heart is embarrassed, he becomes cyanosed, restless and collapsed, with thready pulse and cold extremities ; and unless relief is given, he dies of asphyxia and cardiac failure. Moreover, even if a high-pressure pneumothorax is relieved, the patient may still die if the myocardium fails to stand up to the strain.

As a rule there is no rise of temperature in non-infected pneumothorax. In the less serious types there may be no cough ; if there is, it is usually short and dry. Rarely a little blood-streaked mucus may indicate bleeding from the tear in the lung.

PHYSICAL SIGNS

These depend on whether the pneumothorax is partial or complete ; on the condition of the underlying lung (is it adherent to the chest wall, and if so, how far ; if not, is it fully collapsed or can it still expand with respiration to a more or less degree ; has it a hole which allows air to pass to and fro with respiration, into and out of the pleural space ?) ; on whether or not the mediastinum is fixed ; and on whether or not there is an accompanying effusion.

Partial pneumothorax—Here there is diminished expansion of the affected side of the chest, seen by the eye and confirmed by palpation. If the pneumothorax is of appreciable size—one causing collapse of the lower half of the lung, for example—vocal fremitus is indistinct or absent over it ; the percussion note is resonant by comparison with that of the opposite side ; the spoken and whispered voice sounds are much diminished or absent ; and the breath sounds diminished or absent on the affected side, but exaggerated on the healthy side whenever the opposite lung is expanding more than it does normally, by way of compensation. If the partial pneumothorax is situated in the upper half of the pleural space, failure to note the locally diminished expansion may easily lead to error ; for the resonance to percussion over one apex in comparison with the note over the other may be misinterpreted. Lacking absolute standards of the percussion note normal to a particular patient, the examiner may find himself thinking that the resonance is normal and the healthy note dull by comparison, and so make the mistake of suspecting a lesion, such as tuberculous infiltration, in the wrong lung. Diminished movement and weakened air entry should always suggest the possible presence of a pneumothorax—they may, of course, be due to other causes of collapse of the lung—even when there is difficulty in assessing correctly the resonant percussion note. Moreover, collapse of the lung due to these other causes produces a dull percussion note, easily distinguished from a normal or a hyper-resonant one.

Complete pneumothorax: no positive intrapleural pressure—This produces similar physical signs over the whole affected side of the chest. There is no bulging of the intercostal spaces ; there is markedly diminished expansion, absent vocal fremitus, hyper-resonant percussion note, absent whispered and voice sounds, and silence in place of the normal breath sounds.* Air on the left side may abolish all or part of the normal cardiac dulness.

If there is no displacement of the mediastinum because it is fixed, the trachea and the apex beat of the heart are found in their normal positions. With displacement of the medias- tinum, the trachea and apex beat are found to be pulled over, away from the side of the lesion, by the elasticity of the sound lung.

In both partial and complete pneumothorax the opening into the pleural space is sometimes free, so that air enters and leaves with inspiration and expiration (*open pneumothorax*). Such holes may vary in size in different patients, from the diameter of a probe to that of a silver threepenny bit, and either the margins are rigid with induration of the surrounding tissue or else an adhesion keeps the hole gaping. On percussion of the chest over the side of the lesion, a " cracked pot " sound may occasionally be heard, and on auscultation the air can be heard passing to and fro through the opening, save when it is very small, both inspiratory and expiratory murmurs being distinctly heard. When the hole is small the murmurs, which have a curious but unmistakable metallic quality, may be described as fairly high-pitched amphoric sounds. The larger the hole the deeper the quality of these amphoric breath sounds. Both voice sounds and cough are also heard with a character- istic reverberating metallic echo. It is clear that these metallic and amphoric sounds are likely to be heard in only a limited number of cases of pneumothorax—those with a patent hole in the lung, produced either by ulceration (acute infections such as subpleural pyæmic abscess, or caseous phthisis), or by the mechanical effect of a near-by adhesion which prevents the tear of the lung from closing.

Tension pneumothorax—Owing to the positive intrapleural pressure, the intercostal spaces on the affected side are widened and the normal intercostal depressions obliterated. The whole thorax on that side is immobile and distended, and conse- quently the chest wall looks smooth and bulging. Unless the

* Occasionally the student listening over a pneumothorax may be puzzled to hear an indefinite, distant rustling or rumbling. He is hearing the far-off sounds of the other lung ; let him bear this in mind and listen again, and realise now that it does not come from the underlying lung.

mediastinum is fixed, the trachea and the apex beat are displaced towards the sound side. Vocal fremitus is absent. The percussion note is hyper-resonant or even tympanitic. If the intrapleural tension is very high, however, the note may be somewhat like that heard when a fully inflated football is kicked—a sharp, deadened " punk," recognisable for what it is if the examiner knows that a tension pneumothorax is present, but not always easy to distinguish from an ordinary dull note if he does not. Voice and whispered sounds are absent, and the breath sounds are not heard. The diaphragm may be displaced downwards if the tension of the air is very high. The level of the liver dulness, therefore, may be depressed, and its actual area is diminished also, by reason of the air which collects in the costophrenic space. This is best seen if the patient is lying on his back or on his left side ; if in addition there is a moderate collection of free fluid, it accumulates in the paravertebral gutter, displaces air towards the front and side of the thorax, and so makes it easier to distinguish the resonant area which replaces that of the normal liver dulness. This depression of the diaphragm may occur rarely even in a pneumothorax without positive pressure ; a clinically appreciable degree of it, however, is likely to be found only if the intrapleural tension is very great.

Pneumothorax with effusion—When there is a complicating effusion the fluid is free to move about, and so shifting dulness is found, varying with the position of the patient. Its upper level is horizontal, in contrast to the curved upper limit of dulness in effusion without accompanying air, and there is resonance above it.

Succussion splash, due to the splashing of the free fluid against the walls of the chest, may be heard when the ear is placed against the chest and the patient shaken. He may be seated on a firm stool, or lying on a couch.*

If there is a pleuropulmonary fistula below the level of the fluid, bubbles of air may be heard escaping during inspiration, through the hole and through the fluid, the sounds so produced reverberating in the air-filled portion of the pleural cavity. These sounds vary according to the size of the hole, from the " glou-glou " of the larger bubbles (like the sound of

---

* But not on a water bed ! Obviously this is not a manœuvre to practise on a patient who is very ill.

water poured from a carafe, or wine from a bottle) to the hard metallic tinkles of tiny bubbles.

THE BELL SOUND

Long ago Hilton Fagge * grouped together certain physical signs, " the metallic phenomena," which when they are present point strongly to a diagnosis of pneumothorax. " They are therefore apt," he adds, " to impress inexperienced auscultators with an undue sense of their importance."

Just as a grotto in a rock gives an echo to the voice, or a sharpness to the sound of dripping or splashing water, so a pneumothorax or a large air-filled cavity may give a metallic echo to voice or cough or splashing fluid, and a metallic hardness to any moist sounds (râles) produced either in the lung itself or through fluid outside the lung. The actual conditions under which these sounds may occur in pneumothorax have already been discussed. Near-by sounds, such as the heart sounds or even the note obtained by percussion, may be reverberated with a similar metallic quality ; and a special type of metallic echo, the bell sound or *bruit d'airain* (" the sound of bronze "), has been particularly associated with pneumothorax.

It is usually sought for by listening over the anterior or posterior wall of the chest while a coin placed on the opposite wall is tapped with another coin. In many books it is therefore called the " coin test," but it is better to think of it as " the sound of the bell," for it may also be obtained by using two pieces of wood, or by simple finger percussion. Indeed it was during the course of auscultatory percussion that Trousseau first noted it ; the sound was so intense as to hurt the ear. Probably it got its name because it was like the single half-cracked clang of the bell of some French village church. Until Osler in 1895 reported a characteristic bell sound in a patient with a large, rigid-walled tuberculous cavity, it was thought to be pathognomonic of pneumothorax ; and it is strange (and indeed significant) that Laennec, with his immense experience, did not apparently notice this sign, or if perchance he did, did not think it of importance in the diagnosis of pneumothorax.

It depends on the presence of an air-containing cavity in the thorax, but many a patient with a pneumothorax or cavities in the lung does not show the sign. There must be certain conditions, therefore, which determine the appearance of the bell sound over such a cavity ; and these conditions are as yet not fully understood. It seems to be clear that for its presence the wall of the air-containing cavity must be firm and rigid ; a partial pneumothorax with a rigid pleura may give it, whereas a complete pneumothorax with a comparatively healthy pleura may not. It may—or may not—occur, therefore, in complete pneumothorax or in partial pneumothorax. A high intrapleural tension does not necessarily produce it, yet it may occur even with a negative pressure pneumothorax ; but if it is present, the greater the tension, the more intense the sound.

The student should try the test on many normal chests. He will then realise that the tap of percussion or of the coin may be transmitted in varying degree even in normal patients, and that to hear it very clearly does not constitute a true bell sound. One day he may be lucky enough to find a pneumothorax which does give the true metallic bell sound. He may also find help in understanding what he may expect by half filling a rubber hot-water bottle with water and ensuring that there is plenty of air above the fluid before he screws in the cork. He can then compare the notes given by percussion or by the tapping of the coins over the fluid and then over the upper portion of air as he compresses the bottle from below to make the air tense. Even so, it is only within certain limits of tension that he will obtain the typical sound. During his student career he is not likely to hear the bell sound often, a fact which underlines the truth that while the presence of a *bruit d'airain* is diagnostic of an air-containing cavity, it is absent in many cases of pneumothorax.

---

* *The Principles and Practice of Medicine* (1886).

THE NATURE OF THE AIR IN THE PLEURAL SPACE

Atmospheric air trapped in the pleural cavity soon alters in character. Carbon dioxide passes into it from the pleural capillaries and oxygen passes out; and as carbon dioxide is some twenty times as diffusible as oxygen, it diffuses in more rapidly than oxygen diffuses out, so that in the course of an hour or two after the establishment of a closed pneumothorax the actual volume of intrapleural gas is considerably increased. Later an equilibrium is attained, the sealed pneumothorax having lost much of its oxygen and gained carbon dioxide.

A pleuropulmonary fistula, however, allows the movement of atmospheric air to and fro between the air passages and the pleural space, so preventing the above alteration in the composition of the intrapleural air. With an open hole in the lung, therefore, the amount of oxygen in samples of air removed from the pleural space remains approximately that of normal atmospheric air. Thus, analysis of the composition of the intrapleural air is sometimes used to differentiate between a sealed pneumothorax and one in which there is free communication through a pleuropulmonary fistula.

X-RAY EXAMINATION

The chest should be examined in the oblique or lateral plane as well as the anterior. The extent of the retraction of the lung is seen, together with the collection of air which replaces the normal lung markings by a completely translucent area. Displacement of the mediastinum, if present, is indicated by the displacement of the trachea and the heart towards the unaffected side. Sometimes the customary film, taken in the position of full inspiration, does not show any mediastinal displacement, whereas a film taken at the end of expiration may reveal marked displacement. This striking contrast may occur when there is a tiny bronchopleural fistula. During expiration, air from the intact lung escapes through the puncture into the pleural cavity; during inspiration it is sucked back again. This causes **" mediastinal flutter,"** a to-and-fro movement of the mediastinum during respiration. In this way, radiology may determine the cause of an otherwise unexplained dyspnœa. If there is effusion, the horizontal level of the fluid is clearly seen whatever may be the position of the patient. The films also show something of the condition of the underlying lungs—whether the " sound " lung looks healthy, the extent of collapse of the damaged one, a tuberculous focus perhaps, adhesions from visceral to parietal pleura, or bullæ which stand out in contrast to the denser collapsed lung tissue surrounding them. The film may also reveal depression of the diaphragm.

DIAGNOSIS

As a rule the recognition of complete pneumothorax presents little difficulty. Occasionally, when the onset is accompanied by severe pain, it may be mistaken for perforation of a peptic ulcer, or for cardiac infarction, especially when the pain is attended by severe dyspnœa and a sense of constriction of the chest. When the onset is gradual, and especially when the pneumothorax is but partial, the most likely mistake is to overlook it altogether.

Emphysema gives a resonant percussion note and feeble breath sounds ; but whether it is acute or chronic, both lungs are affected, save on the exceedingly rare occasions when acute unilateral emphysema follows a ball-valve type of obstruction to one of the main bronchi.

An extensive cavity in the lung, a large emphysematous bulla, or a large congenital cyst may on occasion be mistaken for a pneumothorax. So also may a hernia of the stomach and colon through the diaphragm, particularly in crush injuries of the chest. These are all rare conditions, and it is only in the two latter that the clinical signs are really likely to be equivocal. Radiology will usually be of crucial help. It is helpful also in determining the position of the diaphragm, either when it is eventrated, or when a subphrenic collection of air or gas presses it upwards into the thorax ; on clinical examination alone this may be confused with a basal pneumothorax.

PROGNOSIS

In simple benign pneumothorax, where the tear is sealed by the consequent retraction of the lung, the only danger is in the initial shock. The air is absorbed and the lung gradually re-expands, usually in from two to six weeks, according to the amount of air which has escaped into the pleural cavity.

If, however, the lungs are already seriously diseased— from tuberculosis, emphysema, bronchiectasis, silicosis or acute inflammation—the complication of pneumothorax is serious and may be fatal. Very rarely, a patient with unilateral tuberculosis of the lung may be lucky enough to find Nature establishing what turns out to be a successful therapeutic pneumothorax. Tension pneumothorax is always serious, because of its danger to the circulation. The development of an appreciable serous effusion after a pneumothorax almost certainly indicates underlying tuberculosis of the lung or pleura. A complicating pyopneumothorax is exceedingly serious, because it indicates either underlying tuberculosis or some other serious infective process, associated, for example, with lung abscess, suppurative bronchiectasis or bronchial carcinoma.

If the air remains unabsorbed and the condition becomes a **chronic pneumothorax,** it usually means that the hole in the pleura has failed to close ; removal of the air cannot help the lung to expand. Even so, in some of these cases gradual fibrosis in the diseases area may at last obliterate the hole, allowing the lung eventually to expand. Chronic pneumothorax, however, is a rare condition ; most patients with so-called " chronic pneumothorax " are in reality suffering from a large congenital cyst of the lung.

TREATMENT

Whatever may be the cause of the pneumothorax, the immediate treatment depends on the severity of the initial symptoms. The patient should be put to bed, and even the apparently mild case must be watched carefully for the next twenty-four hours, because in some instances a " valvular " tear may produce its serious symptoms only gradually and progressively. A half-hourly pulse, temperature and respiration chart should be instituted as soon as the patient comes under observation. The patient who is frightened or in pain should be given ¼ gr. of morphia at once, and reassured. The medical attendant must try to visualise the condition of the lung and pleura, helped by X-ray films and intrapleural pressure readings, and direct his treatment accordingly. If the case is a benign one, the sealed tear in the lung must be given a chance to heal ; re-expansion of the lung will follow in its own proper time, and meddlesome interference on the part of the doctor, as by attempting to hasten expansion of the lung by drawing off air, may only do harm. The patient should be kept quietly in bed, for movement and activity will cause more rapid absorption of the air, and an undesirable hastening of the re-expansion of the lung. As long as there is no serious respiratory distress, even a slightly positive-pressure pneumothorax will not call for more than rest and the initial dose of morphia ; but if the patient is seriously distressed and dyspnœic, the danger to the circulation outweighs any possible disadvantage of re-expansion of the lung as a result of drawing off air to relieve a tension pneumothorax.

In any patient with a pneumothorax, the intrapleural pressures should be taken as soon as possible, by means of a pneumothorax apparatus. This can be done at the bedside. After preliminary local anæsthetisation with about 1 c.c. of 1 per cent. novocain solution, a refill-needle, connected in the usual way, is inserted through the fifth intercostal space in the mid-axillary line, unless there are obvious reasons for choosing some other site. Readings are taken in inspiration and expiration, and the mean intrapleural pressure calculated. If this is positive, and the patient is distressed, enough air is removed, by using the artificial pneumothorax apparatus in the reverse way, to give clinical relief and to leave a slightly negative pressure. Relief of distress and dyspnœa may, however, be urgent and the apparatus not be available ; after anæsthetisation of the skin and pleura, a large-bored aspiration needle, or a trocar and cannula, should be inserted into the pleural cavity through the fifth intercostal space, and the air allowed to escape. In emergency, even the local anæsthetic may have to be omitted. If the intrapleural tension is high, the air escapes through the needle with a rush and whistle ; with reduction of the tension, the patient is soon comfortable again, and he is propped up with pillows and kept at absolute rest. After the air has escaped, the needle should be attached to a pneumothorax apparatus, the mean intrapleural pressure noted, and reduced farther, if need be, until it is just negative. Administration of cardiac stimulants and of oxygen may then be advisable.

Control of cough by the initial dose of morphia may avoid any further escape of air into the pleural cavity through a valvular rupture of the lung ; often, however, air again enters it, and the intrapleural pressure rises progressively. The severe dyspnœa thus recurs ; it is then advisable to leave the needle or trocar in the pleural cavity, fixed to the chest wall by strapping to prevent its slipping out, and to connect a rubber tube to it, with the distal end led into a bowl of water. This simple water-valve allows air to leave but not to enter the pleura by way of the needle and tube. When a proper water-seal bottle is available, this should preferably be used.

It must be remembered that if the respiratory reserve is already much diminished by reason of underlying disease of the lung, a highly positive intrapleural pressure is not necessary
28

for the production of great distress and dyspnœa. Indeed, a pneumothorax which brings the negative pressure near to zero, while still leaving it slightly negative, may in certain patients with reduced respiratory reserve make all the difference between his just holding his own and being in grave danger. Here the insertion of needle and tube may not be enough, and continuous gentle suction by some such means as a Sprengel's pump attached to a water tap and connected with a manometer may be the only way to give relief.

Once the urgent symptoms of a pneumothorax are finally relieved, the patient may gradually recover uneventfully. On the other hand, there may be subsequent trouble which calls for further treatment.

If the lung fails to re-expand, this is usually due to a persistent pleuropulmonary fistula. Thoracoscopic examination by an expert may reveal the actual condition of the lung at the area of the tear. If there is an adhesion holding the tear open, it may be possible to divide it, and so allow the lung to collapse and heal. With a patent hole, the natural development of a scar may gradually close it. If after some months the lung still does not expand, it used to be the practice to attempt to produce an obliterative pleurisy by injection into the pleural cavity of 5 to 10 c.c. of 5 per cent. gomenol in liquid paraffin, or 20 c.c. of 30 per cent. glucose solution. Direct application, however, of some sclerosing agent such as silver nitrate or tincture of iodine, done under thoracoscopic vision, is far preferable, if the fistula can be located. Dr. Geoffrey Marshall has told me of one of his own patients in whom thoracoscopy was done by R. C. Brock, and revealed not an actual hole in the lung but rather a " leaky area " through which inhaled cigarette smoke could be seen during the examination slowly percolating through into the pleural cavity. Painting the area with a solution of silver nitrate caused enough fibrosis to give an eventual cure, with full expansion of the lung.

If the pneumothorax is complicated by sterile serous effusion, the condition is almost certainly tuberculous. There may be active tuberculosis in the underlying lung parenchyma, or scattered subpleural tuberculous foci. The treatment now becomes that of the underlying tuberculous lesion, and it is important to decide whether this lesion demands the maintenance of an artificial pneumothorax, quite independently of the accident of the spontaneous pneumothorax. An active tuberculous focus in the underlying lung suitable in itself for therapeutic pneumothorax calls for refills which will prevent the expansion of the lung ; and the problem of the fluid is then the same as if it had appeared during the course of artificial pneumothorax treatment. If the foci are tiny and subpleural only, therapeutic pneumothorax is not necessary, and the fluid may be left alone unless it causes pressure symptoms and respiratory distress. The problem of tuberculous effusions is dealt with in Chapter XXIV.

If the pneumothorax is complicated by purulent effusion, then the treatment is that of an episode in some more general and serious disease. Whether the pus arises from an ordinary lung abscess, from suppurative bronchiectasis or from suppuration distal to a bronchial carcinoma, it must be evacuated— at first by aspiration and later, if the patient still survives, by closed suction drainage, except in carcinoma. Even if the infection subsides, a bronchial fistula may remain, to call for surgical treatment later on.

When the underlying trouble is tuberculous, tubercle bacilli may be found in the sputum and in the pus itself. Treatment becomes that of tuberculous empyema ; this is discussed in detail in Chapter XXV.

SPONTANEOUS PNEUMOTHORAX IN CHILDREN

Spontaneous pneumothorax in babies or young children is not common. A large proportion, perhaps half of them, are associated with inflammatory processes, either by rupture of the lung from subpleural ulceration (pyæmic abscess, gangrene) or by rupture of a subpleural emphysematous area in the field of a bronchopneumonia. About one quarter of the cases are due to tuberculous ulceration of the lung and a few to rupture of a congenital cyst.

Clinical diagnosis is not difficult except in certain patients with a partial pneumothorax only, or an encapsulated pyopneumothorax, when the condition may be confused with a large bronchiectatic cavity, a congenital cyst of the lung or a congenital diaphragmatic hernia. Because of the primary inflammatory disease of the lung the accident is usually serious, for already the vital capacity is seriously diminished, and will be even more so if the pneumothorax produces a positive pressure. Moreover, if the child survives the immediate accident, infection of the pleural space with the septic material from the inflamed lung will almost certainly follow.

PNEUMOTHORAX AND AIR TRANSPORT

During the recent war, air transport for the wounded and the sick came to be more often employed. In the normal person anoxia begins and oxygen administration becomes necessary at a height of about 10,000 feet. Obviously, an anæmic patient with less than normal hæmoglobin to carry the oxygen will feel the effects of oxygen lack at lower altitudes than this. The patient with pneumothorax especially is placed in jeopardy by high altitude flights. In accordance with Boyle's law (whereby if the temperature remains constant the volume occupied by a given sample of gas is inversely proportional to the absolute pressure under which it is held), the volume occupied by a pneumothorax increases with ascent, being increased by half as much again at 10,000 feet. Such expansion of air enclosed in the pleural cavity may rupture adhesions and may cause fatal embarrassment to a patient whose cardio-respiratory capacity is already seriously reduced. The hazards of air transport for these patients must be lessened, therefore, by the maintenance of a steady flying height— probably 1,000 feet is the ideal, though it is not always practicable : by the making of ascents and descents as gradually as possible (a too rapid descent reduces the volume of the pneumothorax, allows the lung to expand rapidly, and may thus result in the tearing open of a sealed wound of the lung), and by the provision of medical supervision, so that oxygen may be given if need be, or excessive intrapleural tension may be relieved.

CHAPTER XXVIII

SPONTANEOUS HÆMOTHORAX, HYDROTHORAX, CHYLOTHORAX

SPONTANEOUS HÆMOTHORAX

WHILE traumatic laceration of the lung which involves the larger blood vessels may cause considerable hæmorrhage into the pleural cavity, severe hæmorrhage from spontaneous pneumothorax is rare. The amount of bleeding from rupture of a subpleural bulla, for example, is likely to be at most very small. As air accumulates in the pleural cavity, however, it separates the visceral and parietal pleural layers, and any adhesions between them will be subjected to tension, the more so if the intrapleural pressure becomes positive. If the adhesions are soft, delicate and vascular they may rupture, and blood then oozes into the pleural space from the torn parietal ends. Rarely the ruptured vessels are large enough to determine persistent and occasionally fatal hæmorrhage.

At first the patient shows the symptoms of a spontaneous pneumothorax. As the hours go by, however, and bleeding continues, he becomes pale and faint, and the pulse rate steadily increases. It then becomes clear that he is suffering from a severe internal hæmorrhage. Some patients have abdominal pain, nausea and vomiting, especially if the torn adhesions are attached to the diaphragm. There may be some degree of upper abdominal rigidity also, so that the condition can be mistaken for a surgical abdominal emergency. If a half-hourly pulse chart is kept in every instance of pneumothorax, a rising pulse rate *in spite of the relief of any mechanical consequences of the accumulating air* will suggest, among other possibilities, that of internal hæmorrhage. Within a few hours of the onset of the lesion, pallor is noticeable, there is evidence of pleural effusion, and diagnostic needling of the chest reveals the presence of blood in the pleural cavity.

The early treatment is naturally directed to the initial

437

spontaneous pneumothorax (see Chap. XXVII). Not until later does the problem of the hæmorrhage force itself upon the attention of the doctor. In the majority of patients the bleeding eventually ceases of its own accord, though about a third of these accidents end fatally. As the blood usually comes from the parietal ends of the torn adhesions, re-expansion of the lung will make no appreciable difference to the bleeding, unless it reopens the tear which originally caused the pneumothorax. It may then cause a recurrence of bleeding from the lung also. As long as the patient is not in danger, therefore, it is not wise to aspirate the blood (and so allow expansion of the collapsed lung) for at least forty-eight hours. If the amount is small it may then be withdrawn, but if it is considerable it should be drawn off and replaced simultaneously with air.* If, however, it is causing mechanical embarrassment, partial air replacement should be done at an earlier stage. Meanwhile it may be necessary to give the patient a transfusion of blood.

If it becomes clear that, in spite of complete rest, blood transfusion, and the administration of morphia, the intra-pleural bleeding is continuing, then the situation is grave. It calls for the help of a surgeon experienced in thoracoscopy to determine if possible the cause and site of the bleeding. Usually, however, it is not possible by thoracoscopy to find the bleeding points, and in any event the chest must be opened and the bleeding vessels tied off. At the same time the accumulated blood is evacuated from the pleural cavity.

In patients who survive without operation the blood should not be allowed to remain in the pleural cavity, but should be removed by successive aspirations with the needle and syringe (see also the section on Hæmothorax, Chap. XXXII, p. 483). It is especially important to avoid the organisation of extensive fibrinous deposits on the surface of a collapsed lung, for if this happens the lung may never re-expand, remaining permanently shrunken inside a crust of scar tissue—a condition to which has been given the vivid term " frozen chest." If it becomes clear that residual blood *clot* persists in the pleural cavity, it should be removed by open operation.

* For the importance of secondary effusion due to pleural reaction, see Chap. XXXII, p. 484.

HYDROTHORAX

Hydrothorax is the term given to the accumulation in the pleural cavity of transudate, in contrast to an exudate of fluid resulting from an inflammatory process. The transuded fluid differs from that of an exudate in that the transudate has a lower specific gravity, contains less protein (including fibrin) and very few cells, mainly endothelial in type (see also p. 374). Pleural transudate may occur as part of the generalised dropsy of congestive cardiac failure or of renal disease : it may result from obstruction of the thoracic veins and lymphatics, as by pressure of enlarged glands at the hilum in malignant disease or Hodgkin's disease, or thrombosis of the azygos vein ; or it may be the sequel to the development of excessive capillary permeability such as may be seen in grave nutritional defects.

The factors associated with circulatory disturbances which complicate heart disease are discussed in detail in Chapter XXXI. Congestion and œdema due to heart failure usually begin over the right lung, and remain more intense on this side. For this reason hydrothorax in congestive cardiac failure is as a rule seen first on the right side, later on the left. The hydrothorax of renal and nutritional disease is usually bilateral. That associated with the pressure of glands or other swellings may be unilateral or bilateral, according to the anatomical site of the obstruction.

The treatment of hydrothorax is essentially that appropriate to the primary disease. Nevertheless, the mechanical effects of the fluid may be distressing enough to call for the removal of a sufficient amount to relieve the symptoms.

CHYLOTHORAX

Occasionally, paracentesis of a supposed pleural effusion reveals the presence of opalescent fluid resembling chyle. The fluid may be truly *chylous*, yellowish-white in colour, its specific gravity usually above 1012, showing fat globules in great numbers when examined by the microscope. These globules stain with Sudan III. If the fluid is shaken with ether and a little potassium hydroxide, the fat is dissolved and the opalescence disappears. On the other hand, the opalescence may only be *pseudo-chylous* or *chyliform*, caused by a lecithin-globulin complex which results from the degeneration of cells which have been shed into a pleural effusion. Here the specific gravity is usually less than 1012, refractive granules which do not stain with Sudan III are present, and shaking with ether and potash does not remove the opalescence.

True chylous effusion is rare. It follows rupture or section of the thoracic duct owing to trauma ; or it may follow increased pressure within the duct due to obstruction. The commonest cause of non-traumatic obstruction is invasion and occlusion of the duct by a metastatic malignant tumour or gland. Sometimes the duct may be buried in a mass of glands in Hodgkin's disease, or in a mass of lymphosarcoma. Occasionally the duct is obstructed by tuberculous or syphilitic lesions, or in the thickened tissue associated with polyserositis. Rarely it is blocked by filaria. In these non-traumatic lesions, chylous ascites may also be present.

Occlusion of the duct does not necessarily cause chylothorax. It has been found experimentally that it is only when the collaterals are also occluded that closure of the duct leads to the accumulation of chylous fluid. These collaterals may carry chyle and lymph to the veins when the duct is obstructed ; moreover, the duct itself may communicate with venous channels before it empties into its main vein.

The symptoms and signs in any particular patient depend on the underlying cause of the effusion, and on the amount of chylous fluid which has accumulated. In some patients the presenting signs are those of a massive pleural effusion. Sometimes this is accompanied by chylous ascites. Paracentesis of the chest reveals the presence of chylous fluid. If the patient is given Sudan III by mouth, further paracentesis shows that the fluid has taken on a pink tinge.

In the traumatic type the duct usually remains open and large quantities of chyle escape out of circulation. Emaciation is therefore rapid and profound. This may also occur in the non-traumatic types, but not always, for some of the chyle may pass into the veins by means of the collaterals. Moreover, in the non-traumatic types, the collaterals may become opened up, with the result that chylous fluid does not reaccumulate after paracentesis.

The prognosis depends largely on the underlying cause of the chylothorax. Many instances have a neoplastic origin, and the outlook is hopeless.   In the more benign ones, recovery may take place after one or more aspirations, provided that an effective collateral circulation becomes established.   In the traumatic cases, occasionally the hole is closed by a thrombus, after which recovery may be possible.

The treatment is that of the underlying disease.   If the fluid causes respiratory embarrassment, it must be aspirated, although it will usually reaccumulate rapidly.   Meanwhile the patient should be given a diet rich in protein and carbohydrate, but with restricted fat.

Chyliform effusion is occasionally seen in Bright's disease, hepatic cirrhosis, and in tuberculosis or malignant disease of the pleura.   The nature of the fluid is due to the disintegration products of the cellular exudate and endothelial cells.

CHAPTER XXIX

DEVELOPMENTAL PULMONARY CYSTS

SINCE the development of radiology of the chest, a certain number of instances of " cystic disease of the lungs," regarded as congenital and bronchial in origin, have been recognised. As yet, however, the developmental pathology of these cysts has not been clearly established ; moreover, the characteristics which have been described as differentiating multiple congenital cysts from "honeycomb lung " due to bronchiectasis (see Chap. IX) are not entirely convincing. It is strange that very few examples of the condition have been described in the fœtus ; more certain knowledge should be available in the future, now that developmental anomalies of the lungs are likely to be looked for with more lively interest than in the past. A few examples have been recorded of pulmonary cysts associated with other congenital malformations, such as congenital heart disease or polycystic disease of the kidneys.

Cysts may be solitary or multiple, unilateral or bilateral, and either in communication with bronchi or not. The solitary cyst may be of comparatively small size, up to the size of an orange, and give rise to no symptoms unless secondary infection occurs. Occasionally, however, the communicating bronchus runs a tortuous course in the cyst wall, and owing, maybe, to some mechanical change, such as kinking, it comes to act as a check-valve, allowing air to enter but not to leave the cyst. This progressive inflation produces a " giant cyst " or " balloon cyst." The pressure inside it is positive ; it may displace the mediastinum to the opposite side and by pressing on vital structures inside the thorax threaten the patient's life. These " giant cysts " are usually seen in new-born infants or young children, though if they do not cause early death they may not be recognised until the later years of childhood or even of middle life. A giant cyst is liable to be mistaken for a pneumothorax, especially if the patient is examined shortly after one of the attacks of dyspnœa which are a fairly common complication.

442

The X-ray film shows a clear air space, but usually the costo-phrenic angle is not translucent as in pneumothorax, and careful inspection may reveal faint trabeculæ or " lung markings " crossing the clear space. If a needle has been inserted to draw off air, or to take pressure readings, the wall of the cyst may be torn, and a subsequent X-ray film may show a true pneumo-thorax between the thin wall of the partially collapsed cyst and the wall of the thorax.

It is difficult in any particular patient to know whether small multiple cysts are congenital or are forms of acquired saccular bronchiectasis ; in either event the problem of treat-ment is the same. In a certain number of cases (the proportion cannot yet be estimated) the cysts become *secondarily infected*. The solitary cyst then gives the symptoms and signs of empyema, or of lung abscess, according to its size and site ; infected multiple cysts show the clinical picture of suppurative bronchiectasis. When the infected cyst or cysts communicate with a bronchus, X-ray films show a fluid level in them ; if they do not communicate the cyst is shown as a dark rounded shadow. Other complications besides infection are hæmoptysis: cough and dyspnœic attacks if there is pressure by the cyst on adjacent lung tissue : and cerebral abscess (as in infected bronchiectasis).

The *differential diagnosis* depends to a great extent on the X-ray appearances. If the cyst contains air, and is solitary and large, it has to be differentiated from pneumothorax, from large emphysematous bullæ, and from diaphragmatic hernia (here a " barium swallow " will help) ; the smaller solitary cyst, from thin-walled tuberculous cavities (when tubercle bacilli are likely to be found in the sputum). If the cyst is full of fluid, or contains fluid and air, it has to be distinguished from empyema (interlobar or otherwise), from lung abscess, from hydatid cyst, or from solid tumours. Multiple cysts cannot easily be distinguished from saccular bronchiectasis.

Treatment of the tension cyst is similar to that of the valvular pneumothorax emergency, namely, to relieve the tension by withdrawing air, a manœuvre, however, which is likely to give but temporary relief. Until the extent of the risk of secondary infection can be assessed with certainty, it is doubt-ful whether excision (where feasible) of the cystic portion of the lung is justifiable in the absence of symptoms either of pressure or of secondary infection ; probably the wisest course then is to adopt prophylactic measures against respiratory infection, to watch the patient carefully, and to be ready to adopt surgical measures if infection supervenes. If suppuration occurs, it may be necessary to undertake preliminary drainage of a solitary cyst, and later perform lobectomy or pneumonectomy. Multiple cysts are treated on the same lines as bronchiectatic dilatations.

If the cysts are bilateral, palliation of symptoms is in most instances all that can safely be undertaken. The principles of treatment are then much the same as those applying to bronchiectasis (see Chap. IX).

A congenital abnormality which needs mention is that of **transposition of the heart.** In true dextrocardia the heart lies in the right side of the thorax, the apex beat being found in the fourth or fifth right intercostal space, $4\frac{1}{2}$ in. from the middle line—a mirror image, as it were, of the normal position. The electrocardiogram shows an inversion of the P, R and T deflexions, but is otherwise normal. Often other organs are transposed also, the great vessels for example, and the abdominal viscera. The condition gives rise to no abnormal symptoms. If, however, it coincides with such other congenital abnormalities as a patent cardiac septum, there are obvious symptoms and signs of serious disability.

Acquired dextrocardia merely means that there has been *displacement* of the heart towards the right side, by reason of right-sided fibrosis of the lung, left-sided pleural effusion, or the pressure of a large left-sided tumour. Here the apex beat still remains the extreme left part of the heart, whatever its position may be. Radiograms will reveal whether the heart is transposed or merely displaced.

CHAPTER XXX

ASTHMA

THE ancient physicians used the word "asthma" to mean dyspnœa, and any breathless patient was called asthmatic. Nowadays the term has been narrowed to describe a condition characterised by transient paroxysmal attacks of laboured breathing, especially in the expiratory phase. The difficulty of breathing is caused by a narrowing of the smaller bronchi and bronchioles due to contraction of the circular plain muscle of the bronchi, accompanied by swelling of the bronchial mucous membrane, and later by the exudation of sticky mucus.

The bronchial muscle is innervated by the vagus nerve (parasympathetic), stimulation of which causes constriction of the smaller tubes. This same mechanism of bronchial spasm, combined with swelling of the mucous membrane, may occur in anaphylactic shock. The vagal constrictor fibres can be reflexly stimulated by afferent impulses reaching the medullary centre from various parts of the body, as, for example, the higher cerebral centres, the nose and nasal sinuses, the alimentary tract, the uterus, or the bronchi themselves. Dilator fibres to the bronchi are supplied by the sympathetic, stimulation of which causes relaxation of the bronchial muscle ; this action is also brought about by the injection of adrenalin. The vagus contains also broncho-secretory fibres, stimulation of which produces the secretion of mucus.

The immediate results of the partial bronchial block typical of asthma are essentially the same as those seen in emphysema (see Chap. XVI). Both inspiration and expiration are interfered with, and the accessory muscles of respiration are brought into play. Expiration, being much less powerful than inspiration, cannot easily overcome the obstruction and expel air from the lungs ; it is therefore embarrassed and greatly prolonged. The lungs become overdistended with air which cannot escape, and soon the shape of the thorax corresponds to the position of full inspiration. The impairment of alveolar ventilation leads to deficient oxygenation of the pulmonary blood, to an increase of reduced hæmoglobin in the circulating blood, and therefore to cyanosis. In the periods between attacks the patient is apparently normal, provided that secondary changes have not become established.

THE ASTHMATIC ATTACK

Uncomplicated asthma is characteristically paroxysmal. As a rule the attack comes on suddenly, often in the middle of the night, though it may occur also in the daytime. The patient wakes up with a sense of oppression in the chest, which quickly develops into great distress of breathing. Sometimes there are premonitory symptoms such as sneezing, flatulence or drowsiness. He has to sit up, wheezing and fighting for breath, and he may feel such a sense of suffocation that he hangs his head out of the open window in the attempt to get fresh air. As a rule expiration is the more urgent difficulty, and the greater part of his energies are directed towards expelling air from the lungs. He grasps the mantelpiece, or sits with his elbows resting on the table, bending over them, so fixing the shoulders and tensing the abdominal muscles, to aid respiration. Nevertheless he feels it almost impossible to expel air and to empty the chest ; his anxiety increases and the whole expression is one of anguish. The face is cyanosed, the skin is covered with perspiration, the eyes protrude and the extremities are cold. He is so distressed with trying to breathe that he can hardly speak or move. After a time he begins to cough a little, bringing up with difficulty a few grey, viscid pellets of mucofibrin. The ability to expectorate usually indicates that the bronchial spasm is beginning to pass, and gradually the symptoms subside. The duration of the attack varies considerably from patient to patient ; generally it lasts an hour or two, unless it is cut short by effective treatment. As it subsides, the dramatic symptoms and signs disappear and the sufferer falls into an exhausted sleep. He may wake up next morning apparently well. Sometimes, however, attacks are maintained for several days, merging one into the other, with perhaps a slight degree of relief in the daytime ; sometimes the paroxysms are so continuous as to merit the description of *status asthmaticus*.

Examination of the patient during an attack shows that the breathing is slower than normal in both its phases, expiration being greatly prolonged. While wheezing may accompany inspiration, it is so pronounced during expiration that it is easily heard even at a distance. The shape of the chest is that corresponding to deep inspiration. Though the accessory respiratory muscles are seen to be in action, and the abdominal muscles in particular are taut with the effort to assist the expulsion of air from the lungs, the amount of expansion and of recession of the chest is very small. The lungs are over-distended, and the hyper-resonant percussion note over them encroaches appreciably on the normal area of heart and liver dulness. On auscultation the vesicular murmur is hardly audible, partly because of the poor respiratory excursion, partly because it is overshadowed by sonorous and sibilant rhonchi.

Some light has been thrown on the pathology of the asthmatic attack by bronchoscopy, for occasionally the bronchoscopist has been able to describe the appearance of the bronchi during an attack which has interrupted the normal course of his examination. They are seen to be much contracted, and although they may vary slightly from time to time they never relax to their normal calibre. The mucous membrane is thickened and congested, and in the bronchi which are accessible to bronchoscopic vision small muco-fibrinous plugs are seen adhering to the much-reddened walls.

These small plugs form the grey pellets which are eventually coughed up ; unrolled, they appear as spiral structures (*Curschmann's spirals*). They originate as mucous casts of the smaller bronchi, and their spiral form is probably due to the way in which they are forced forwards towards the trachea and mouth in corkscrew fashion. When allergy is an important factor in the attack, eosinophils are present in considerable numbers both in the blood and in the infiltrated bronchial walls, and many escape into the sputum. At the same time, the so-called Charcot-Leyden crystals, colourless and octahedral, can be recognised in the sputum; their chemical nature is unknown, but they appear to be associated only with true allergic attacks.

If the patient has suffered from asthma for many years, or if there is underlying inflammatory lung disease, it is likely that secondary infection, most commonly chronic bronchitis, will complicate the picture ; some degree of chronic emphysema may also be present. The bronchitis alters the character of the expectoration, so that a certain amount of purulent sputum may be coughed up during the attack ; it may also determine the production of moist râles (coarse and medium crepitations). In the presence of chronic emphysema the acute asthmatic attack may be dangerous by increasing the strain on the heart and leading eventually to left ventricular failure. Acute pulmonary œdema follows, and the sputum becomes copious and frothy and may be tinged pink with blood. Frank hæmoptysis is very rare and indicates sudden laceration of pulmonary tissue or acute rupture of alveoli.

The typical severe asthmatic attack already described does not always occur ; the intensity of the attacks may vary from time to time, and in some more fortunate patients they can never be described as more than mild. Moreover they may be greatly modified by appropriate treatment.

THE FACTORS PRODUCING THE ASTHMATIC ATTACK

The asthmatic patient reacts to particular stimuli in wholly different fashion from non-susceptible persons. He possesses a " diathesis," an abnormal sensitivity to some foreign sub-stance or to a particular reflex stimulus ; the bronchial centre in the medulla is oversensitive, and reacts abnormally to blood-borne irritants such as foreign proteins and bacterial toxins, and to peripheral and psychical stimuli. The patient is like dry gunpowder, ready to explode. Some spark, how-ever, is necessary to fire the powder ; in the asthmatic it may be either an extrinsic or an intrinsic factor, or both.

The **constitutional factor** is often inherited. Parents or grandparents may have suffered from hay fever, urticaria or asthma. The patient himself in early life may have shown manifestations of abnormal sensitivity other than asthma ; as, for example, infantile eczema, urticaria, migraine or hay fever.

The **extrinsic factors** which may precipitate the attack can enter the body by *inhalation*, by *ingestion* or by *injection*. The most common pathway is by inhalation, and innumer-able kinds of dusts have been incriminated—pollens from grasses and flowers : animal dusts from fur, feathers or hair : vegetable dusts of all kinds, as, for example, flour, or the orris-root constituent of face powders : industrial dusts, such as those from cotton or leather : and house dust, which may be a mixture of fluff and hair and a host of other ingredients. Foods and other ingested substances are less important ; they contribute more commonly to the asthma of children than to that of adults. Eggs, wheat, milk and various types of shell-fish are the main foods implicated, other foods and drugs being only occasional precipitating factors. The subcutaneous or parenteral pathway is but rarely involved, as by the injection of therapeutic serum or even during the course of skin testing for allergic sensitivity.

On the other hand, it may be an **intrinsic factor** which lights up an attack. The products of bacterial infection of the respiratory tract or elsewhere may determine an *allergic reaction* which results in an asthmatic paroxysm. Toxic infectious foci, including inflammatory changes in the nose, nasal sinuses, tonsils or lungs, may initiate *reflex stimulation of the vagal nerves* ; as also may vasomotor rhinitis, nasal polypi, pelvic abnormalities (including pregnancy), and gastro-intestinal upsets (a heavy meal at night may determine an attack). Purely *psychological stimuli* may be the spark which touches off the explosion. The important rôle of emotion is well illustrated by a story which Trousseau, himself an asthmatic, tells in his *Lectures on Clinical Medicine.* " The worst fit of asthma which I ever had myself," he wrote, " came on under the following circumstances. I suspected my coachman of dishonesty, and in order to assure myself of this I went upstairs to the loft one day and had the oats measured in my presence. Whilst this was being done I was all at once seized with a fit of dyspnœa and oppression at the chest so great that I had scarcely the strength to get back to my apartment ; my eyeballs protruded out of their sockets and my pale and turgid face expressed the deepest anxiety. I had only time to pull my tie off and to rush to the window, which I opened in search of fresh air. I am not a habitual smoker but I then had a cigar and took a few puffs ; in eight or ten minutes the paroxysm was over.

" What had caused this fit ? Doubtless it was the dust from the oats which were being measured that penetrated into my bronchi. But it was unquestionable also that this dust was not enough to bring on of itself such an extraordinary attack, or

29

the cause at least was quite out of proportion to the effect produced. I have a hundred times in the streets, or on the boulevards of Paris or on the high roads, been exposed to an atmosphere of dust considerably thicker than the one which I had then breathed for a very short time, and yet I had never felt anything approaching to this. There must, therefore, have been something special in the cause, and it had besides acted on me whilst I was in a peculiar state. My nervous system was shaken from the influence of mental emotion caused by the idea of a theft, however trifling, committed by one of my servants, and a cause, very slight in itself, had acted on my nerves with extreme intensity." This account emphasises in striking fashion the fact that there may be a *summation of several factors*, constitutional, nervous and allergic, in determining the initiation or the intensity of the attack.

The symptoms and signs of the typical asthmatic paroxysm have already been described. The dramatic nature of the attack must not, however, overshadow our interest in the **asthmatic patient** himself, for whom the attacks are only part of a constant and harassing disability. He lives on the edge of a volcano which is always liable to erupt. His life becomes more or less disturbed, and schooling or work may be seriously interrupted. Many patients with but a mild degree of the disease can live a fairly normal life, punctuated by periodic inconvenience ; for others, anything like a normal life of work and social activity becomes impossible. A nurse undergoing her hospital training, for example, may find that she cannot work in the operating theatre or in a surgical ward without being made helpless, for days at a time, by asthmatic attacks determined by a sensitivity to cotton-wool protein. A man finds that he cannot carry on a particular occupation because he is susceptible to the dusts which accompany it. Others dare not sleep in a strange bed, or come in contact with animals. A simple cold in the head, by starting a series of attacks, may lay some patients low for weeks. Many sufferers come to learn what are the contacts which inevitably bring on an attack, and a conditioned reflex may be established. The classical example is that of the patient who had an attack of asthma whenever she smelt a rose ; eventually she developed an attack whether the rose was real or artificial. Any emotional stress or strain may be devastating ; the sufferer may be unable to face an awkward interview, or a school examination or a difficult family situation, without the sure and certain anticipation of a disabling attack.*

Often a vicious circle is established. The patient is only too well aware of his disability and that he cannot work as well and constantly as he might otherwise do. An anxiety neurosis is established ; he fears the disabling attacks and may also unconsciously use his illness as an excuse for possible failure. The schoolboy, for example, whose parents are too obviously fussy, or who show their anxiety that he will do well in an examination, may have attack after attack, persuading himself and them that if perchance he fails to pass, the asthma is clearly the determining cause.

Complications of the disease are few. Rarely, during the acute attack, spontaneous pneumothorax may occur ; it is usually due to the rupture of a small subpleural bulla in an already scarred lung (see Chap. XXVII). In old-standing, chronic cases emphysema may develop. Those patients in whom bronchitis, bronchiectasis, fibrosis of the lung, silicosis or, rarely, tuberculosis are determining factors may suffer from the usual complications of these diseases. The **prognosis** of the acute attack is usually good. It is sometimes said that no one ever dies from an asthmatic attack, but this is not entirely true. Occasionally the strain of a series of paroxysms in a patient with emphysema or chronic fibrosis of the lung leads to acute myocardial failure, from which he does not recover. Occasionally pneumonia follows collapse of a part of the lung, due to bronchial occlusion by mucus. The long-term outlook is largely dependent on the discovery of the causal factors, and on the removal of them when possible. The inherent predisposition remains, however, and while long periods of *relief* may follow appropriate treatment, it is impossible to speak of a *cure* for asthma.

DIAGNOSIS

The diagnosis is made clear mainly by the characteristic, periodic attacks of wheezing dyspnœa with, especially, marked expiratory embarrassment ; in between the paroxysms the

* *The Life of H. R. L. (Dick) Sheppard,* by Ellis Roberts, is worth reading not only for its own intrinsic interest but also because it gives an insight into the difficulties and trials of the confirmed asthmatic.

patient may be comparatively well. The condition must be differentiated from the inspiratory stridor or wheezing of tracheal or bronchial obstruction, such as is seen, for example, when there is an impacted foreign body, or bronchial neoplasm : and from other types of grave dyspnœa, such as that of cardiac failure, chronic emphysema or renal insufficiency. Myocardial damage determines a dyspnœa which, if it is severe enough to simulate asthma, is persistent : so also is the breathlessness of emphysema, dependent as it is on a progressive organic lesion. It should always be borne in mind that true bronchial asthma seldom arises for the first time in elderly patients. When elderly persons become " asthmatic," therefore, the doctor should be particularly on the look out for other causes of paroxysmal dyspnœa—left ventricular failure, for example, or uræmia, or bronchial neoplasm. The situation is thus somewhat similar to that of an epileptic attack occurring for the first time in the elderly ; it is seldom " idiopathic."

Correct diagnosis of the asthmatic nature of the attack is not enough. The determining factors must also be investigated and if possible tracked down in detail. The family and personal history may throw light on the constitutional nature of the disease. Blood examination may reveal an eosinophilia. Skin tests should be made to discover any specific sensitivities ; the solutions put up by Bencard are useful and reliable for this diagnostic investigation. Radiological examination of the lungs, together with sputum tests, will help to reveal associated organic pulmonary changes. Foci of infection or abnormalities in the nose and throat must be diligently looked for ; chronic disease of the nasal sinuses is especially liable to be overlooked. Infection elsewhere, as in the abdomen or urinary tract, may be a contributory factor, and the appropriate routine investigations should be made. The patient's temperament and psychological history should be assessed, together with his environment ; fussy parents or an unhappy home, for instance, may make all the difference between persistence of, and freedom from, attacks.

TREATMENT

1. Of the attack—In all but the milder forms of attack the patient should be put to bed and propped up in the position which he finds most comfortable. A sturdy bed-table on which he can rest his arms is useful. *Adrenaline* is the drug of choice ; it relaxes the bronchial spasm, and if given immediately after the onset it may abort or greatly reduce the duration and intensity of the paroxysm. To ensure this the patient should be taught to give the initial injection to himself. As a rule the later it is given the less effective it is and the greater the dose required to give relief. As early as possible, therefore, 2 minims of a recently made 1 in 1000 solution are injected subcutaneously, care being taken not to puncture a superficial vein. Adrenaline injected into the circulation may cause startling symptoms—tremor, intense head-throbbing, faintness, palpitation, or even collapse ; a slight withdrawal of the piston of the injection syringe will reveal whether the needle is in a blood vessel or not. If the attack persists, the doctor should be called and he should repeat the injection (3 to 5 minims) every half-hour until the attack subsides. If this dose fails, a combination of adrenaline and $\frac{1}{2}$ to 1 c.c. of pituitrin (" asthmo-lysin " is a convenient preparation) may succeed. If the attacks are continuous (status asthmaticus), the adrenaline must be given continuously. The needle of a 1 c.c. hypodermic syringe is inserted into the skin and both needle and syringe are strapped firmly *in situ*. The syringe should previously have been filled with adrenaline solution ; 1 minim of this is injected every minute until there is relief. It may be necessary to reload the syringe several times before this aim is achieved. Thereafter 1 minim is given every quarter of an hour for the first hour, each half-hour for the second hour, and then hourly for two or three hours until it becomes clear that further attacks are unlikely. In all but the severest attacks, phenobarbitone is an adequate and safe sedative, if a sedative is necessary. Morphia is dangerous, and may be deadly.

For milder attacks the patient himself frequently adopts the form of treatment which he has previously found efficacious, without calling upon the doctor's aid. Ephedrine tablets (in $\frac{1}{4}$ or $\frac{1}{2}$ gr. doses), or nasal sprays containing ephedrine, or various proprietary sprays, are used with more or less success. The inhalation of the fumes of burnt powders should not be encouraged, as they frequently irritate the bronchi and produce bronchitis.

Once the acute attack has subsided the patient can be

given a hot drink, made comfortable and allowed to sleep. During severe attacks some patients are much comforted by a kaolin or linseed poultice on the chest ; if the nursing facilities are available, so that the poultice can be put on skilfully, quickly and without undue disturbance of the patient (see p. 184), it should be done. After a severe attack it may be necessary to keep the patient in bed for a day or two ; after any attack he should take an antispasmodic mixture, such as

Sod. iodid.	.	.	.	gr. v
Tr. stramon .		.	.	℥xv
Ext. glycyrrhiz. liq.		.	.	℥xv
Aq.	.	.	.	to ℥ss

t.d.s., with the addition of ¼ gr. of ephedrine hydrochlor. if the attack has been more than mild.

2. General treatment of the patient—The management of the patient in the intervals between attacks is of paramount importance, and much depends on discovering the factor or factors involved. The various possible factors have already been described, and experience of asthmatic patients shows clearly that a combination of them is frequently necessary to precipitate an attack. Granted the constitutional basis, together with an allergic or reflex precipitating stimulus, it is nevertheless surprising to find how often a patient loses his attacks during a stay in hospital, or after a change of treatment to some new form of therapy for which doctor or patient has enthusiasm. Even the omission of a wonted flavouring agent (coffee essence, for example) from the usual " successful " medicine may be sufficient to determine a relapse.

In a large number of patients, therefore, the *psychological factor* is most important. The asthmatic is usually highly strung, over-conscientious and sensitive. His whole temperament is overtensed ; it is not surprising that the bronchoconstrictor centre should be hypersensitive and at the mercy of stimuli which would not affect a normal person. One of the most striking aspects of asthma is that eight out of every ten asthmatic children cease to have attacks as soon as they come into hospital, and start them again when they go out. Clearly, this cannot be due to differences between hospital and domestic food or dust. Rather is it strong proof of the psychological basis of asthma.

The influence of psychological factors on the determination of asthmatic attacks emphasises the great part which the family doctor must play both in assessing the factors involved and in the general management of the patient. The following example affords an illustration of this :—

A clever girl of 15, who since childhood had been a " martyr to asthma," belonged to a home which lacked nothing of material comfort yet in which serenity was notably absent. The father was a fussy, meticulous business man with apparently little capacity for affection. The mother was an over-intellectualised managing woman who did her utmost to live other people's lives for them. Whenever she was seriously frustrated she herself had an attack of asthma. The parents had spent a small fortune on the " cure " of the daughter ; they had consulted all the best specialists, native and foreign, and possessed a formidable dossier of reports, opinions and suggestions for treatment.

The war came, and the father had to take up special work elsewhere. The family moved house and came under the care of a wise old practitioner, who sized up the situation and managed to subdue the girl's asthma sufficiently to persuade her parents to allow her to be sent to a boarding school. She had no attacks there after the first week until just before she was due home for the holidays ; then she had a severe and continuous attack which made her unable to travel. The mother rushed off post haste, and brought her home in an ambulance. Once home, the girl was bedridden with continuous attacks. The mother, who was almost winning the war off her own bat by the multitude of her outside activities, swept in and out of the sickroom like a tornado, instructing doctor and nurse in her spare moments exactly how to treat the patient. The father had the dossier out to study, referring the doctor to various memoranda which seemed to him of vital importance to the present series of attacks ; and at all times he radiated gloom and despondency, for the war had destroyed any faith he might have had in the future of mankind, of himself or of his child.

The practitioner, fortified by the opinion of a consultant, transferred the girl to a nursing home, the parents consenting reluctantly, for they were sure that no one would understand their daughter's case as they did themselves. There her attacks ceased almost at once. For the remainder of the month she was there she had but one attack ; it occurred as she was being skin-tested for sensitivity. She proved highly sensitive to house dust inhalants, and application of the test solution intradermally caused widespread urticaria as well as a startlingly severe asthmatic paroxysm. In contrast to the attacks at home, this one subsided with surprising rapidity.

It was clear that the restless, insecure home atmosphere was a far weightier factor than any sensitivity to house dust. Treatment, therefore, comprised much more than an attempt at desensitisation and the giving of antispasmodics ; it necessitated the management of the whole family, for a large part of the patient's disability was a subconscious protest against her home environment. The parents were told kindly and firmly the truth about the illness, and of their own part in it, a delicate operation only made possible by the old doctor's good-humoured understanding of men and women. He arranged that the girl should continue to go to boarding school despite her asthma, and entered into a discreet conspiracy with the child whereby she realised that he was on her side in relieving her from much of the pressure of the home circle. At school she was happy and had hardly any attacks.

As a rule the family doctor is in the best position to assess the psychological factors and to bring common-sense advice to bear upon them ; occasionally, however, the problem may be so difficult as to call for the help of an experienced psychotherapist. The patient himself would be less liable to alternations of optimism and pessimism if he accepted the truth that while in most instances he can do much to avoid asthma or can treat it when it comes, he will still remain an asthmatic. The doctor on his part should encourage the hope of relief, but should be chary of using the word " cure." It is when hopes of some particular therapy are pitched too high, and relapse follows an initial success, that the patient is liable to lose faith in his doctor ; and sometimes, because the patient does not continue to respond according to plan but relapses badly, the doctor may lose interest in his patient.

The *overexcitability of the vagal centre* in the medulla is still further increased by overstrain and fatigue. The asthmatic should therefore try to keep a steady level of good health and fitness, by means of adequate rest, relaxation and holidays. Under circumstances of excessive strain a sedative such as phenobarbitone may be given at nights to an adult, or chloral to a child.

The presence of an *allergic factor* is usually revealed by the patient's history and by skin tests. Exposure to the particular allergen should be avoided if possible, whether it be a food or an inhalant ; the patient may have to forgo sleeping on a feather bed, for example, or associating with dogs, cats or horses. Injections of therapeutic sera into asthmatics should be made only after the most careful preparations against an anaphylactic reaction. On the results of skin tests it may be possible to desensitise the patient by a graduated and lengthy series of injections of the specific substance to which he is allergic.* It must be remembered, however, that the allergic factor may not be the only or even the principal one which determines the asthmatic attack. Failure of this form of therapy does not necessarily mean that the attempt is worthless ; success may sometimes be due more to the encouraging mental effect of the injections than to desensitisation. Non-specific desensitisation may be attempted by means of injections of peptone, or of tuberculin, or by auto-hæmotherapy ; careful and detailed skin tests with reliable test solutions, however, should make these cruder methods superfluous.

Infectious foci, acute or chronic, may produce either bacterial allergy or reflex vagal stimulation, and should be treated as early and efficiently as possible. Theoretically, vaccine

* I usually use the desensitising solutions made up by C. L. Bencard, Ltd.

therapy might seem to offer a means of desensitisation ; but clearly it can be no substitute for drainage of a suppurating nasal sinus, removal of infected tonsils or the extirpation, if feasible, of an infected bronchiectatic portion of lung. It is not surprising, therefore, that vaccines have proved to be of limited value in this disease.

Nasal abnormalities may be infective, mechanical, allergic or a combination of more than one of these. Cauterisation of the sensitive, so-called " asthmagenic area " in the nose may give temporary relief, by lowering its irritability. Any decision to undertake radical surgical measures should primarily depend not on a hope of curing the asthma but on the necessity of dealing surgically with the particular lesion which is present. Where a nasal factor is suspected, conservative rather than radical principles are more likely to forward the best interests of the asthmatic patient.

Reflex vagal stimulation may arise from *gastro-intestinal disturbances*. Flatulent dyspepsia and chronic constipation are especially to be avoided. Diet should be simple, digestible and not excessive, and the evening meal should be light. Flatulence is seldom due to the fermentation of food ; in the great majority of patients it is caused by air swallowing, associated either with some degree of neurosis or with constipation, and treatment of the primary cause is essential.

The use of *nebulæ*, applied to the nose by means of a finely spraying atomiser, is often preferred by the patient suffering from the milder forms of attack ; the apparatus is immediately available as soon as the attack starts, and the necessity for auto-injection with adrenaline is avoided. A solution of 1 per cent. ephedrine in 4 per cent. glucose saline is satisfactory, though many patients rely on proprietary preparations.

Remedial breathing exercises are of great importance, for as a rule the asthmatic needs to learn how to breathe properly.* The patient should be instructed by a qualified physiotherapist. The exercises are aimed at mobilising the chest, at making fully effective the power of expiration, at training the diaphragmatic as well as the costal breathing, and at correcting any defective posture, especially of the thorax. In early cases

---

* Suitable exercises are described in a pamphlet published by the Asthma Research Council (King's College, Strand, London, W.C.2), *Physical Exercises for Asthma.*

they help to prevent the change to the permanent form of barrel-shaped chest ; in chronic cases they help to restore the chest to its normal size and shape. The patient must be prepared to persevere diligently and faithfully with them if he is to reap full benefit.

CHAPTER XXXI

CIRCULATORY DISTURBANCES OF THE LUNGS

THE lungs have a dual circulation. The major one, from the right ventricle, is concerned with the oxygenation of the blood : the much smaller one, from the left ventricle via the bronchial arteries, serves for the nourishment of the lung tissue. Circulatory disturbances in the lungs are almost wholly disturbances of the right ventricular blood stream, and are of special importance on account of the peculiar position of the lungs between the right and left ventricles, and of the special anatomical features of this circulation.

The pulmonary artery has only a short course, with a rapidly widening bed as its branches divide and follow closely the branches of the bronchial tree. The pressure in the pulmonary arteries is only one-sixth that of the systemic arteries : the arterioles contain but a small amount of muscular fibre in their walls, and their diameter is relatively large : the capillaries are kept comparatively dilated, owing to the influence of the intrathoracic negative pressure : and changes in the calibre of the blood vessels are largely determined by alterations in the intrathoracic pressure during the phases of respiration. While vasoconstrictor fibres are known to be present in the lungs, their activity is not yet fully understood. Peripheral resistance, by comparison with that of the systemic system, is negligible, and from the circulatory aspect the lungs can be regarded as resembling erectile tissue.

The alterations in the calibre of the blood vessels during respiration allow of considerable variations in the blood content of the lungs. During expiration this amounts to some 6 per cent. of the total blood of the body, while at the height of inspiration the proportion rises to over 8 per cent.—a difference, therefore, between an expiratory content of some 300 c.c. and an inspiratory content of over 400 c.c. Moreover, the active capillary bed may vary greatly under different conditions. Under certain circumstances the quantity of blood in the pulmonary vessels may increase to 20 per cent. or more of the total blood volume. The lungs must accept and oxygenate all the blood brought to them. This they do partly by adjusting the breathing, and partly by letting the increased blood flow spread passively through a capillary bed which is sufficient to carry all the blood which can be sent to it even under the most extreme conditions of cardiac output. As in the kidneys, the number of actively functioning capillaries (that is, capillaries through which blood is flowing) may at any given time be only a small fraction of the whole. This allows for a considerable capillary reserve, whereby extra blood may be temporarily accommodated in the lungs without undue disturbance.

If, however, such general engorgement were to persist or to become excessive, it would reduce the pulmonary elasticity by making the lung tissue more rigid, and so intensify the Hering-Breuer reflex. Breathing would become rapid and shallow, vital capacity would be reduced, and the power of pulmonary ventilation would be appreciably diminished.

Furthermore, engorgement of the lung not only renders it more rigid : the blood and œdematous exudate which fill and distend the alveolar walls and escape into the alveolar spaces interfere with the normal exchange of gases, with the result that oxygenation of the blood is impaired and anoxia develops, its degree depending on the diminution of the effective respiratory surface.

Tissue œdema and serous transudates result from a disproportion between the rates of inflow and outflow between the capillaries and the tissue spaces. This may be caused (i) by increase in the hydrostatic pressure in the capillaries ; (ii) by injury to the capillary walls, with resulting excessive permeability ; and (iii) by alterations of osmotic pressure on one side or other of the endothelium of the capillaries. Drinker has expressed the normal conditions obtaining in the lung by means of a diagram (Fig. 128). It will be seen that the hydrostatic pressure is much less than the osmotic pressure of the blood proteins. This makes for the absorption of water, and for dryness of the lungs. Normally this would mean little leakage of fluid from the capillaries, and therefore no need for lymphatics. Yet the lung has a profuse supply of lymph vessels. One reason for this provision is the increase of lung lymph which results from any condition which causes an appreciable increase in the intrathoracic negative pressure (as by severe exercise, or by abnormal resistance to breathing). Moreover, any anoxia alters the permeability of the capillaries towards increased leakage.

The lungs are thus organised to rid themselves of excess

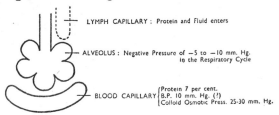

FIG. 128

To show the normal conditions in the lung alveoli, blood capillaries and lymphatics. (*After Drinker.*)

water. An abnormal resistance to the flow of blood through the lungs (as in mitral stenosis) also tends to make them œdematous, while at the same time an increase in the blood

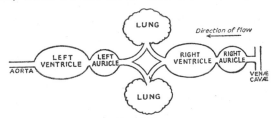

FIG. 129

The relation of the lungs to the circulation.

pressure in the capillaries (see Fig. 128) will prevent the absorption of the excess fluid.

In clinical medicine the terms " congestion " and " œdema " are liable to be regarded as indicating two distinct conditions. The differentiation, however, is only a matter of degree, and the fundamental factors in both conditions are those concerned with the relations between the circulating blood and the fluid which occupies the tissue spaces. The problem of pulmonary congestion and pulmonary œdema involves, therefore, the physiology and pathology of œdema in general, applied in this instance to a particular organ, the lungs.

One of the most important examples of œdema seen in the lungs is that due to **left ventricular failure.** Between the two separate pumping units of the heart (the right and left ventricles) is placed the vascular sponge of the lungs, which can take up varying amounts of blood, and plays an important part in the mutual adjustment of the two sides of the heart. In the healthy individual the output of the left ventricle is nicely adjusted to prevent excessive or persistent engorgement of the lungs. Any increase of venous inflow into the right side of the heart, with resulting increase in the amount of blood discharged thence into the pulmonary circulation, is met by a proportionate increase of output on the part of the left ventricle. When for any reason this delicate balance fails, so that the left ventricle cannot keep pace with the right, blood accumulates in the lungs, pulmonary engorgement and œdema develop, and the important respiratory changes already described become established.

Failure of the left ventricle to maintain a normal output in the presence of a normal filling pressure arises either by overstrain of, or by damage to, the left ventricular pump. The common causes are therefore hypertension (the most frequent factor), aortic disease, and myocardial ischæmia from coronary arteriosclerosis.

When the reserve functional capacity of the left ventricle is impaired in comparison with that of the right, it only needs sufficient physiological stress to determine a serious imbalance between the functioning of the two ventricles, the onset of which may be extremely rapid. According to the degree of this imbalance, the congestion and œdema may be slight, or it may be so severe as to produce gross waterlogging of the lungs. The clinical manifestations vary correspondingly from the **paroxysmal dyspnœa** of minor attacks of pulmonary congestion to the grave syndrome of **acute pulmonary œdema.**

The dyspnœa of paroxysmal pulmonary congestion is sometimes given the name of " cardiac asthma," but the condition is not true asthma, and the term might well be discarded in favour of some such phrase as " paroxysmal cardiac dyspnœa." In mild attacks the physiological stress may be determined by the patient's slipping down in the bed from the pillows which propped him up when he fell asleep. He wakes up in the night with a sense of oppression in the chest, or with cough and slight wheezing. If he sits upright his symptoms soon subside.

Apart from a sudden cardiac accident such as rupture of an aortic valve cusp or coronary thrombosis, severe attacks may be precipitated by the stress of a too strenuous day, or by an injudicious evening meal.   Oppression in the chest is intense and the patient is soon fighting for breath. Before long the lungs are bubbling with œdematous fluid, and profuse expectoration of pink (blood-stained) frothy sputum is the rule. Asphyxia supervenes, with cyanosis and collapse, the blood pressure falls, and the patient becomes semi-comatose. If he recovers, the pulmonary œdema may persist for days or even weeks.

Even with mild degrees of congestion and œdema the excess of blood and fluid takes some time to subside.   Repeated attacks of paroxysmal dyspnœa may lead, therefore, to the progressive deposition, in the tissue spaces, of fibrin which is later invaded by fibroblasts and organised into fibrous tissue.   There is thus produced an induration of the lung, which in the past was termed " induration pneumonia."

Occasionally the œdema involves the interstitial tissue only, with the result that while the patient suffers from dyspnœa and a low vital capacity, crepitations are not heard over the lungs.

If in addition to left ventricular failure right-sided heart failure supervenes, it brings a certain degree of relief to the lungs, in that the previous imbalance between the two ventricles no longer operates.   Nevertheless, the lungs are still congested and œdematous (and therefore more rigid), as part of the general manifestations of congestive cardiac failure. The breathing is persistently shallow and rapid, and cyanosis is common.   Hydrothorax (see Chap. XXVIII) may add further mechanical embarrassment to the breathing.

Paroxysmal pulmonary congestion is predominantly nocturnal by reason of the influence of the recumbent posture in aggravating pulmonary congestion and diminishing the vital capacity (see p. 50).   Sometimes, however, the attack is provoked by effort or excitement during the daytime.   Certain patients suffer from chronic pulmonary congestion without paroxysmal attacks, even though they present no evidence of congestive cardiac failure.   They are apt to be regarded as " chronic bronchitics " ; later they are liable to develop nocturnal orthopnœa and occasional hæmoptysis.

Radiograms show not only alterations in the cardiac shadow characteristic of the particular lesion which may be present (enlargement of the left ventricle, or prominence of the pulmonary trunk, or dilatation of the right heart), but also the resultant changes in the lung fields. These vary from the increased size and density of the pulmonary arterial tree in simple congestion to the bilateral and roughly symmetrical shadowing of pulmonary œdema. In left ventricular failure, this shadowing is, as a rule, most intense in the hilar regions. Dense hilar shadows are surrounded by a " foggy " zone, leaving only the periphery of the lungs clear. Later, the œdema gravitates to the bases, and hydrothorax may also occur. In general heart failure, on the other hand, the development of symptoms is not usually so rapid and alarming, and by the time a radiogram of the chest is made the œdema has become mainly basal. With recovery the œdema, and therefore the pulmonary shadowing, gradually disappear.

According to the distribution and character of the radiological shadows, the appearances may simulate tuberculosis (miliary or other types), pneumoconiosis, or (when there is dense shadowing close to the root of the lungs) neoplasm, or even aneurysm. A careful, complete clinical history and examination will in most instances already have made the *differential diagnosis* clear. An intensely acute onset of pulmonary œdema may follow some such striking lesion as rupture of a syphilitic aortic cusp, or coronary thrombosis. A patient may have had a high blood pressure, with an obvious history of previous attacks of left ventricular failure. Cardiac manifestations such as tachycardia, gallop rhythm, pulsus alternans and an abnormal electrocardiogram may be present. The difficult problems are those in which pulmonary congestion, due to excessive left ventricular strain, is the only objective sign of the cardiac failure. Such patients are often diagnosed as having bronchitis or asthma. Any man over fifty, therefore, who for the first time develops " bronchitis " or " asthma," should be regarded as possibly suffering from myocardial failure, and hypertension, myocardial damage or aortic disease should be carefully looked for. If the cough and dyspnœa occur mainly at night, and particularly if there is orthopnœa or hæmoptysis, a cardiac basis for the symptoms is likely. Radiograms then reveal the cardiac enlargement and the pulmonary œdema, while at the same time they exclude chronic lung disease, especially neoplasm.

Sometimes, however, it is extremely difficult to differentiate between true bronchial and " cardiac " asthma.   In such patients the estimation of the **circulation time** is of great help. The test is somewhat rough, but accurate enough for clinical purposes.   There are certain substances which when carried in the circulating blood to the tongue and throat produce characteristic sensations.   Dehydroxycholic acid, for example, or saccharine give a characteristic taste under the tongue.   Calcium gluconate produces a sensation of heat at the back of the tongue and throat.   Injected into the antecubital vein, they are carried to the right side of the heart, and thence via the pulmonary circulation to the left side of the heart, and into the systemic circulation.   The time taken for the injected substance to reach the tongue (arm-to-tongue time) can thus be measured. In normal individuals this averages about fifteen seconds, with lower and upper limits of roughly ten to twenty seconds. In the presence of pulmonary congestion this time is considerably prolonged.   A reading of, say, thirty seconds can be regarded as well outside the limits of experimental error.   The dose of dehydroxycholic acid given is 5 c.c. of a 20 per cent. solution, injected through a wide bored needle in two or three seconds.

A volatile substance like ether, injected into the antecubital vein, is recognised by its odour as soon as it reaches the lungs. The normal arm-to-lung time, obtained after the injection of 5 minims of ether, is four to eight seconds.   While the arm-to-tongue time is always increased in left ventricular failure, the arm-to-lung time is prolonged only with gross pulmonary engorgement.   The difference between these two times gives a crude but useful index of the pulmonary circulation time (lung-to-tongue), which is invariably prolonged in left-sided heart failure.   In lung disease and in asthma it is usually normal.

As might be expected, these times are also prolonged in congestive cardiac failure.   Here the systemic congestion is revealed by an appreciable increase in the venous blood pressure, whereas in pure left ventricular failure the systemic venous blood pressure is as a rule normal, though occasionally it may be slightly raised when there is gross pulmonary congestion.

The *treatment* of left ventricular failure has as its immediate aim the allaying of the patient's apprehension, and the relief of the restlessness which increases muscular effort.   To reduce

30

this effort is to decrease the return of venous blood to the right side of the heart. The resumption of a comfortable upright position, fresh air from a wide open window, and the administration of morphia ($\frac{1}{4}$ gr.) as early as possible in the attack, will all contribute towards relief. The morphia may be repeated if necessary. Adrenaline should not be given.

If there is gross engorgement of the lungs, with cyanosis, venesection should be performed, 15 to 20 oz. of blood being withdrawn. The presence of cyanosis calls for the administration of oxygen (see Chap. XIII). In the acute stage of paroxysmal dyspnœa digitalis is useful, and should preferably be given intravenously, provided that the patient has not been taking digitalis for at least a week previously. Digoxin ($\frac{1}{2}$ to 1 mg. dose) is a convenient preparation.

Improvement in the patient's condition is usually apparent in an hour or so after these measures, if they are going to be effective. For persistent pulmonary œdema, mercurial diuretics (mersalyl, for example) have been found of great value, in that they dehydrate the lungs and appreciably increase the vital capacity within twenty-four hours of injection. They should not be given if there is obvious renal disease.

Within a few days after recovery from the acute attack the patient may feel fit and able to get up. His myocardial reserve, however, is minimal, and absolute rest in bed for at least three weeks should be insisted upon. Thereafter he must lead a quiet and well-ordered life under medical supervision.

Other causes of congestion and œdema have already been mentioned earlier in this chapter, and some have been dealt with in detail in previous chapters—for example, local or diffuse engorgement in acute infections such as the pneumonias or tuberculosis, and the lesions caused by irritant gases. Pulmonary stasis may also result from interference with the normal outflow of blood from the lungs into the heart, as by mitral stenosis, pressure on the pulmonary veins by tumour or by a tension pneumothorax, thrombosis of the pulmonary vein, or chronic pulmonary disease such as fibrosis or emphysema. Cyanosis and dyspnœa are prominent, the conus arteriosus and the right side of the heart become dilated, and the end result is right heart failure. If the obstruction is prolonged the pulmonary arteries may become grossly dilated and atheromatous. It is probable that the pulmonary arteriosclerosis which has been regarded as a special entity, and given the name of Ayerza's disease when accompanied by cyanosis and polycythæmia, is but an example of this process.

PULMONARY EMBOLISM

Of all the forms of embolus, only the common one, namely, blood clot, will be considered in any great detail. Such emboli may arise from the veins of the leg (especially the deep veins in the calf muscles) or pelvis, following operative or other trauma, or blood stasis. Infection and carcinoma near to the path of the vein are contributory factors, while obesity, blood diseases, cardiac disease, and varicose veins (that is, conditions which on the whole affect older persons) also increase the tendency to embolism. They may also arise from mural thrombi in the right ventricle in cardiac infarction of the areas supplied by the anterior descending or posterior branches of the coronary artery : from vegetations on the valves of the right side of the heart : and from thrombi in the right auricle in mitral stenosis. A striking example of the effect of stasis was seen in the increased number of deaths from pulmonary embolism among elderly people with some degree of varicosity of the lower-limb veins during the period of the heavy air raids on London. They sat for hours on deck chairs in the shelters, with the wooden cross-piece obstructing the circulation about the middle of the thighs. As soon as the provision of sleeping bunks became more general, the number of these deaths was greatly diminished.

The blood clot reaching the pulmonary circulation may be large or small. It may be several inches in length, and is then found coiled up in the main pulmonary artery. It may be small, blocking one of the lesser branches. It may be split up into numerous tiny emboli which are not arrested until they reach the terminal ramifications of the arterial tree. These emboli may be overlooked at necropsy unless the pulmonary artery is opened and its branches followed right up to the periphery of the lungs.

Major pulmonary embolism is a comparatively uncommon catastrophe which is encountered as a rule some seven to fourteen days after childbirth or operation. The patient is suddenly seized with severe pain in the chest and intense dyspnœa. He goes blue, loses consciousness and dies within a few minutes. If the clot obstructs only one branch of the artery, he may survive a little longer, and operation, undertaken within twenty minutes of the onset, may give him a chance of survival. It must be rare, however, for skilled surgical help to be available at the opportune moment.

Pulmonary embolism of catastrophic onset is, however, the exception and not the rule. Warning symptoms, such as a rise of temperature or of the pulse rate, frequently precede the attack. Moreover, it is common for there to be a non-fatal attack before the later fatal one. In other words, pulmonary embolism is often multiple, and in addition it may be preceded by detectable peripheral thrombosis. *Latent* thrombosis may sometimes be detected by observation of an increase in the diameter of one of the lower limbs (measurements being taken at the level of the malleolus, the calf, and the middle of the thigh). The normal measurements should be noted, for comparison, before operation or parturition. There may be associated pain in the calf muscles, produced by squeezing them gently, or by hyperextension of the foot.

In non-fatal attacks of embolism, in addition to the symptoms of dyspnœa and pain in the chest, the patient is apprehensive, deathly pale, and perspiring. The pulse is small and rapid, and the blood pressure low. Later, the temperature rises, there may be hæmoptysis, and signs of local or diffuse pulmonary œdema may be found in the lungs and noted in radiograms. True infarction occurs only if the lungs are already congested. The attack may be mistaken for one of cardiac infarction, but there are certain electrocardiographic differences in the chest lead tracings which help in the differentiation.

Death in pulmonary embolism other than that of the massive type is not due to obstruction of the circulation by the clot, but to vagal reflexes set up by the embolus. Thus, even comparatively small emboli may be fatal, although they do not cause gross obstruction.

After a non-fatal attack of pulmonary embolism the patient may recover completely, or he may remain more or less incapacitated. Disability results when there is organisation of the emboli and cicatricial stenosis of the vessels wherein they lodge. Consequently, there is a progressive obstruction of the pulmonary arteries, which is liable to lead to secondary thrombosis and recurrence of the attack.

In the prophylaxis of thrombosis or embolism there are three obvious steps which can be taken when a patient is submitted to an operation. These are the avoidance of immobilisation and stasis, and of sepsis in the operation field ; the reduction of operative trauma to a minimum ; and the restoration of blood, fluid or salt lost from the body. Recently some evidence has been brought forward to show that in patients, after operation, a fibrinolysin is present in the blood plasma. This is activated less by trauma than by anxiety ; the motto for the patient about to face an operation, therefore, should be, " In quietness and confidence shall be your strength ". For patients who have survived one embolic attack, or who have peripheral thrombosis, continuous heparinisation for at least ten days offers the most useful safeguard.

Fat embolism may arise by the setting free into the circulation of fat globules from the bone marrow, as in fractures of bone, or from laceration of the fatty tissues. The embolus interferes with the pulmonary circulation, causing dyspnœa, cough, cyanosis and a fall of blood pressure. As a rule some of the globules pass through the lungs, to produce emboli in the systemic circulation. Pulmonary manifestations appear a few hours after the trauma, and a few hours afterwards the patient may become comatose from cerebral fat embolism. Globules of fat may be detected in the urine.

Air embolism occasionally follows operations on the neck, owing to puncture of one of the large veins, with sucking-in of a considerable quantity of air. It can arise also from trauma of the prostatic venous plexus, or during insufflation of the Fallopian tubes. The air is churned up in the right ventricle, and the resulting air bubbles obstruct the pulmonary circulation as they are forced into the pulmonary artery and its branches. Pain in the chest and distress of breathing are the salient symptoms. According to the severity of the condition the patient may recover, or he may die of right heart failure.

PULMONARY INFARCTION

It is extremely difficult to produce an infarct in a healthy lung. The organ has a double vascular supply, from the pulmonary and bronchial arteries. The latter anastomose with the lung capillaries, and the blood from both arteries is returned by the pulmonary veins. The pulmonary arteries anastomose very freely, through the wide capillaries. If one pulmonary artery is ligated in a healthy experimental animal the bronchial arterial stream is able to keep the tissue alive (though it eventually contracts and becomes scarred).

In general, it may be said that infarction takes place in the lung only when the outflow of blood from it is impeded (" chronic passive congestion "). For this reason infarction is most commonly a complication of cardiac disease. Mitral stenosis, for example, lowers the output of the left ventricle, and diminishes the pressure in the bronchial arteries. At the same time it obstructs the venous outflow from the lungs. If a branch of the pulmonary artery is now occluded by an embolus, the anastomotic flow of blood must depend on the already lowered bronchial artery pressure, working against a high venous pressure. The flow is insufficient to maintain the normal life of the tissue, though it does not always die. The high venous pressure forces red blood corpuscles through the walls of the damaged capillaries and alveoli, so that the affected zone of lung becomes stuffed with red blood corpuscles (*in-farcire* means " to stuff "). The result is a hard, dry, red infarct, which tends to be pyramidal in form, and extends to the surface of the lung. Over the bulging surface of the infarcted area is seen a fibrinous deposit due to plastic pleurisy. When the embolus is infected, as in pyæmia, the zone of inflammatory necrosis may liquefy and form a lung abscess, provided that the patient lives long enough for this to develop.

In mitral stenosis the source of the embolus is commonly a piece of clot from the right auricle. When no obvious residual clot is found there at autopsy, it is generally assumed that the infarction has been caused by thrombosis in a pulmonary vein. This is less likely than that the original clot in the right auricle was tiny and was wholly set free, so that no residual clot is left there for the pathologist to see ; or that, in a patient bedridden with mitral stenosis and congestive cardiac failure, the embolus came from a thrombus in one of the peripheral limb veins.

The *symptoms* of pulmonary infarct depend largely on the size of the occluded blood vessel, and therefore of the infarct. In addition to shock and collapse (the severity depending on the extent of the infarction), the salient features are pleural pain, dyspnœa and hæmoptysis. Temperature and pulse rate rise, the breathing becomes rapid and shallow, and cyanosis may develop. After about twenty-four hours there is a hard, dry cough, which soon becomes productive. The sputum is then copious, frothy and pink, from the pulmonary œdema associated with the lesion, or it is heavily blood-stained. As the hæmoglobin in the alveoli becomes chemically altered, the sputum becomes brownish or rusty.

The *signs* also depend on the size of the infarct. After the first day pleurisy is evident (pleural rub), and medium and fine crepitations reveal the pulmonary œdema surrounding the infarct. If the infarct is large, signs of consolidation are elicited.

The *diagnosis* is not usually difficult, in that there is usually a history, together with the appropriate signs, of cardiac disease. Differentiation must be made from coronary thrombosis (see earlier in this chapter) ; from lobar pneumonia (see Chap. XVII) ; from pulmonary collapse (see Chap. VII) ; and from pulmonary tuberculosis with hæmoptysis. Radiograms will be of special help in excluding the two latter diseases.

The immediate *treatment* is directed to the relief of pain and of the collapse. Morphia is not contraindicated either by dyspnœa or by cyanosis. Absolute rest in bed, warmth, oxygen administration and nikethamide should be used to combat collapse. Later, treatment becomes that of the primary disease.

CHAPTER XXXII

CHEST INJURIES *

GENERAL CONSIDERATIONS

INJURY to the thoracic cage and its contents assumes a special importance in so far as it interferes with the vital cardio-respiratory mechanisms. The older the patient, the less his cardio-respiratory reserve is likely to be, and the more serious, therefore, the consequences of a chest injury. The elderly civilian with chronic bronchitis, wounded in an air raid, succumbed to injuries such as the healthy young soldier was able to survive.

The thoracic cage may be injured without damage to its contents. On the other hand, young resilient ribs may give without breaking, even to great force, so that extensive laceration of the thoracic contents may occur without fracture of the cage. In most instances, however (apart from damage by blast), any but trivial injuries are likely to involve both cage and contents, whether the damage is by crushing, flying splinters, bullet wounds, or fragments of high explosive.

Seeing that the dome of the diaphragm projects high into the thorax, it is not surprising that chest wounds often involve the abdomen as well (Fig. 18, p. 22), or that blood in the pleural cavity may sometimes come from a wound of the liver.

Injury to the bony framework of the thoracic cage may tear blood vessels (especially the intercostal and internal mammary vessels), with resulting hæmothorax. It may also drive pieces of bone or of clothing into the lung, lacerating its substance, and often carrying in infection. Laceration of the lung leads to the coughing up of blood, and to the escape of blood and air into the pleural space. Persistent hæmorrhage (as a rule from

---

* For a detailed account of this subject, see *War Injuries of the Chest*, edited by H. Morriston Davies and Robert Coope (Edinburgh, 1942, E. & S. Livingstone) and Tudor Edwards' chapter in Hamilton Bailey's *Surgery of Modern Warfare*.

the chest wall) and tension pneumothorax are two paramount thoracic emergencies, immediate relief of which is a matter of life or death. To these must be added the open chest wound and the " stove-in " chest, which will be described later.

The parietal pleura and the periosteum of the ribs are richly supplied with pain nerves. Even a superficial bruising of the chest wall makes it painful to cough or to breathe deeply. Most chest injuries are accompanied, therefore, by distressed breathing, which is quick and shallow. If it continues for long, dangerous anoxia and cyanosis may result. Furthermore, voluntary repression of the cough reflex because of the pain leads to failure to clear the air passages of secretions or of blood, with the result that absorption collapse of the lung is common.

In many chest injuries the diaphragm is paralysed and rises high into the thorax, owing to concussion or laceration of the phrenic nerve. In injury of the lower thorax the pain may be referred to the abdomen via the lower intercostal nerves. Moreover, immobility of the injured side of the thorax may be accompanied by reflex abdominal rigidity. This makes it difficult sometimes to decide whether or not there is an abdominal injury also. With an abdominal injury, however, the rigidity is usually bilateral, whereas if the lower thorax alone has been damaged it is confined to the same side as the injury and subsides when the patient is relieved of his pain.

The victim of a serious chest injury, then, is not only shocked but also dyspnœic. The pain and distress of breathing and the sense of suffocation often lead to an agony of apprehension. Many cough up blood. All are in danger of anoxia. Those with continuous bleeding, or a tension pneumothorax, or a " stove-in " chest, or an open wound of the thorax, are in immediate jeopardy of their lives. Even apparently simple wounds may suddenly develop grave complications. Finally, there may be associated injuries elsewhere, such as in the abdomen or the head.

THE EXAMINATION OF THE CHEST CASUALTY

The doctor should note the general appearance, the colour of the mucous membranes, and the presence (or absence) and type of cyanosis. He should watch the breathing, observing its rate and depth, whether both sides of the chest move equally, or whether one side is immobile or is moving paradoxically (see p. 479). The character of the cough may indicate that the air passages contain fluid : a dry, half-smothered, racking cough suggests pleural irritation. Blood in the sputum points to bleeding from the lung ; copious, thin, frothy expectoration tells of œdematous exudation into the alveoli and bronchi.

Rapid inspection and gentle palpation of the body are made to see what external wounds or injuries are present, and whether they are multiple. If there is a hole in the chest wall, the continuous escape of bright arterial blood, or the sound of air sucking through the opening, or the gurgling of frothy blood, are important indications of injury to a systemic vessel, of a tear in the pleura and a sucking pneumothorax, or of laceration of the lung.

Detailed clinical examination of the back of the chest should be reserved until resuscitation measures have succeeded, since enough practical information can, as a rule, be gained in the first instance if the front of the chest and the axillæ are carefully examined. The injured side shows much less expansion than the sound one. Very occasionally, when there is a large collection of air or fluid in a pleural cavity, that side of the thorax may be obviously distended. Surgical emphysema nearly always means that there is an underlying pneumothorax. The position of the apex beat (which should be marked with a skin pencil) and of the trachea is of prime importance to show whether the mediastinum has been displaced away from a pleural effusion or pneumothorax, or drawn towards a zone of absorption collapse of the lung. Periodic observations will show whether the displacement is increasing or diminishing.

Percussion must be very gentle. It may reveal the dulness of fluid (blood, at this early stage) or the resonance of pneumothorax. Finer differences of note have little helpful significance, especially as injury to the thoracic cage greatly alters it as a percussion instrument.

The most important auscultatory finding is a normal vesicular murmur, for it tells of air entering the lung under examination. Its absence or diminution is of little practical help in the diagnosis of such conditions as hæmothorax, pleural effusion, pneumothorax, or collapse of the lung, for in *any* injury the affected side of the chest may hardly expand, so that normal respiratory sounds are not heard. Moist adventitious sounds are very common in the injured chest, both on the affected and unaffected sides, but they do not enable the examiner to distinguish between the accumulation in the air passages of blood or of œdematous fluid. Pleural or pericardial friction may occur early from bruising, or later from infection. The other routine thoracic physical signs are not particularly helpful. For example, the bell sound (*bruit d'airain*) is seldom heard in pneumothorax, while to attempt to elicit succussion splash in the critical early stage of injury is positively harmful. The presence of subcutaneous emphysema masks the usual physical signs : it gives a resonant note to percussion, and unfamiliar and often bizarre crackling noises on auscultation.

By this time it should be possible to decide whether any of the grave thoracic emergencies previously mentioned need attention. If so, no time should be lost in dealing with them. The examiner has also to ask himself whether the gravity of a patient's condition is due to the wound of the chest, or whether injuries elsewhere are the more important. Abdominal viscera may be lacerated. Injuries of the head or secondary cerebral embolism may be the reason for a failure of resuscitation measures, and disturbances of respiration may have a central origin. The heart or pericardium may be directly injured. Deep-seated intractable pain may result from fracture of, or the impaction of, a missile in a vertebra. The spinal cord may be concussed or lacerated.

Once resuscitation is under way and the patient is recovering from the initial shock, a more detailed examination can be made in order to assess the full nature and extent of the injuries, with a view to further treatment. The medical officer will especially wish to ascertain the track of the missile : the damage it has done to the thoracic wall, the pleura, the lung and elsewhere : whether fragments of it still remain in the body, and if so, where : and whether there is a collection of blood or air in the pleural cavity.

Both clinical and radiological examinations are necessary to obtain a true clinical picture. The larger the entrance wound, especially if bones have been splintered, the more likely it is that fragments of bone, clothing or debris have been driven into the chest. If there is no wound of exit, the missile is still somewhere in the body, unless by rare chance it has been coughed up meanwhile. Small wounds of entrance, however, do not justify the assumption that the internal injuries are trivial.

So long as the patient is distressed, and until the cardio-vascular system has recovered, he should be carefully turned towards the sound side whenever examination of the back is made. This is not so satisfactory a position as the vertical : when, however, a patient sits forward in bed his breathing is cramped. As soon as the stage of recovery permits, it is pre-ferable that he should sit on the edge of the bed with his legs dangling down and the thighs well away from the abdomen : in this posture the diaphragm is not embarrassed. A nurse or orderly sits beside him and supports the trunk, while another stands in front and supports the two hands firmly. The doctor can then carry out a more leisurely examination.

It is the custom in some clinics to X-ray the chest casualty immediately on admission, on his way to the resuscitation ward. This seems an unnecessary risk, for at this stage only thoracic emergencies call for operative attention, and these should be discovered by clinical examination. Nothing, therefore, is lost by waiting until resuscitation measures have been undertaken. The only occasion for urgent radiology is when the medical officer suspects but is not certain of a perforating wound of the stomach or bowel. Here early operation is imperative, and X-ray films may reveal a missile, together with gas, in the abdominal cavity. As soon, however, as the patient is fit for it, anterior and lateral chest films of good quality should be taken. From them much valuable information will be obtained of the site and size of a retained foreign body, of fractures of the thoracic cage, of the presence of a lung hæmatoma, of pulmonary collapse, or of the extent of a hæmothorax or pneumothorax ; of, in addition, the presence or absence of changes in the lung on the uninjured side. When the patient is out of immediate danger, screening of the chest becomes both justifiable and advisable.

TYPES OF INJURY

The accepted clinical differentiation of thoracic injuries into two main groups, (1) non-penetrating and (2) penetrating, is useful in that it indirectly emphasises the importance both of damage to intrathoracic organs and of infection carried, from without, into the pleural cavity or the lung. Such a rough classification does not absolve the student from thinking of injuries in terms of their detailed pathology. An empyema, for example, may arise from an infected hæmothorax due to a piece of shell entering the chest ; on the other hand, it may result from a blow on the chest which caused bruising of the chest wall and pleura, followed by pleural exudate which may or may not have contained blood, and was eventually secondarily infected from the lung.

Simple bruising or laceration of the soft tissues or of the bones of the chest wall are of special significance only if the lesion extends into the thoracic cavity or involves its contents. Contusion of surrounding areas, hæmatoma, hæmorrhage, splintering of bones and involvement of nerves (intercostals, or branches of the brachial plexus) are all possible complications of such injuries. Open wounds of the chest wall which do not penetrate the pleura are " non-penetrating " ; such a wound, caused by a bullet, is spoken of as a " non-penetrating gunshot wound."

Fractures of ribs may arise from the impact of blunt missiles, from compression of the chest, or, rarely, from muscular action (as in the convulsive treatment of mental disease, or even severe coughing). They tend to be multiple. There may be no accompanying laceration of the skin or soft tissues. Because of the elasticity of the bony cage of the thorax, especially in children, severe laceration of the underlying viscera may take place without rib fracture, even in severe crush injuries.

When the fracture is caused by compression antero-posteriorly, the ribs are liable to break outwards in the axillary plane, and laceration of the lung is much less likely to happen than when a broken end or fragment of bone is driven inwards into the thorax. Injury to the underlying lung may cause hæmoptysis, localised surgical emphysema of the chest wall, and the escape of air and blood into the pleural cavity. Tension pneumothorax may then develop if the laceration is of the valvular type (see Chap. XXVII). The broken ends of the bone may tear an intercostal artery and cause a hæmatoma of the chest wall or a rapidly accumulating hæmothorax.

Pain over the site of the fracture, limited expansion of the affected side of the chest, difficult breathing, and palpable bony crepitus are the salient clinical manifestations. Anterior and lateral radiograms will usually reveal the site and extent of the fractures. Treatment is by immobilisation by means of 2-in. Holland strapping applied in full expiration, and made to extend to at least 3 in. on to the sound side of the chest, front and back. Union nearly always takes place, even when it is not possible to obtain complete immobilisation of the fragments. If the fragments are displaced, some deformity occurs, and as the callus also may be considerable, persistent intercostal pain may result from pressure on the intercostal nerve.

Surgical emphysema, though distressing to the patient, is rarely serious, as the air will be absorbed when the supply is cut off. Treatment, therefore, is that of the primary injury.

Fractures of the costal cartilages are more liable to occur in young adults. The cartilage may be torn from the rib at the costochondral junction, or dislocated from its attachment to the sternum, or broken across at any point. Pain in true fracture may be severe : instead of crepitus, a typical click associated with movement is common. Unless there is calcification of the cartilage, the lesion is not visible in radiograms. **Fracture of the sternum** is rare. If due to a direct blow the force is transmitted to the mediastinum and may cause cardiac trauma.

" **Stove-in** " **chest** is the term given to a lesion in which a number of ribs or cartilages are fractured in two or more places. It is usually produced by a diffuse blow on the chest, such as a crush by a fallen beam or compression by a vehicle. It is a serious injury, often accompanied by grave damage to underlying thoracic viscera. If a large vessel or the heart is ruptured, death is almost instantaneous.

The main symptom is dyspnœa. This is caused partly by damage to the underlying lungs, but the greatest factor is the paradoxical movement of the loose mobile section of ribs lying between the fractures. This detached segment, instead of moving outwards with the rest of the thoracic cage in inspiration, is sucked inwards as the intrapleural negative pressure increases (Fig. 130). During expiration the thoracic cage contracts, the intrapleural pressure becomes less negative or even positive, and the mobile rib segment is squeezed outwards (Fig. 131). With the phases of respiration the mediastinum moves to and fro (*mediastinal flutter*),

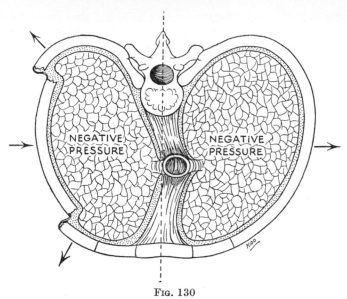

Fig. 130
" Stove-in " chest.   Inspiration.

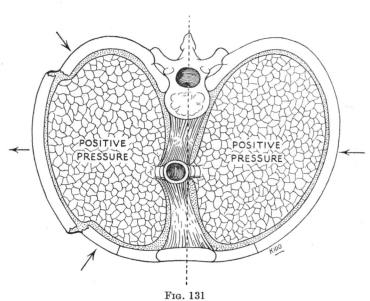

Fig. 131
" Stove-in " chest.   Expiration.

Note the paradoxical movement of the loose fragment, and the
mediastinal shift.

causing serious embarrassment to the heart and great vessels. During respiration pulmonary ventilation on the injured side is incomplete. If the mobile segment is extensive, the lung on that side may actually become smaller on inspiration, some of its already deoxygenated air being pressed out into the bronchi, whence it is inspired into the contralateral expanding lung. During expiration the normal retraction of the lung on the sound side forces this vitiated air back into the lung of the injured side. This it does at the expense of fresh air inhaled into the lungs : the normal intake is diminished by the amount displaced from one lung to the other. Hence the normal oxygen exchange is embarrassed, with consequent anoxia and cyanosis.

The injury, as has been said, is serious, and lesions in the underlying lungs are common. The lung parenchyma may be torn, with resulting hæmoptysis. Pulmonary œdema may be prominent. The extensive damage to the thoracic cage makes effective coughing difficult or impossible : secretions accumulate in the bronchi, and absorption collapse, either on the same side as the injury or contralaterally, is a frequent complication. Sometimes there is cardiac trauma, either myocardial bruising, or rupture of a valve, or rupture of the heart itself. The chest itself may not be the only part of the body injured. Damage to abdominal viscera, for example, is often associated with crush injuries of the chest. Occasionally, reflex dilatation of the stomach or paralytic ileus follow multiple rib fractures.

Treatment aims at recovery from the severe shock : at correction of the respiratory disability which arises from the paradoxical movement of the mobile section of the thoracic cage : and at relief of pain and dyspnœa, together with measures to prevent the onset of complications. The loose fragment must be fixed by Holland strapping applied over a pad of wool during expiration and carried completely around the chest. Recently, W. D. W. Brooks has had notable success by placing the patient in a mechanical respirator.

Pain should be controlled by morphia as well as by fixation of the fragment. It is essential for the patient to empty his lungs of blood and secretions in order to lessen the danger of absorption collapse and of anoxia. In the acute stage immediately following the injury, a nurse should be in constant attendance to help him with cough and expectoration, firmly supporting the sides of the chest in order to restrain the sudden, painful expanding movement of the chest wall at each expulsive effort. By reducing the pain, morphia will make it easier for him to get up the accumulated secretions. Some degree of anoxia is inevitable, and oxygen administration should be started at the earliest possible moment after the injury. It must be continued until there is no further need for it. The symptoms, signs, and treatment of absorption collapse have been described in Chapter VII ; those of tension pneumothorax in Chapter XXVII.

" **Traumatic asphyxia** " — sometimes called " traumatic cyanosis "—is caused by violent but temporary compression of the thoracic wall, and is associated with severe crushing injuries. It is characterised by a diffuse blue ecchymosis of the face, neck and upper thorax. The discoloration is the result of the sudden, intense rise of intrathoracic pressure, which compresses the thin-walled veins of the mediastinum, and forces blood out of the thorax into the veins of the head and neck. Venules are ruptured, with the formation of numberless tiny venous hæmorrhages under the skin and conjunctivæ. In places where the skin vessels are supported, as by a collar or a cap, white bands of normal skin are seen. Sometimes retinal vessels are involved to the extent of producing blindness, which may be temporary or permanent. Rupture of cerebral veins may give rise to coma. The skin discoloration usually subsides in two to three weeks, with the typical colour changes of an ecchymosis.

Bruising of the chest wall may be extensive enough to cause **contusion of the parietal pleura,** with resulting dry pleurisy or a mild serofibrinous effusion. The manifestations are pain on breathing, pleural rub, and sometimes slight fever due to the absorption of protein or blood from the injured area. The main point in treatment is to immobilise that side of the chest by strapping.

Puncture or laceration of the pleural membrane is inevitable in penetrating wounds. With small missiles the wound in the pleura often seals itself immediately. An effusion may develop, however, serofibrinous if the wound in the pleura and lung seals itself early and is not infected, purulent if there is associated infection. Hæmorrhage from vessels in the chest wall or lung may lead to hæmothorax. If the laceration is extensive

31

and exposes the pleural cavity to the atmosphere an open chest wound is established.

The **open chest wound** must be regarded as one of the grave thoracic emergencies. The inroads which it makes into the cardio-respiratory reserve have already been described in Chapter XXV (p. 393). The lung collapses, and with each respiration air enters and leaves the pleural cavity through the external wound. The bigger the wound opening the more air will go through it and the less through the glottis. Given a large hole and a poor vital capacity, the results on respiratory exchange are catastrophic.

With a large opening little or no air enters the collapsed lung on the affected side during inspiration ; indeed, the expanding sound lung sucks over into itself some of the stagnant deoxygenated air left in the lung on the affected side, collapsing it still farther. At the same time, because there is no opposing balanced action of the affected side, there is an increase in the shift of the mediastinum to the sound side, thus farther reducing the vital capacity. During expiration, air from the sound lung is propelled not only up the trachea but also into the opposite lung, partially re-expanding it, and the mediastinum now moves again towards the wounded side (see Figs. 119 and 120, p. 394). Thus, even the blood coming from the sound lung is imperfectly oxygenated, because of the reduced vital capacity and the deficiency in oxygen of the air which enters it. Equally serious is the see-saw movement of the heart and great vessels during the mediastinal flutter. This interferes with the venous return and causes a marked irregularity in the cardiac output. All these factors help to increase the gravity of the anoxia.

It is imperative to close an open wound of the chest (" sucking wound ") as soon as possible, either by one or two temporary sutures or by a pad of vaseline gauze covered with a layer of plain gauze and wool, fixed and made airtight by overlapping strips of elastoplast. In emergency a handkerchief or a portion of shirt may have to be utilised.

Contusion and **laceration** of the lungs are frequent results of external injuries. High velocity bullets may produce **through-and-through wounds,** which are often strangely free from complications. The slight degree of pulmonary retraction in these injuries effectively seals torn vessels and small air passages, though there is always some intra-alveolar hæmorrhage around the track of the missile. These hæmorrhages are irregular in extent, and are surrounded by zones of serous effusion beyond which a mild compensatory emphysema of the alveoli is noticeable. Radiologically, therefore, the track and its surrounding collar of infiltration may stand out as a dense shadow. **Hæmatoma** of the lung may follow a blow on the chest, or a penetrating wound ; in either instance there is considerable intrapulmonary hæmorrhage, and the blood in-filtrating the alveoli bursts their walls and forms a localised mass of blood clot. Occasionally pulmonary contusion or hæmatoma occurs in the contralateral lung by *contrecoup*.

Pulmonary contusion is fairly common, and the essential change is hæmorrhagic infiltration without necessarily other gross injury. The diagnosis is based on the presence of hæmoptysis, mild fever, signs of consolidation if the lesion is extensive, and radiological evidence of a dense shadow which slowly resolves. Expectant treatment should be adopted, provided that there is no retained foreign body.

HÆMOTHORAX

Hæmothorax may be an immediate or a later complication of almost any chest injury—a direct blow, a crush, stabs, bullets, bomb fragments, or splinters, including glass, resulting from explosions. In non-penetrating injuries of the chest wall the hæmothorax is usually due to a tear of an intercostal artery or of the lung by a fractured rib ; it can also result from lacera-tion of the lung without bone fracture. When the lung is torn some quantity of air as well as blood escapes into the pleural cavity ; if a rib is fractured the air may make its way into the subcutaneous tissues. Lacerations of the large intrathoracic blood vessels are rapidly fatal and beyond the help of treatment.

Apart from the shock and severity of the initial injury, hæmothorax becomes dangerous to life (i) when there is much loss of blood ; (ii) when it compresses the lungs and the great vessels ; and (iii) when it becomes infected.

Bleeding from a torn intercostal or internal mammary artery may cause death unless it is recognised in time, and checked. Bleeding from the lung parenchyma is much more often arrested naturally. The pressure in the pulmonary circula-tion is about a sixth only of that in the systemic ; moreover, as the lung retracts before the accumulating blood and air, the wound tends to close, unless it is held out by a splintered rib. Nevertheless, the bleeding, though not of itself sufficient to cause death, may turn the scale in an already severely shocked patient. An appreciable escape of air into the pleural cavity adds to the pressure inside the thorax, and is especially dangerous if the tear in the lung acts as a valve and produces a tension hæmopneumothorax.

The symptoms of progressive bleeding are pallor, restlessness, thirst, an increase in the rate and a reduction in the volume of the pulse. Periodic recording of the pulse rate and the blood pressure is therefore of the first importance. Pressure on the large veins is accompanied by a sense of tightness in the chest, a greater increase in the threadiness of the pulse, a progressive quickening and shallowness of the breathing, cyanosis and, later, engorgement of the veins of the neck.

The cardinal sign is the displacement of the apex of the heart. The importance of marking the position with a skin pencil has already been stressed. It enables progressive displacement to be readily detected, especially valuable if there has been a change in symptoms. Next in importance is the " stony " dulness to percussion over the fluid. Difficulty may sometimes arise if there is an extensive hæmatoma of the lung, especially if the diaphragm is temporarily paralysed and raised ; dulness may be marked, and differentiation certain only after diagnostic needling of the chest. As has been pointed out earlier, alteration of the normal breath sounds and voice sounds are of little diagnostic help when the chest has been injured. Most of these patients cough up blood at some time or other, but this indicates only that there has been damage to the lung and gives no further clue to the presence or absence of a hæmothorax.

Blood is irritating to the mesothelial lining of the pleural cavity. In consequence, **secondary pleural effusion** is common at any time after the first twenty-four hours. This effusion, added to the blood already present, will produce a rapid increase in the intrapleural pressure which may lead to dangerous compression symptoms. Moreover, when under tension it will cause pyrexia, which (unlike that due to sepsis) does not remit, is associated with only mild constitutional symptoms and subsides as soon as the intrapleural tension is relieved. The onset of secondary effusion frequently explains sudden deterioration in the general or local symptoms, and it must always be kept in mind as an important phase in the management of hæmothorax.

Unless a foreign body has been introduced and remains there, or unless there is sepsis, blood in the pleural cavity does not clot. When a clot forms it is impossible to remove it completely by a needle and syringe. Even when the hæmothorax remains uninfected there is a gradual deposition of fibrin together with endothelial and blood cells, and a still further enrichment by fibrin when the secondary effusion develops. If the blood is allowed to remain in the pleural cavity the deposited fibrin and cellular debris eventually become organised, with the inevitable result that both visceral and parietal membranes become encased in fibrous tissue. A " shell " of organised exudate (" clotted haemothorax ", " frozen chest ") prevents the lung from expanding, resulting eventually in an immobile contracted chest with crowding of the ribs and severe scoliosis.

While the blood at first has certain bactericidal powers owing to its contained antibodies, macrophages and leucocytes, these cease to be effective after a few hours. The hæmothorax then becomes an excellent medium for the growth of organisms. The danger of infection is much greater with penetrating wounds, though even with non-penetrating injuries a tear of the lung may introduce bacteria from the air passages.

On all counts, therefore, and whether there are compression symptoms or not, the blood should be removed as soon and as quickly as is consistent with safety and comfort. This will minimise the dangers of secondary effusion, of infection and of the later crippling fibrosis.

Treatment—In the early stages death may result from bleeding from a systemic vessel. If the bleeding is from the lung the loss of blood volume is usually insufficient to cause death, save when one of the large vessels is torn. Nevertheless, death may result from compression of the lungs and vessels, early if there is an added pneumothorax, and later when the volume of intrapleural blood is markedly increased by the secondary effusion.

If in the first few hours after the injury the symptoms and signs indicate continuous bleeding (increasing pallor, progressive fall of blood pressure in spite of measures of resuscitation, progressive displacement of the heart apex), it must be assumed that a systemic vessel has been torn, and immediate operation is called for. The transfusion of blood is continued, enough intrapleural blood is aspirated to reduce the intrapleural pressure to a point which relieves compression, and the bleeding vessel is found and ligatured as rapidly as possible. The operation is an emergency one, and should be reduced to the minimum necessary to stop the bleeding. Later, when the patient has recovered from the loss of blood the wound and the hæmothorax can be dealt with under quieter and more favourable conditions.

Provided that there are no manifestations of compression from an associated pneumothorax, a hæmothorax which originates from the lung should be left undisturbed for at least twenty-four hours in order that the tear in the lung through which blood and air have escaped may become sealed. Meanwhile anti-shock and other treatment is given, and radiograms are taken, especially with the aim of detecting any retained foreign bodies. Thirty-six to forty-eight hours after the injury, according to the condition of the patient, the whole of the intrapleural blood should be evacuated, not only for the reasons already enumerated but also to encourage the expansion of the lung and the obliteration of the pleural cavity.

Pulmonary re-expansion helps to limit pleural infection and restore respiratory efficiency. Damage to the lung either from a large penetrating wound or from a non-penetrating injury which nevertheless causes a pulmonary contusion, hæmatoma or laceration, delays re-expansion of the lung and greatly increases the risk of pleural infection. This is especially true if an upper lobe is damaged and collapsed, with resulting " total " hæmopneumothorax. The longer blood remains in the pleural cavity, the more likely is pleural thickening to occur and " freeze " the lung in a position of incomplete expansion.

Early pulmonary re-expansion, therefore, is the ideal at which to aim. Evacuation of blood and clot helps this by lessening the chances of pleural fibrosis. If there has been a small penetrating wound which has produced a hæmothorax without the presence of an appreciable amount of air in the pleural cavity, the likelihood is that damage to the lung itself is not serious, and that the lung will probably re-expand when the blood is withdrawn. The hæmothorax should therefore be aspirated, and penicillin instilled into the pleural space in order to combat the possible development of local infection. A large penetrating wound, however, is likely to result in considerable damage to the lung, the escape of a considerable amount of air as well as of blood into the pleural cavity, and almost inevitable infection. Early operation ("surgical toilet" of the injured chest wall or pleura or lung) is therefore advisable.

Provided that the hæmothorax has been attended to early and that the underlying lung is not badly damaged, re-expansion is usually complete in four to six weeks. In the earlier stages, secondary effusions may occur even after removal of the blood. These must be evacuated as they arise and not allowed to interfere unduly with lung expansion.

Aspiration of the hæmothorax, however, may fail to induce proper expansion of the lung, either because there is a mass of clot and debris in the pleural cavity, or because the damaged portion of the lung remains collapsed. Clotting of the blood in the pleural cavity is usually an indication of infection, though it may occur in a sterile hæmothorax around a sterile foreign body. The heat of metal fragments may sterilise them, and may even sterilise small pieces of cloth which they carry in with them. The presence of clot should be suspected if it is found impossible to aspirate blood through a needle inserted into the lower zone of a hæmothorax, while the fluid withdrawn from a higher level is serous or sero-sanguineous in character. Radiograms will reveal a shadow of uniform opacity after aspiration of the supernatant fluid. If the clot is infected it may not necessarily produce any constitutional symptoms until the organisms which are within it reach the surface and infect the pleural cavity.

Because of the danger of infection in a clot, and because it will organise and perhaps calcify if it is allowed to remain even though sterile, removal with the least possible disintegration is essential. This should be done through a free inter-costal incision, penicillin being afterwards instilled into the pleural cavity, and the wound then completely closed. If an effusion develops subsequently, it must be aspirated ; if infection occurs, an airtight drain will become necessary.

Collapse of the upper lobe of a lung is as a rule much more troublesome to overcome than collapse of a lower lobe. With collapse of an upper lobe, whether pneumothorax is associated with the hæmothorax or not, the sooner operative removal of the clot and debris can be performed safely, the better for the patient. If, however, the upper lobe is well expanded, open operation may (by the inevitable introduction of air) result in a total pneumothorax and collapse of that upper lobe. For a purely basal mass of clot, therefore, it is well to defer operation until the pleural layers at the apex are firmly adherent to each other, combating infection meanwhile by penicillin therapy.

It is clear, then, that if the lung does not expand satisfactorily the possible causes are (i) extensive damage to the lung, with subsequent fibrosis ; (ii) fibrinous deposits on the pleura, and the subsequent organisation of these while the lung is still collapsed ; and (iii) the recurrence of effusions or their non-removal.

Early and efficient treatment of the damaged lung will ensure speedier healing and return of function. The recognition of a " frozen lung " at a stage before organisation of the deposit by firm fibrous tissue has taken place will allow of satisfactory decortication and re-expansion of the lung. The detection and aspiration of effusions as they develop will guard against the disabilities which follow neglect of them.

INFECTED HÆMOTHORAX

Infection of a hæmothorax may arise from spread of infection from the track of the wound, especially if excision of an infected wound has been late or imperfect ; it may be carried in by the missile ; it may spread from the air passages in lacerated lung tissue or from the blood stream ; carelessness of technique during treatment may be the cause. The first two sources are by far the commonest ; hence the comparatively high incidence of infection in hæmothorax due to penetrating wounds as compared with non-penetrating injuries.

Diagnosis—Evidence of infection can appear within a few hours of the injury, or it may occasionally be delayed for some weeks. The change from an apparently sterile hæmothorax to an infected one often occurs with dramatic suddenness. This may be because, as has been pointed out earlier, the organisms have not infected the pleura until they reach the surface of a mass of intrapleural clot. The onset of severe constitutional symptoms, together with a rise in the pulse and respiratory rates, and a change from continued to a remittent pyrexia should serve to differentiate infection from a secondary irritative pleural effusion, both of which may give rise to a sudden increase in intrapleural pressure and the appearance of symptoms of compression. A blood count may show a rise in the number of polymorphonuclear leucocytes. The only certain evidence of infection is to find organisms in smears or on culture of the aspirated fluid. Anærobic organisms produce an offensive odour and a purplish colour of the fluid, and they may determine such a rapid formation of gas that relief of dyspnœa by intercostal drainage becomes urgent. Whenever there is the slightest doubt as to the character of the fluid, or the smallest possibility that infection has supervened, a diagnostic puncture must be made.

If infection is suspected, it is not wise to wait for bacteriological confirmation. The sulphonamides which have hitherto been given prophylactically (see p. 496) should be increased in dosage, preferably in the form of sulphathiazole or sulphadiazine ; all the fluid obtainable from the pleura should be aspirated and treatment by penicillin should be instituted if the organisms are penicillin-sensitive.

If infection has supervened in spite of early and efficient treatment of the original chest injury, it is wise to have X-ray films of deep penetration taken again. A foreign body may easily be hidden behind the heart shadow when the films are not of sufficient penetration. If so, the likely cause of the infection is revealed, and the condition will probably not subside until the foreign body is removed.

If treatment has been inadequate or delayed, blood clot, sloughs, debris and perhaps foreign bodies may still be within the pleural cavity, and thoracotomy through an intercostal incision may be necessary. Meanwhile, the treatment is to keep the pleura as dry as possible by means of successive aspirations, not only with a view to diminishing the toxæmia but in order to ensure that the ultimate localised empyema is a small one which will heal rapidly when eventually it is drained by rib resection.

The frequency of aspiration is determined initially by the amount of fluid present, and later by the rate of its reaccumulation and also by the recurrence of toxic symptoms. With a large empyema, aspiration will be necessary twice a day until the pleural cavity diminishes in size sufficiently to be emptied at less frequent intervals. If the empyema is total and of some days' or even weeks' standing, with markedly thickened visceral pleura, removal of the fluid will produce a high intrapleural negative pressure, with painful drag on the unyielding lung and mediastinum. Under these circumstances it may be possible to control the infection with penicillin, and then free the lung by decortication, so allowing it to re-expand.

After a few days of successive aspirations the fluid will either become less turbid or more purulent. In the first instance, aspiration should be continued ; in the latter, particularly if gas-forming organisms are present, an airtight intercostal drain should be inserted and connected to a water-seal bottle. Once there is a localised empyema cavity, with the mediastinum fixed by adhesions and the pus thick, open operation is called for. In nearly every instance of infected hæmothorax rib resection will eventually be necessary if there is to be perfect healing in the shortest time and with the minimum of disability. The principles of post-operative management directed towards the achievement of this result are described in Chapter XXV (p. 398).

Chronic empyema may follow inefficient drainage, re-infection, or a retained foreign body. It is discussed in detail in the earlier chapter on Empyema (p. 402). Its crippling nature underlines the cardinal importance of early diagnosis and of immediate and efficient treatment of the acute infection.

Throughout the course of treatment of an infected hæmothorax, everything should be done to support the patient's general condition—good nursing, blood transfusion when necessary, large amounts of fluids including glucose drinks, nourishing food and fresh air. If there is infection by gas-forming organisms, polyvalent gas-gangrene antitoxin (20,000 to 30,000 units) should be given intravenously every six hours, combined with full doses of sulphonamide and penicillin.

PENETRATING AND OPEN CHEST WOUNDS

Penetrating wounds may result from all types of missile— bullets, pieces of shrapnel, shell fragments, and fragments of stone, glass, wood or metal as the result of high explosive damage to buildings, roads or other objects. Bomb and shell fragments are responsible, as a rule, for the most serious injuries, owing to the widespread destruction of tissue caused by their irregular shape. Any missile may carry with it into the chest pieces of clothing, splinters of bone and various forms of dirt and debris ; these increase the extent of the laceration and the danger of infection. By reason of their irregular shape and slower velocity, shell and bomb fragments are retained in the chest more often than bullets. Although bullets and shrapnel balls may produce small, and often relatively clean, wounds, the explosive effect of a bullet which has been set spinning by a ricochet may determine wounds of entry and exit even more extensive and lacerated than will a shell fragment of similar size. If the bullet strikes bone and is thus set spinning after it has entered the chest, only the exit wound shows this disruptive effect. Moreover, particularly as their speed lessens, metal fragments and bullets may be deviated by their impact with bony structures, so that they run an angular course through the body. They may even run round the chest, along the fascial planes. In these instances a straight line drawn from the entrance to the exit wound will not give a true indication of the track. For the same reason a missile which is retained in the body may eventually be located in an unexpected situation.

Purely parietal injuries, such as the non-penetrating gunshot wound, have already been mentioned. As a rule, they are the least serious of chest injuries. Sometimes, however, they cause bruising of the pleura or of the lung. Wounds which lacerate the muscular masses of the back and of the scapular region are more serious, in that they are liable to cause severe hæmorrhage, or deep suppuration, or anærobic infection. Through-and-through bullet wounds which cleanly traverse the periphery of the lung, and tiny bomb fragments which penetrate and are retained in the lung, may cause surprisingly little damage. The elasticity of the pleural membranes and the local collapse of the lung seals the small hole made by the wound, and there is no appreciable escape of blood or air into the pleural cavity. The patient may expectorate a small amount of blood, and radiograms may show the shadow of infiltration around the wound track. Sometimes a localised pulmonary hæmatoma is formed. In some instances, however, a moderate hæmothorax or pneumothorax results.

More serious are the penetrating wounds in which an opening through the parietal pleura is established, so exposing the patient to the dangers of an **open chest wound** ("sucking pneumothorax"); or in which the lung is badly lacerated, with or without involvement of the large vessels or bronchi. The seriousness of the open chest wound has already been described earlier in this chapter. Severe laceration of the lung leads to hæmothorax, pneumothorax, collapse of the lung and mediastinal displacement, and conduces to later pleural and pulmonary infection. If one of the main bronchi is torn, or if a pneumothorax is associated with a tear in the mediastinal pleura, air may escape into the mediastinum (**mediastinal emphysema**). Its gravity lies in the fact that it compresses the great veins, so interfering with the flow of blood to the heart (see Chap. XXXIII).

A missile which penetrates the chest may injure the œsophagus or the thoracic duct. Early recognition of these injuries is not easy, for œsophageal contents or chyle in the pleural cavity are usually overshadowed by the blood which also accumulates there. A bullet passing through the chest may hit the vertebral column and cause spinal concussion, or it may directly lacerate the spinal cord.

The *treatment* of these penetrating wounds is primarily that of the shock and hæmorrhage, together with immediate attention to the thoracic emergences of an open chest wound or a tension pneumothorax. As soon as the patient is fit for it, radiological studies should be made to determine the number and situation of any retained foreign bodies, and the condition of the lungs and pleural cavities.

As soon as resuscitation measures have succeeded and radiograms have been taken, most patients with thoracic wounds will need to be submitted to operation. The earlier the excision of a wound after injury the greater is the chance of avoiding later sepsis. Even the more trivial wounds of the chest wall should be excised : if the patient is not operated upon within six or at most twelve hours of his wound, drainage should be provided.

More extensive operative exploration is not, as a rule, necessary for small penetrating wounds, with or without hæmothorax. Wounds which call for a full exploration of the chest, either through a deliberately enlarged wound of entrance, or through a planned thoracotomy opening, are sucking wounds ; gutter wounds and those with splintered bone ; extensively lacerated wounds with an open pleural cavity and lacerated viscera ; wounds accompanied by intrathoracic foreign bodies larger than the nail of the little finger, especially if the X-ray film shows a diffuse infiltration of the wound track or a pulmonary hæmatoma ; wounds which have caused a tear of the bronchus and mediastinal emphysema ; and wounds associated with damage to the diaphragm, pericardium or heart.

These indications apply only if the patient is seen reasonably early after his wound, for once infection or suppuration is established, or secondary inflammatory changes supervene in the lung, large operative measures are not practicable —though with the advent of penicillin, much more can be undertaken with safety. The aim of operation is to examine thoroughly the intrathoracic structures, to excise lacerated, non-viable tissue, together with any foreign body, and to suck out debris and effused fluid from the pleural cavity. Patients seen late after their wound present the problem of intrathoracic infection and suppuration, and their treatment is based on the general principles which underlie the treatment of pulmonary, pleural and mediastinal infections (see Chaps. XVII to XIX, XXV and XXXIII).

FOREIGN BODIES IN THE CHEST

If a foreign body is allowed to remain in the lung it inevitably causes an inflammatory reaction. If it is infected, pus forms round it, and it comes to lie in a small abscess cavity. The abscess may extend, and sooner or later drain through a bronchus ; the missile then becomes gradually enclosed in a capsule of fibrous tissue. This may occur also if the initial infection was of low grade without the formation of pus. A metal fragment may remain innocuous for many years, yet eventually (by reason of infection in its vicinity or the re-awakening of infection by organisms previously imprisoned in its capsule) produce hæmorrhage from ulceration of a blood vessel, or lung abscess, or bronchiectasis. A foreign body left in the mediastinum may finally ulcerate into one of the great vessels, or if it is close to the posterior aspect of the heart, may cause persistent tachycardia and arrhythmia.

A retained foreign body is therefore a menace, especially if it is of any size. If it is larger than the little finger nail, and especially if it is jagged, it will almost certainly have carried dirt or clothing in with it. If the surgeon can safely remove it, therefore, he should do so. If not removed at the original operation within a few hours of the wound it should be left alone for at least six weeks, until the secondary inflammatory changes in the lung or elsewhere have had time to subside. As a preliminary to this delayed operation, a prophylactic course of sulphonamide or penicillin should be given during the three preceding days, and if the injury was sustained more than three months previously, antitetanic serum (3000 units) should be readministered. The methods used for localising foreign bodies and the technical details of operation are beyond the scope of this book.

ABDOMINO-THORACIC WOUNDS

Wounds and injuries involving both the abdomen and the thorax in the same patient have a high mortality. They may be caused by separate missiles. A missile may pass from the chest to the abdomen, or from the abdomen to the chest, with damage to the structures immediately above and below the diaphragm. They may arise from tangential wounds in which the missile and the indriven fractured ribs tear through the diaphragm. Crush injuries of the chest may also lacerate abdominal organs or rupture hollow viscera.

Shock is always severe, overshadowing the relevant symptoms and often masking the signs of abdominal hæmorrhage. Yet in these early hours after this type of injury operation is imperative, and must be done as soon as the patient can be made fit for it. The surgeon has to assess the case as best he may, knowing that in many instances a tentative diagnosis only can be made before operative exploration. The position of the entrance and exit wounds may suggest that both thorax and abdomen have been traversed ; or radiograms of a patient with an entrance wound only in the thorax may reveal a foreign body in the abdomen ; or there may be bilateral immobility and rigidity of the abdomen and absence of the normal liver dulness in a patient with a chest wound ; or a single wound of entry in the abdomen may be associated with dyspnœa and hæmoptysis. Save when the main symptoms are those of abdominal injury and the chest symptoms suggest that no gross thoracic injury is present, it is advisable to explore the chest first. Often it is possible to enlarge the diaphragmatic wound and then to repair injuries in the upper abdomen. When the missile has entered or left the abdominal cavity low down, a separate abdominal incision will be necessary after the diaphragm has been repaired and the chest wound has been closed. The aim of operation is to excise the edges of the tear in the diaphragm, to deal with the intrathoracic injuries on the general principles already described in this chapter, and with the abdominal injuries according to their special indications—all with a view to saving the patient from what is in any event an almost desperate situation.

CARDIAC AND PERICARDIAL INJURIES

Wounds which result in laceration of the heart or great vessels are nearly always immediately fatal. Crush injuries or direct blows which result in cardiac or pericardial bruising may produce transient damage only ; or they may cause rupture of a cusp or of the heart muscle itself. Contusion of the myocardium may cause pain of an anginal type, cardiac dilatation, irregular rhythms, and an electrocardiogram similar to that of coronary thrombosis. It may also result in pericardial effusion, serofibrinous or hæmorrhagic. Occasionally, when the contusion extends to the endocardium, an intracardiac thrombus is formed, with resulting emboli into the systemic or pulmonary system, or both, according to the chambers involved.

Pericarditis, with or without effusion, may also follow bruising of the pericardium, or the penetration of a foreign body through the lung and near to the heart. In the latter instance, it is presumably due to inflammatory reaction to the trauma of tissue in the vicinity, or to low-grade infection. Extension of severe infection, as, for example, from an infected hæmothorax, will cause suppurative pericarditis. The accumulation of fluid in the pericardium, whether it is an effusion, or blood which escapes from a laceration of the heart, compresses the heart, progressively reduces the venous return and thereby the cardiac output, and lowers the arterial blood pressure while at the same time increasing the venous pressure. The condition is given the name **cardiac tamponade.** The more rapid the accumulation the less time there is to bring into play certain compensatory mechanisms, and the greater the danger. If there is a wound into the pericardium which is still open, it will allow the blood or fluid to drain away without compressing the heart.

The patient with acute cardiac compression becomes intensely restless. He has a sense of oppression over the præcordium ; he feels that he is suffocating. The veins of the neck are distended, he is cyanosed, the skin is cold and clammy, the heart sounds are less and less distinct, the pulse rate becomes ever more rapid and the volume less, until finally, unless the condition is quickly relieved, the heart fails entirely.

Pericarditis, with or without effusion, does not call for direct treatment unless it is causing distress or producing cardiac compression, though careful nursing and complete rest are obviously essential. When the effusion is progressive and is embarrassing the heart, aspiration should be carried out under local anæsthesia, through the angle between the xiphisternum and the left costal margin. If, however, the lesion is a hæmopericardium following injury, aspiration should not be done save as an urgent emergency preparatory to open operation, in which examination and cleaning of the wound track is carried out according to the usual principles. Operation is the more urgent when fragments of shell are retained, owing to the dangers of infection. Open operation with drainage is necessary also for suppurative pericarditis.

PROPHYLAXIS AGAINST INFECTION

In addition to the routine administration of antitetanic serum, patients with chest or other wounds should be given prophylactic doses of sulphonamide as early as possible after the injury. In order to obtain rapid absorption the first dose should be 1·5 gm. dissolved in hot 1 per cent. citric acid, followed by 0·5 gm. two hours later, and then 0·5 gm. at four-hourly intervals for a period of about four days. If the patient is not seen for several hours after his injury, the first few doses should be doubled. It should be borne in mind that sulphonamides may cause methæmoglobinæmia and cyanosis (see p. 224). This may lead occasionally to confusion with more serious causes of cyanosis following chest injuries. As has been said earlier, the administration of penicillin makes surgical intervention much safer when infection has been established ; but it must never become a substitute for sound surgical principles.

" BLAST LUNG "

The effect of blast upon the lung has been studied particularly in relation to air raids on land and to depth charges at sea. There is fairly general agreement upon the nature of the injuries, but some difference of opinion about the mechanism of their production. On the whole, it appears to be clear that they are due mainly to the wave of intense compression of the air which constitutes the blast, and less (if at all) to the subsequent wave of negative pressure or suction which follows immediately upon the compression, provided that the latter has space in which to dissipate itself. The generally accepted opinion is that the intense damage to the lung is due to direct and sudden compression of the chest rather than any direct action on the interior of the lung.

The pulmonary lesions may be accompanied by trauma to the chest wall, but often they are found unassociated with any damage whatever to the bony or soft parts of the thoracic cage, particularly in young adults and children with resilient bones. The surface of the lung commonly shows well-defined rib markings which may be a quarter of an inch or more in depth. On the pleural surfaces there are ecchymoses and petechiæ, and intra-alveolar hæmorrhage is invariable. Indeed, the fundamental lesion is a hæmorrhagic exudate into the alveolar and interstitial tissue. These traumatic hæmorrhages may be localised to the side facing the explosion, provided that the victim is sufficiently far away from it. The lesions may become confluent, characteristically so at the costophrenic angles and (according to some observers) at the hilum. In this way, wedge-shaped, consolidated areas are produced. On section of the lung, multiple diffusely distributed points of hæmorrhage are seen. According to Shaw Dunn they are due to inhaled blood and are therefore secondary (Fig. 132).

Shock is severe. Most of the bleeding comes from the

32

capillaries of the pulmonary artery which lie relatively un-protected in the walls of the alveoli. There is evidence that the bleeding is apt to continue for some time. This explains why, in patients who survive the immediate shock of the explosive, marked respiratory symptoms may not develop for forty-eight hours or more. These consist of cough, expectoration, hæmoptysis, severe dyspnœa and cyanosis. Radiograms reveal the shadows due to those confluent hæmorrhages which are of a size large enough to be visible on the film. Pyrexia often marks the irritation caused by blood in the interstitial tissue. Later,

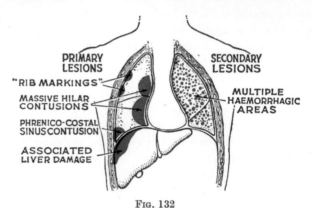

FIG. 132

The principal lesions found at necropsy in blast injuries of the lungs. (*After Shaw Dunn.*)

the lesions may become secondarily infected, with the pro-duction of patches of true bronchopneumonia. Treatment is by rest, small doses of morphia ($\frac{1}{6}$ gr.), and oxygen. Trans-fusions of blood or fluid must be given with caution and constant watchfulness lest they restart the alveolar bleeding or cause pulmonary œdema. If there is much pulmonary œdema and cyanosis—the former a reaction to infiltration of the interstitial tissues with blood—venesection is indicated. Secondary bronchopneumonia will be treated according to the usual methods.

Carbon monoxide poisoning—Patients removed from the cellars of bombed buildings or other confined spaces after an explosion may be suffering from varying degrees of carbon monoxide poisoning (see also p. 361). Like victims of blast lung, they are poor subjects for surgery if they happen to have chest injuries which ordinarily would call for surgical intervention.

THE AFTER-CARE OF PATIENTS WITH CHEST INJURIES

These patients are likely to be best cared for in a chest unit where a specially trained nursing and medical personnel is available. Apart from the detailed care after operation and the instructed watchfulness to prevent (or, if necessary, to deal with immediately) various complications such as absorption collapse of the lung or tension pneumothorax, planned re-habilitation is of the first importance. The chest casualty has usually a prolonged and tedious stay in hospital before he can be made fit for discharge. Muscles become soft, the respiratory mechanism has lost its capacity to cope with hard work and exertion, and the patient often becomes dispirited. As soon as the condition of the wound and recovery from toxæmia permit, his re-education must begin. At first, this takes the form of special breathing exercises and massage, while he is still confined to bed. They aim at teaching him to regain the *balanced* use of the respiratory muscles. When, by reason of a unilateral injury, one side of the chest is left functioning badly or not at all, those unilateral muscles must be selectively trained. When he is able to get up, the exercises are controlled by radiological observations. Adhesions, for example, to one dome of the diaphragm may be found to be restricting movement ; periodic X-ray screening will show if concentration on that side brings about improvement.

As recovery progresses, occupational exercises bring more muscles into use at the same time and keep the patient interested. Later, physical training, walks, occupational interests, recreation and rest periods are added in a rehabilitation centre where he is one of a community of men who are getting back to normal. All the time he is under the care of trained observers who can determine *on medical grounds* how much he can and should do without undue strain upon the heart and lungs. Throughout the whole period the medical supervisor controls his progress, not only by clinical observation but also by vital capacity and other tests. It is remarkable how often a man who has had a serious chest injury can be restored to a normal life by patient and skilled rehabilitation.

CHAPTER XXXIII

MEDIASTINAL LESIONS

FROM the clinical standpoint there are two salient anatomical features of the mediastinum. In the first place, it contains certain structures (phrenic nerve, left recurrent laryngeal nerve, œsophagus, superior vena cava, azygos veins, thoracic duct, vagus nerve, trachea and main bronchi, and heart and pericardium) which when pressed upon by a swelling or invaded by a new growth result in characteristic " pressure symptoms and signs " (see p. 138).

The second important feature is the division of the mediastinum by the fascial layers into various compartments, the most important of which are prolongated into the neck. The **anterior visceral space** extends from the pharynx and larynx above to the bifurcation of the trachea below (Fig. 133). It contains many lymph nodes and vessels, to which infection from the nose, throat or ear can extend ; and along it cellulitis of the neck may readily make its way. The **posterior (retrovisceral) space** is continuous from the base of the skull to the diaphragm. Behind it is the prevertebral fascia, in front the pharynx and œsophagus, and laterally the carotid sheaths. Infection can thus travel along this space from a retropharyngeal abscess, or from perforation of the posterior pharyngeal or œsophageal walls either by a foreign body or as the result of ulceration of an œsophageal growth. Behind the sternum is another space, but it is walled off from the neck by the attachment of the cervical fascia to the posterior surface of the manubrium sterni. It is infected as a rule only by injury or infection of the anterior chest wall at the level of the first and second costal cartilages.

The loose areolar and connective tissue of the mediastinum does not encourage the formation of a protective barrier to the spread of inflammation. Infection usually spreads rapidly and widely. *Diffuse suppurative mediastinitis* is therefore a fulminating and fatal disease.

Localised pyogenic abscesses do, however, occur. They are always secondary, and the student must go carefully into the

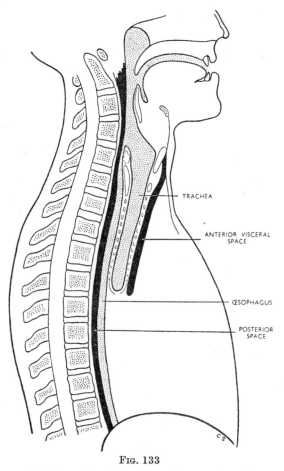

Fig. 133

Sagittal section of thorax showing anterior and posterior spaces.

history and the clinical features in order to discover the primary lesion which causes them. Acute *abscess in the anterior visceral space* arises as a rule from infections in the neck, larynx or lung. In the *posterior space* it usually follows perforation of the œsophagus or suppuration of the lymph nodes.

In addition to the manifestations of general toxæmia, pain is a prominent symptom. In abscess of the anterior space it is usually substernal and throbbing ; in posterior abscess it is felt particularly on swallowing and coughing, and it may radiate from between the shoulder blades forwards along the intercostal nerves. With anterior abscess the symptoms and signs of mediastinal pressure may be conspicuous, whereas posterior abscess, pressing upon œsophagus, trachea and maybe the lungs, produces symptoms (dysphagia, cough) rather than signs. Radiograms may reveal air in the mediastinum if there is an œsophageal perforation, or the displacement forwards of the trachea by an abscess in the posterior space.

Rarely a mediastinal abscess will rupture into the lung or a main bronchus, and so drain itself spontaneously. Since mediastinitis is usually only part of a more widespread infection, the prognosis in any event is serious and the death rate high. Nevertheless, when the abscess is the outstanding lesion, its recognition and early drainage by surgical measures will give the patient a chance of recovery.

Chronic abscess may result from tuberculous disease of the vertebral bodies. The pus collects between the bone and the prevertebral fascia, but only rarely does it burst through into the posterior space.

Chronic diffuse mediastinitis may be syphilitic, tuberculous or associated with rheumatic pericarditis. The two latter examples give the clinical picture of adherent pericardium, a term which signifies not merely symphysis of the pericardial layers but a true mediastino-pericarditis. The indurative lesion eventually causes pressure symptoms and signs, venous obstruction being the most constant of them. Once the condition is established there is no specific treatment, save for the syphilitic patients. Surgical attempts to free the heart from the adhesions which embarrass its free action have been undertaken in selected cases, with not too damning an operative mortality, and with reasonable benefit to some 40 per cent. of the patients.

MEDIASTINAL EMPHYSEMA

Air may escape into the mediastinum not only from perforation of the trachea or œsophagus, but also from rupture of overdistended alveoli and from pneumothorax accompanied by rupture of the mediastinal pleura. Air which escapes from ruptured alveoli into the interstitial tissue travels along the vascular sheaths towards the root of the lung. It will continue to accumulate as long as the channel of air remains open, will eventually compress mediastinal structures, particularly the blood vessels, and will track into the retroperitoneal space and upwards into the root of the neck and into the axilla.

The main symptom is pain, which may be anginal in type if there is severe compression of the large arterial trunks. Air in the sheath of the aorta may lead to an erroneous diagnosis of coronary thrombosis. Dyspnœa is also prominent if the accumulation of air is considerable. Subcutaneous emphysema may be seen in the neck, and a tympanitic note is elicited over the mediastinum, sometimes with obliteration of the cardiac dulness. On auscultation, crepitations are heard and the heart sounds are distant or inaudible. Occasionally a peculiar crunching sound is heard along the left border of the heart, synchronous with systole (" systolic clicks ").

Treatment should be directed to the underlying cause of the emphysema, for as soon as the supply of air is cut off, that already accumulated will be gradually absorbed. If the patient's condition is serious by reason of intense mediastinal pressure, an incision into the subcutaneous tissues at the root of the neck may give an opportunity for the escape of air, and therefore for the relief of the symptoms.

Mediastinal tumours have been described in Chapter X.

CHAPTER XXXIV

DIAPHRAGMATIC LESIONS

OWING to the cardinal importance of the diaphragm as a respiratory muscle, disturbance of its action is serious, whether by damage to its nerve supply or by alteration in the balance of the pull of the various muscles of respiration.

Primary inflammation is rare. It appears to be a favourite site, however, for trichinæ, a fact which explains the diaphragmatic pain and the dyspnœa found at times in trichiniasis. Infection and suppuration in its vicinity have been discussed in Chapter XXVI.

Spasm of the diaphragm is comparatively common. *Hiccough* is due to an involuntary contraction of the diaphragm which sucks in air so suddenly that the vocal cords are drawn together. It may be caused by local or reflex irritation— diaphragmatic pleurisy, upper abdominal peritonitis, irritation of the gastric mucosa. It may result from excitation of the respiratory centres in the medulla, as by local vascular lesions such as thrombosis, by tumours, by the toxins of uræmia, or by encephalitis. In epidemic encephalitis, hiccough is but one expression of the myoclonic spasms which are a frequent feature of the disease.

Treatment is primarily that of the underlying cause. In the mild, simple examples, holding the breath or diluting the irritating gastric contents is usually sufficient to give relief. When the hiccough is persistent, gastric lavage, inhalation of carbon dioxide, administration of morphia, or anæsthetisation by chloroform may have to be tried. In intractable instances, accompanied by general exhaustion, the establishment of a temporary phrenic paralysis may bring relief.

Tonic spasm occurs in epilepsy, tetanus, strychnine poisoning and eclampsia. It is accompanied by marked dyspnœa, and, if prolonged and associated with intercostal spasm also, is likely to end in asphyxia. Treatment of the local condition is by counter-irritation, by sedatives such as chloral, or by anæsthetisation by ether or chloroform.

Paralysis of the diaphragm is now most commonly due to deliberate surgical interference with the phrenic nerve. Phrenic nerve palsy may arise also in diphtheria, poliomyelitis, or by involvement in local inflammation, injury or new growth. The latter is more common on the right side (see p. 139). With bilateral phrenic paralysis the consequences to respiration are serious if other respiratory muscles are paralysed, or if there is considerable pulmonary infection.

Paralysis of the diaphragm is best revealed by radiology. The dome on the affected side rises high into the thorax : there is paradoxical respiration (the paralysed leaf is pushed upwards by the intra-abdominal pressure in inspiration, and descends in expiration—the reverse of the normal movements seen on the sound side)—and there is exaggerated paradoxical movement on sniffing (sniff test).

DIAPHRAGMATIC HERNIA

Embryologically the anterior part of the diaphragm is formed from the septum transversum, a mass of mesoblastic tissue which begins its growth up towards the head, and gradually descends. From the primitive dorsal mesentery will arise the crural portions of the muscle. The pleuroperitoneal membranes will form the lateral portions, growing inwards to fuse with the dorsal mesentery (Fig. 134). The periphery is formed by infolding of the lateral walls of the torso. Fusion may be incomplete, leaving a gap : this is more common on the left side. On the right side the liver guards the abdominal aspect of the right dome. Centrally and anteriorly the pericardium and heart form a solid mass. The left side and the posterior part in the mid-line are least protected, and are therefore the commonest sites of hernia.

For clinical purposes diaphragmatic herniæ may be classified into (i) congenital and (ii) traumatic. In addition, there are certain non-traumatic acquired hernia which could hardly arise unless the diaphragm had been previously weakened by developmental defect or local muscular trauma.

Large congenital herniæ are usually due to imperfect fusion

of the septum transversum and the pleuroperitoneal membranes. They may be compatible with life, though many of them are recognised only at necropsy after death in early infancy. The stomach is the most frequent organ to be found in the hernia, though on occasion omentum, spleen, colon and small intestine may also be found in the thorax.

The condition may be surprisingly symptomless, or it may cause dyspnœa and cyanosis from encroachment on the lungs. The leading symptoms, on the other hand, may be digestive, owing to mechanical embarrassment of the herniated stomach. Physical signs may be somewhat bizarre, and radiology is essential to establish the diagnosis (including a barium meal, and, if need be, a barium enema). When the hernia contains air-filled portions of stomach or intestines, the differentiation has to be made from localised pneumothorax and from basal cavities or cysts.

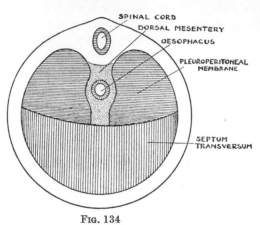

FIG. 134

To show development of diaphragm.

The most common form of congenital lesion is the **periœsophageal (hiatus) hernia.** Here, a knuckle of stomach protrudes into the thorax through a defect adjacent to the œsophageal foramen. It has to be distinguished from a diverticulum of the stomach or of the œsophagus, and from " thoracic stomach " (in which the œsophagus is shortened, and ends in the thorax).

This type of hernia is sometimes symptomless, but more often there is evidence of intermittent but progressive incarceration and obstruction of the stomach. There may be attacks of dysphagia, vague discomfort, or pain after meals. The pain is relieved by the escape of gas when the patient changes position, as by lying down. This picture of pain or discomfort associated with belching may be mistaken for that of cholecystitis. There may be periodic vomiting, again with relief of the pain. The mucous membrane is liable to become congested from pressure at the neck of the sac, and hæmatemesis is therefore a frequent symptom. Later, the pain becomes more severe, owing to associated spasm of the diaphragm and of the cardiac end of the œsophagus.

Many of these patients are suspected of having a peptic ulcer. When they are X-rayed the hernia is revealed by radiograms taken in the prone position, in which the barium defines the contours of the cardiac end of the stomach. It is important to define the lower end of the œsophagus and its relationship to the diaphragm and to the herniated portion of the stomach.

Traumatic hernia may result from perforating wounds, or from crush injuries of the lower thorax. In the latter, any tear in the diaphragm is likely to be extensive.

In **" thoracic stomach,"** the œsophagus is shortened and ends in the thorax, with the result that part of the stomach is situated above the diaphragm. The condition is therefore not a true hernia.

Eventration of the diaphragm signifies an abnormally high position of a dome or of part of a dome, owing to a defect whereby the muscle is thinned out to what is little more than a fibrous sheet. It is distinguished from phrenic paralysis in that the muscle moves normally, in contrast to the paradoxical passive movements of a paralysed dome.

Treatment—In patients with a small diaphragmatic hernia and no symptoms, active treatment is not indicated. Where the hernia is of moderate size, the stomach the only organ involved, and the symptoms mild, regulation of diet (frequent small meals, rest in the recumbent position after meals) and reduction of weight may be sufficient to keep the symptoms under control. If, however, the lesion is progressive in spite of medical measures, operation should be performed unless the patient's general condition contraindicates it.

In a certain number of patients phrenic paralysis will give considerable though not as a rule complete relief by abolishing secondary spasm of the diaphragm and so reducing the pressure on the neck of the hernia. It may also be used as a preliminary to radical operation, or as a palliative when the patient is unfit for a serious major operation. If the colon or small intestine is contained in the hernia, there is danger of eventual intestinal obstruction, and early radical operation is all the more advisable. The diaphragm can be approached from the abdomen or from the thorax : some surgeons are impressed with the frequency of post-operative thoracic complications and choose the abdominal route, while others choose the thoracic approach because it gives an excellent exposure.

In patients with a shortened œsophagus, either congenital or as the result of cicatrisation, it may be impossible to bring the stomach back into the abdomen, even after relaxation of the diaphragm by phrenic paralysis.

APPENDIX I

NOTES ON THE PRESENT POSITION OF CERTAIN CHEMOTHERAPEUTIC AGENTS

SULPHONAMIDES

IN order to combat infection in the body, it is necessary that the infecting organism (i) should be susceptible to concentrations of the therapeutic agent which do not damage the patient's tissues, and (ii) come into contact with enough of the agent (that is, the necessary *effective* concentration). Thus, the best conditions for effective therapeutic action are found in a spreading lesion such as lobar pneumonia, in which there is no necrosis of tissue and no cutting off of the blood supply, in the earlier stages at least. Here, the drug can gain adequate access to the infecting organisms. In the presence of pus and necrotic tissue, however, the sulphonamides are particularly ineffective ; staphylococcal lesions, in which there is a central area of pus and necrotic tissue, afford an example of this, for it is clear that adequate contact at the site of infection is not easy to achieve.

Sulphapyridine and Sulphathiazole can now be discarded in the treatment of systemic infections ; not only are they often not well tolerated by the patient, but they also produce lower levels of concentration in the blood than do Sulphadiazine, Sulphamezathine and Sulphamerazine.

RESISTANCE

Unfortunately, nearly all species of organisms can become habituated or *resistant to sulphonamides*, though this occurs more readily in some species than in others. The gonococcus, for example, has developed a large and increasing percentage of resistant strains ; at the other extreme, the meningococcus has remained outstandingly vulnerable and sensitive. In between, come the pneumococcus and the haemolytic streptococcus ; here, resistant strains have appeared, though they are not common—perhaps because penicillin and other antibiotics may be used successfully against them when sulphonamides have failed.

Resistance to penicillin is also troublesome in infections by the gonococcus and by staphylococcus pyogenes. So far, however, no such change appears to have developed among pneumococci and haemolytic streptococci.

Resistance to streptomycin is much more serious. All species of bacteria can become highly resistant to the drug, in many instances with startling rapidity. Tubercle bacilli may acquire resistance more slowly, for their growth is slower than that of other bacteria; happily, it has been found that simultaneous administration of para-amino-salicylic acid greatly lessens the frequency of this change.

Newer antibiotics such as chloramphenicol (chloromycetin) and aureomycin were originally thought to be free from this disadvantage, but already there is some evidence that acquired resistance to them can develop, though slowly and only of moderate degree. Terramycin is said to behave similarly.

Other difficulties have been encountered. Under certain conditions, penicillin, streptomycin and chloramphenicol may actually make a patient worse—by reason of the development of what is known as *dependence*. Certain strains of bacteria may come to depend nutritionally upon drugs which are normally lethal to them. Sometimes, indeed, they are actually stimulated to growth by these drugs, if and when the concentration of drug in the blood is lower than that required to inhibit growth.

Penicillin. This is a directly bactericidal agent; it has an optimum concentration for its antibacterial effect—" not too little, not too much." The concentration necessary depends partly on the sensitivity of the infecting organism, and partly on the number of bacteria which need to be killed (and this in turn depends on the stage of the infection). More penicillin will be needed, the more established or extensive the infection.

It has been found that to maintain an effective blood level of penicillin—for it is rapidly excreted via the kidneys—relatively high doses must be given : 25,000 units three-hourly, 100,000 units six-hourly, 250,000 units eight-hourly, or 500,000 units twelve-hourly.

Preparations of penicillin are now available in which absorption is delayed by the use of oily suspensions, or of powders (suspended in water before injection) containing procaine penicillin. A really high blood level is not attained ; but an effective level, lasting for 24 hours, is achieved by an injection of 250,000 units. These preparations are useful, therefore, in treating patients in their own homes, or in reducing the number of needle pricks necessary. They will not produce a high blood level, however, and therefore are ineffective against relatively resistant organisms. When a high blood level is aimed at, large doses of sodium penicillin should be given.

The purity of modern penicillin allows it to be given subcutaneously as well as intramuscularly, without ill-effects. Given orally, much larger doses are necessary (say, 10 times the intramuscular dose), and even so, the effects are uncertain. Nevertheless, there is a place for oral administration, on an empty stomach, to babies and to patients to whom the hollow needle may be unduly distressing.

Being an ideal antiseptic (lethal to bacteria, harmless to tissue), penicillin may be simply and effectively used by local application. It may be injected, for example, into an empyema cavity; a large empyema will need about 100,000 units in order to keep up a high concentration in the fluid for 24 hours.

Infections of the upper respiratory passages may be treated either with a penicillin spray, or a snuff containing 5000 units of calcium penicillin per gram of sulphathiazole. Infections of the bronchi may be treated by inhalation—100,000 units in concentrated solution being administered several times a day via an efficient inhaler. Penicillin is especially useful for infections by streptococcus pyogenes, and for pneumococcal infections which are either severe or resistant to sulphonamides. For streptococcal infections, sulphonamides are not very effective, and to penicillin, resistant strains are becoming more prevalent. If high doses of penicillin fail, aureomycin is advisable.

Streptomycin must be given by intramuscular injection, the daily dose being commonly 1 gramme. Though it is a bactericidal agent, bacteria may rapidly and permanently acquire a high degree of resistance. It also has the disadvantage of a toxic effect on the eighth nerve (vertigo, occasionally deafness), if higher doses than the above are used for long periods. Its main indications are in rapidly extending tuberculous lung infections and in ulcerative tracheo-bronchitis. It is also useful in making surgical intervention for tuberculous lesions feasible and safer. In chronic disease, especially with cavitation, its value is much more limited and its use then depends on the assessment of the individual case. While the danger of establishing streptomycin resistant tubercle bacilli is considerable, p-amino-salicylic acid given orally (12 grammes daily) and in combination, reduces the incidence of the resistance; at the same time, it is in itself a useful drug against the tubercle bacillus.

Other infections for which streptomycin is valuable are those due to Friedlander's bacillus and to H. influenzæ. It has also been applied locally in tuberculosis of the pericardium and in tuberculous empyema, in the hope that it may reduce the severity of the infection, in preparation for later surgical intervention.

Aureomycin and **chloromycetin** (the synthetic product is given the name *chloramphenicol*) are purely bacteriostatic. They are given by mouth, the dose of each drug being 2 to 4 capsules three or four times a day—each capsule contains 250 mgm. Both substances appear to be valuable in certain virus diseases. In respiratory infections, aureomycin is preferable, and is effective against all forms of pneumonia—those due to pneumococci, streptococci, staphylococci, Friedlander's bacillus, H. influenzæ, and the viruses of psittacosis and " primary atypical pneumonia." At present, aureomycin is not only expensive, but is not generally available ; it may, however, be possible to obtain supplies from a Ministry of Health supply depot.

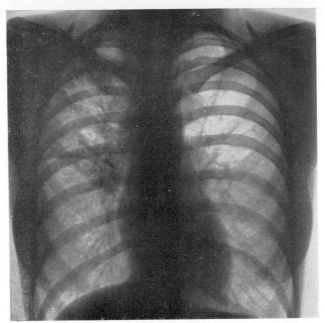

PLATE 3—Unilateral exudative pulmonary tuberculosis affecting right upper lobe.   There is a small apical cavity.

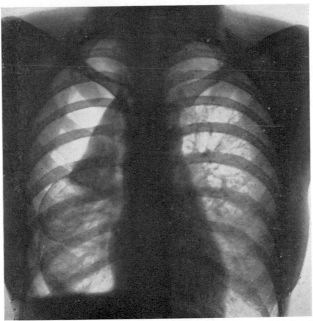

PLATE 4—Same case four months after the induction of artificial pneumothorax. A good selective collapse has been secured.   There is a small pleural effusion.

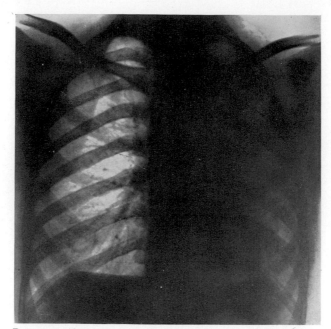

PLATE 5—Chronic fibroid unilateral pulmonary tuberculosis. There is notable retraction of the mediastinal structures towards the diseased side.

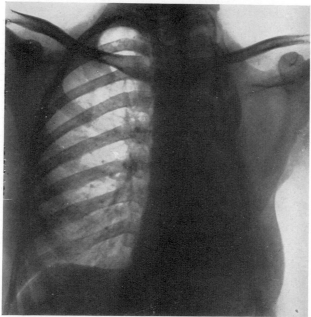

PLATE 6—Same case two years after an extensive thoracoplasty. Patient is well and working.

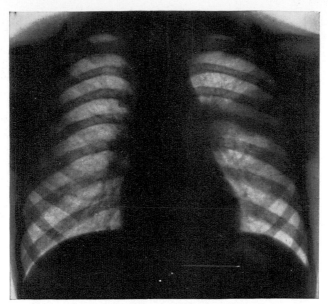

PLATE 7—A large primary focus in the left upper lobe associated with hilar lymphadenitis.

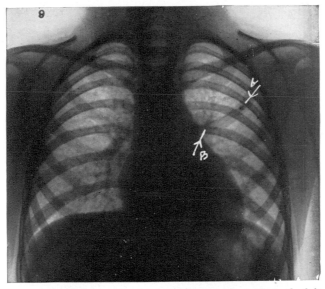

PLATE 8—A primary (Ghon's) focus of tuberculosis (A) in the left lung with involvement of the hilar gland (B). Both lesions show early calcification.

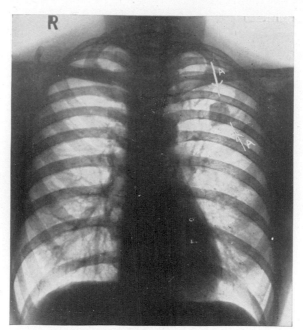

PLATE 9—A secondary (Assmann's) focus of tuberculosis (A) in the left subclavicular region.

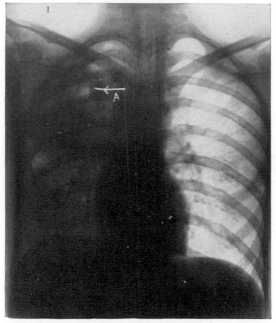

PLATE 10—Tuberculous pneumonia involving nearly the entire right lung. Excavation is just beginning at A.

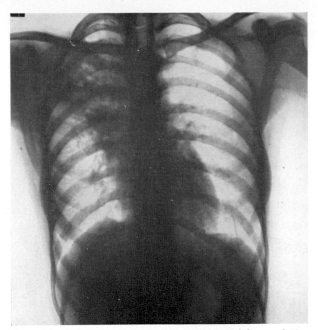

PLATE 11—Pulmonary tuberculosis, right upper lobe, exudative type with cavitation. A case suitable for attempt at collapse therapy by artificial pneumothorax.

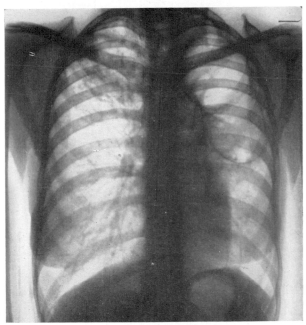

PLATE 12—Pulmonary tuberculosis both upper lobes: large cavities in left upper lobe.

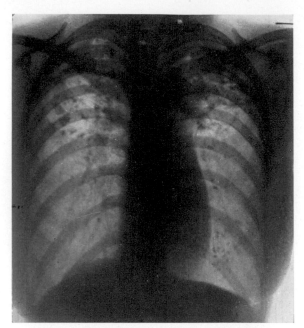

PLATE 13—Healed calcified bilateral tuberculosis.

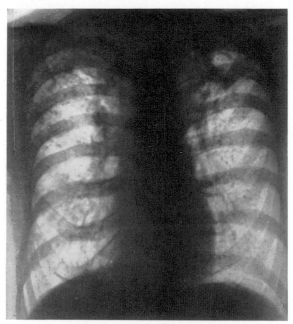

PLATE 14—Pulmonary tuberculosis: cavity left upper lobe:
calcified nodules of miliary distribution.

518

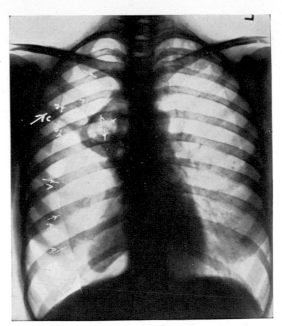

PLATE 15—Right artificial pneumothorax showing the
lung edge (A) and an uncollapsed cavity (B) in the right
upper lobe held out by adhesions (C).

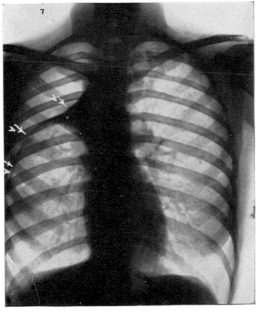

PLATE 16—The same case after the adhesions have
been divided. The lung edge is visible at A. The
diseased area shows complete selective collapse.

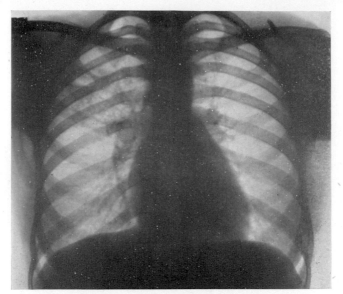

PLATE 17—Pulmonary tuberculosis, right upper lobe, with small cavity. Tubercle bacilli found in sputum. Please compare with Plate 33.

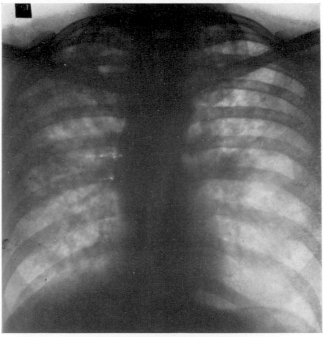

PLATE 18—Acute caseating pulmonary tuberculosis. This patient was sent to a surgeon with the tentative diagnosis of carcinoma of the stomach (see p. 288).

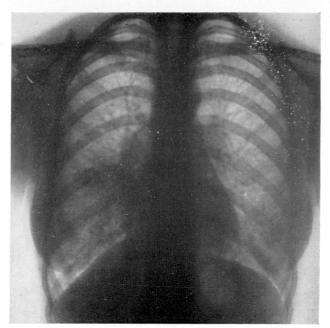

PLATE 19—Bilateral bronchiectasis : ordinary anterior film : see Plate 20 for the lipiodol bronchogram.

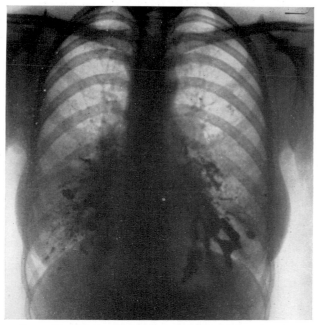

PLATE 20—Bilateral bronchiectasis : lipiodol bronchogram. Same patient as Plate 19.

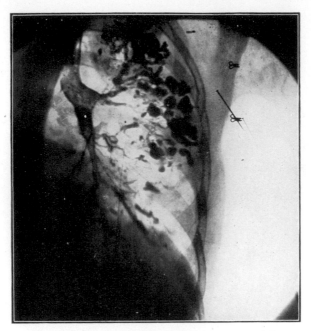

PLATE 21—Bronchiectatic cavities in the upper lobe
filled with lipiodol.

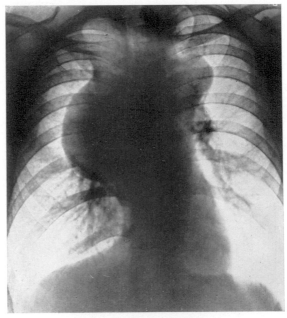

PLATE 22—Aortic aneurysm.

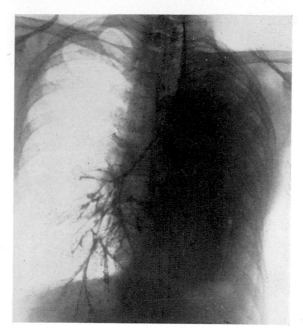

PLATE 23—Complete obstruction of left main bronchus by carcinoma, shown by lipiodol bronchogram. Note the collapse of the whole of the left lung, the displacement of the trachea and the heart to the side of the lesion, and the "crowding" of the ribs.

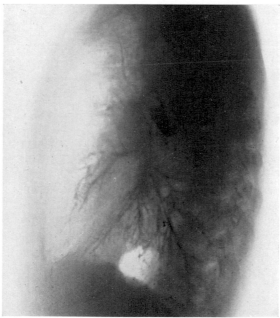

PLATE 24—Same patient as Plate 23. Lateral view. The lipiodol has flowed into the bronchi of the opposite lung.

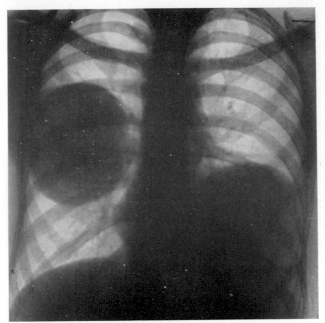

PLATE 25—Hydatid cysts. Anterior view.

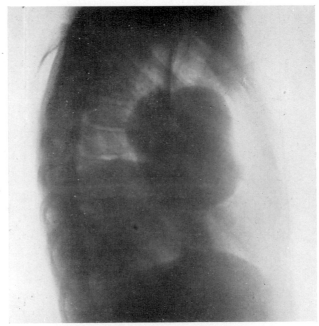

PLATE 26—Same patient as Plate 25. Lateral view.

524

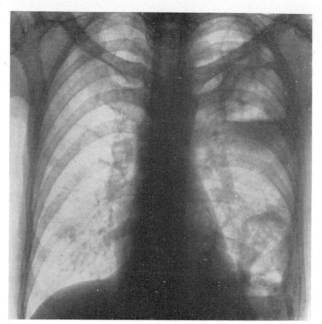

PLATE 27—Multiple lung abscesses. There are two cavities in the left upper lobe, and one in the left lower lobe. Note the horizontal "fluid level."

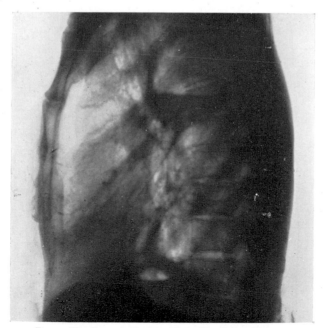

PLATE 28—Same patient as Plate 27. Lateral view.

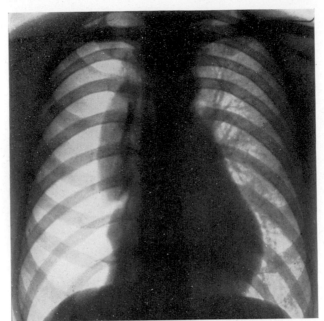

PLATE 29—Right-sided spontaneous pneumothorax.

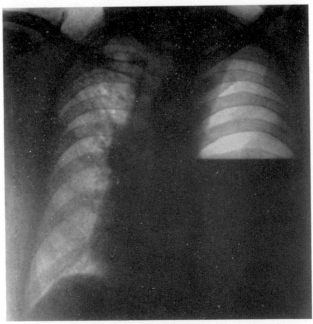

PLATE 30—Left-sided hydropneumothorax.   Note the
displacement of the heart towards the right.

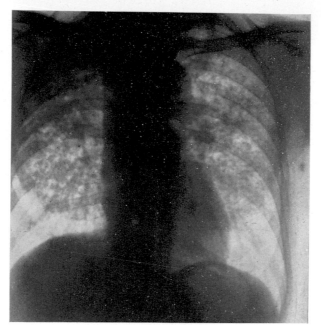

PLATE 31—Silicosis. Note distribution of shadowing, the bases
being comparatively clear.

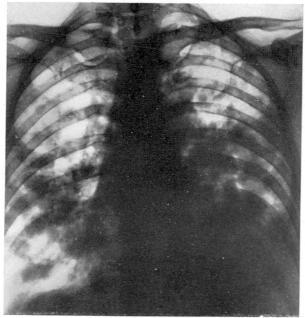

PLATE 32—Secondary carcinomatous deposits.

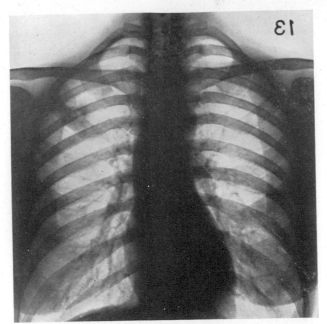

PLATE 33—Lung abscess. Note small cavity right upper lobe.
Compare with Plate 17.

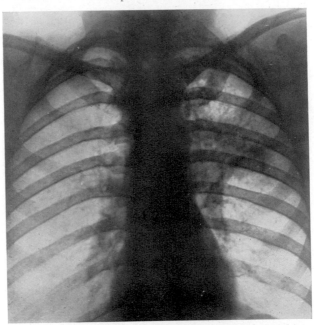

PLATE 34—Necrotising bronchopneumonia, which developed into
a lung abscess. Radiologically this picture could also be one
of pulmonary tuberculosis, or of pneumonia secondary to a
bronchial carcinoma which is not completely obstructing the
upper lobe bronchus.

These two plates underline the fact that diagnosis depends on the whole clinical
picture and not merely on radiograms. In both patients the history of the illness,
especially the expectoration of foul sputum, led to the diagnosis (see Chapter XIX).

INDEX

A

Abdominal pain in chest injury, 473
 in pleurisy, 371, 425
 rigidity in chest injuries, 473, 495
Abdomino-thoracic injuries, 480, 494
Abscess of lung, 98, 232, 246, 397, 401, 413, 420, 493
 and bronchial carcinoma, 143
 chronic, 254
 clinical course of, 254
 diagnosis of, 255
 embolic, 246, 251, 470
 following bronchial obstruction, 98
 following subdiaphragmatic infection, 413
 Friedländer's bacillus infection, 236
 pathology of, 246
 prognosis of, 257
 putrid, 232, 248, 322, 323
 " reactionary effusion " in, 247, 256, 372, 383
 signs of, 253
 staphylococcal, 235, 420
 streptococcal, 234, 257
 surgery of, 259
 symptoms of, 251
Accessory muscles of respiration, 10, 196, 237, 447
Acidosis and respiration, 16
Actinomycosis, 325, 402
" Acute abdomen," diagnosis from pneumonia, 217
 diagnosis from pneumothorax, 425
Adenoma, bronchial, 148
Adhesions, pleural, 300, 302, 363, 368, 413, 421, 422, 437
Adrenaline in asthma, 453
Ægophony, 81, 382
After-care and chest injuries, 499
 and pulmonary tuberculosis, 314
Age and prognosis in pneumonia, 219
Air embolism, 300, 302, 389, 469
 in pleural space, nature of, 430
 replacement, 387, 399, 407, 438
 sacs, 13
 transport and pneumothorax, 436
Albuminuria in pneumonia, 219
Alcoholism and pneumonia, 210, 218
Alexander, 409
Alkalosis and respiration, 16
Allergic infiltrations of the lung, 323
Allergy in asthma, 449, 456

Allergy—*contd.*
 in pulmonary tuberculosis, 266, 268, 270, 274
 to cotton, 346
Alveoli, 13
 œdema of, in influenzal broncho-pneumonia, 167 (see also *Pulmonary œdema*)
Aminophylline in emphysema, 200
Ammonia, inhalation of, 353
Amœbic abscess, 411
Amphoric breath sounds, 80, 427
Anærobic infection of hæmothorax, 489, 490
Anaphylactic shock, 445
Aneurysm of aorta, 150, 464
Anginal pain in mediastinal emphysema, 503
Anoxia and asthma, 446
 and chest injury, 473, 480, 482
 and emphysema, 198
 and high altitudes, 436
 and pneumonia, 219, 237, 240, 242
 and war-gas poisoning, 355, 358
 causes of, 51, 172
Anthracosis, 344
Anthrax of lung, 346
Antitetanic serum, 494
Aortic aneurysm, 150, 464
Apex beat of heart, 18, 59, 474, 484
 collapse of lung and, 96
 fibrosis of lung and, 364
 pleural effusion and, 377, 484
 pneumothorax and, 427 (see also *Mediastinum*)
Aphonia, 44
 and bronchial carcinoma, 139
 functional, 44
Arsenical ducts, 348
Arseniuretted hydrogen, 348
Artificial pneumothorax, 111, 260, 299, 385, 387, 407
 bilateral, 301, 420
Asbestosis, 342
" Asbestosis bodies," 343
Aspergillosis, 346
Asphyxia, following inhalation of foreign body, 112
 " traumatic," 481
Aspiration of hæmothorax, 486
 of pericardial effusion, 496
 of pleural effusion, 382, 386, 388, 398, 408, 416, 489

34

PRINTED IN GREAT BRITAIN
BY R. & R. CLARK, LTD., EDINBURGH